LIVER-DIRECTED THERAPY FOR PRIMARY AND METASTATIC LIVER TUMORS

Cancer Treatment and Research

Steven T. Rosen, M.D., *Series Editor*

Kurzrock, R., Talpaz, M. (eds): *Cytokines: Interleukins and Their Receptors.* 1995. ISBN 0-7923-3636-4.
Sugarbaker, P. (ed): *Peritoneal Carcinomatosis: Drugs and Diseases.* 1995. ISBN 0-7923-3726-3.
Sugarbaker, P. (ed): *Peritoneal Carcinomatosis: Principles of Management.* 1995. ISBN 0-7923-3727-1.
Dickson, R.B., Lippman, M.E. (eds.): *Mammary Tumor Cell Cycle, Differentiation and Metastasis.* 1995. ISBN 0-7923-3905-3.
Freireich, E.J, Kantarjian, H. (eds.): *Molecular Genetics and Therapy of Leukemia.* 1995. ISBN 0-7923-3912-6.
Cabanillas, F., Rodriguez, M.A. (eds.): *Advances in Lymphoma Research.* 1996. ISBN 0-7923-3929-0.
Miller, A.B. (ed.): *Advances in Cancer Screening.* 1996. ISBN 0-7923-4019-1.
Hait , W.N. (ed.): *Drug Resistance.* 1996. ISBN 0-7923-4022-1.
Pienta, K.J. (ed.): *Diagnosis and Treatment of Genitourinary Malignancies.* 1996. ISBN 0-7923-4164-3.
Arnold, A.J. (ed.): *Endocrine Neoplasms.* 1997. ISBN 0-7923-4354-9.
Pollock, R.E. (ed.): *Surgical Oncology.* 1997. ISBN 0-7923-9900-5.
Verweij, J., Pinedo, H.M., Suit, H.D. (eds.): *Soft Tissue Sarcomas: Present Achievements and Future Prospects.* 1997. ISBN 0-7923-9913-7.
Walterhouse, D.O., Cohn, S. L. (eds.): *Diagnostic and Therapeutic Advances in Pediatric Oncology.* 1997. ISBN 0-7923-9978-1.
Mittal, B.B., Purdy, J.A., Ang, K.K. (eds.): *Radiation Therapy.* 1998. ISBN 0-7923-9981-1.
Foon, K.A., Muss, H.B. (eds.): *Biological and Hormonal Therapies of Cancer.* 1998. ISBN 0-7923-9997-8.
Ozols, R.F. (ed.): *Gynecologic Oncology.* 1998. ISBN 0-7923-8070-3.
Noskin, G. A. (ed.): *Management of Infectious Complications in Cancer Patients.* 1998. ISBN 0-7923-8150-5
Bennett, C. L. (ed.): *Cancer Policy.* 1998. ISBN 0-7923-8203-X
Benson, A. B. (ed.): *Gastrointestinal Oncology.* 1998. ISBN 0-7923-8205-6
Tallman, M.S. , Gordon, L.I. (eds.): *Diagnostic and Therapeutic Advances in Hematologic Malignancies.* 1998. ISBN 0-7923-8206-4
von Gunten, C.F. (ed.): *Palliative Care and Rehabilitation of Cancer Patients.* 1999. ISBN 0-7923-8525-X
Burt, R.K., Brush, M.M. (eds): *Advances in Allogeneic Hematopoietic Stem Cell Transplantation.* 1999. ISBN 0-7923-7714-1
Angelos, P. (ed): *Ethical Issues in Cancer Patient Care* 2000. ISBN 0-7923-7726-5
Gradishar, W.J., Wood, W.C. (eds): *Advances in Breast Cancer Management.* 2000. ISBN 0-7923-7890-3
Sparano, Joseph A. (ed.): *HIV & HTLV-I Associated Malignancies.* 2001. ISBN 0-7923-7220-4.
Ettinger, David S. (ed.): *Thoracic Oncology.* 2001. ISBN 0-7923-7248-4.
Bergan, Raymond C. (ed.): *Cancer Chemoprevention.* 2001. ISBN 0-7923-7259-X.
Raza, A., Mundle, S.D. (eds): *Myelodysplastic Syndromes & Secondary Acute Myelogenous Leukemia; Directions for the new Millennium.* 2001. ISBN 0-7923-7396-0.
Talamonti, Mark S. (ed.): *Liver Directed Therapy for Primary and Metastatic Liver Tumors.* 2001 ISBN 0-7923-7523-8
Stack, M.S., Fishman, D.A. (eds.): *Ovarian Cancer.* 2001 ISBN 0-7923-7530-0

LIVER-DIRECTED THERAPY FOR PRIMARY AND METASTATIC LIVER TUMORS

edited by

Mark S. Talamonti, M.D.
Northwestern University Medical School
Chicago, IL

with

Sam G. Pappas, M.D.
Northwestern University Medical School
Chicago, IL

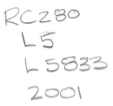

KLUWER ACADEMIC PUBLISHERS
Boston / Dordrecht / London

Distributors for North, Central and South America:
Kluwer Academic Publishers
101 Philip Drive
Assinippi Park
Norwell, Massachusetts 02061 USA
Telephone (781) 871-6600
Fax (781) 681-9045
E-Mail <kluwer@wkap.com>

Distributors for all other countries:
Kluwer Academic Publishers Group
Distribution Centre
Post Office Box 322
3300 AH Dordrecht, THE NETHERLANDS
Telephone 31 78 6392 392
Fax 31 78 6546 474
E-Mail <services@wkap.nl>

 Electronic Services <http://www.wkap.nl>

Library of Congress Cataloging-in-Publication Data

A C.I.P. Catalogue record for this book is available
from the Library of Congress.

Printed on acid-free paper.   Printed in the United States of America

To my wife, Anne, for her unwavering love,
to my family for their encouragement and support,
and for my children, Brittney and Jason
who have given me my greatest joys in life.

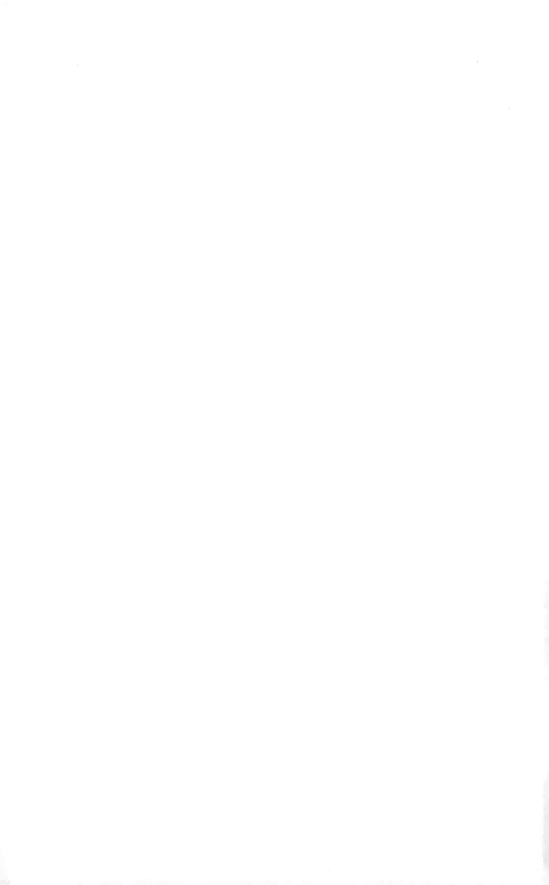

TABLE OF CONTENTS

Preface

A comprehensive text book examining tumors of the liver. In addition to chapters examining traditional surgical techniques, there are specific chapters dealing with novel and evolving treatments including transplantation, radiofrequency ablation, and chemo-embolization. Also unique to this book are chapters discussing the incidence, etiology and biologic characteristics of primary and secondary liver tumors. Other interesting chapters include a chapter providing a comprehensive review of radiology procedures and imaging studies that provide state of the art radiologic staging of liver tumors. Also included are chapters examining the role of interventional radiology and interventional gastroenterology in the treatment of liver tumors. It will appeal to surgeons because of the comprehensive examination of strategies, techniques and outcomes. Other specialists who treat liver tumors will also find it to be valuable because of the unique and comprehensive chapters examining the biologic and epidemiologic factors involved into the development and progression of primary and secondary liver cancers. Interventionists in Radiology and Gastroenterology will also value the text for its review of new and unique non-surgical strategies used to treat liver tumors.

1

CLINICAL FEATURES OF PRIMARY AND METASTATIC HEPATIC MALIGNANCIES

Sam G. Pappas, M.D., Jacqueline S. Jeruss, M.D., and Mark S. Talamonti, M.D.

Northwestern University Medical School, Chicago, IL

INTRODUCTION

In the United States, it is estimated that 1,268,000 new cancer cases will be diagnosed in the year 2001. Approximately 550,000 cancer-related deaths will occur in the same time period (1). Cancers with the liver as a major site of disease involvement will constitute a significant portion (16,200 new cases) of these new cancer cases. Of concern is the typically poor response of primary liver tumors and hepatic metastases to conventional therapies. However, more aggressive operative strategies and the expanding use of regional and systemic chemotherapeutic approaches have led to more treatment options for tumors of the liver.

Management of hepatic malignancies continues to evolve rapidly. The high incidence of both primary and secondary metastatic tumors of the liver makes the subject of their appropriate management an important medical concern. The treatment of primary and metastatic hepatic malignancy markedly differs and will be discussed in the subsequent chapters. This chapter will focus on the more common forms of liver and biliary tract cancer, the suspected etiologies of these diseases, and the commonly encountered clinical features of each.

Worldwide, primary liver cancer is considered the fifth most significant cancer in terms of number of cases (437,000, or 5.4% of new cancer cases) but fourth in terms of mortality (427,00 deaths, 8.2% of the total) (2). The small difference in incidence and mortality reflects the extremely poor prognosis of liver cancer.

PRIMARY HEPATIC MALIGNANCY

Hepatocellular Carcinoma

Primary cancers of the liver include hepatocellular carcinomas, cholangiocarcinomas and rarely tumors of the intrahepatic vasculature, such as hemangioendothelioma, hemangioblastoma, angiosarcoma, and undifferentiated primary sarcoma (3).

Hepatocellular carcinoma (HCC) is the most common primary malignancy of the liver. The overwhelming majority of primary liver cancer cases are found in developing countries. Of concern is the rising incidence of HCC occurring in the United States over the past twenty years. Furthermore, the age specific incidence of this cancer has progressively shifted towards younger people (4). Of note, the incidence of HCC is also increasing in certain Asian and European countries as well as in Mexico (5,6).

The broad geographic distribution of HCC points towards a multifactorial causation, however certain demographic features are consistent. Overall, the incidence of HCC is higher in men than in women, and higher in blacks than in whites. Patients diagnosed with HCC are generally older, yet this trend is not uniform. In areas where HCC is hyperendemic, patients tend to be younger at diagnosis, whereas in average to low incidence areas the age at diagnosis approaches seventy (7).

HCC typically presents in the setting of severe parenchymal liver disease (3). A large variety of underlying disease states, as well as multiple natural and synthetic carcinogens have been implicated in HCC pathogenesis. Undoubtedly, the incidence of HCC is high in areas of prevalent chronic hepatitis infection and cirrhosis. Chronic infection with the hepatitis B virus (HBV) is a strong risk factor for HCC. The epidemiologic evidence for this is very convincing (8). In a prospective study of over 20,000 men in Taiwan, the risk ratio for HCC was greater than 100 for those who were HbsAg positive at the start of the study (9). The age of HBV acquisition appears to be significant in the development of HCC. The younger the age of HBV infection, the greater the chance of a person becoming a chronic HBV carrier (10). Chronic infection with hepatitis C virus (HCV) appears to increase the risk of HCC at about the same rate as chronic HBV infection does (8). In places of low incidence of chronic hepatitis infection, like in the US, alcohol-related cirrhosis constitutes a major risk for the eventual development of HCC. Aflatoxins have also been suspected as an environmental contaminant important in the oncogenesis of HCC (8,11).

HCC typically presents as a right upper quadrant abdominal mass, a decline in the overall health of a patient with a history of cirrhosis, or as an incidental finding on a radiologic examination. When HCC presents as a mass (as it commonly does in sub-Saharan Africa), abdominal pain, malaise, and inanition are frequent accompanying signs and symptom (8). HCC that infiltrates a cirrhotic liver often severely compromises already impaired hepatic function (8).

Since the development of hepatocellular carcinoma tends to occur in a definable population and because the outlook for those with advanced disease remains poor, it is tempting to postulate that screening cirrhotic patients may yield individuals who could receive successful therapy for HCC early in their disease. Proposed screening strategies have mainly included periodic ultrasound (every six months) or computed tomography examination of the liver or periodic monitoring of tumor related proteins (alpha fetoprotein AFP, des-γ-carboxyprothrombin) or a combination of the two.

Cottone and others (12) prospectively screened a series of patients with well-compensated cirrhosis (Child's Class A) who if found to have HCC were potentially treatable by surgery or alcohol ablation. They screened 147 patients in an eight-year surveillance program with testing by ultrasound and AFP every six months. They showed that the cumulative incidence of HCC in cirrhotics might be higher than previously reported. The report also found that periodic ultrasound was of value in detecting treatable tumors. Finally, intermediate AFP values (>50 and <400 ng/ml) may indicate the presence of undetectable cancers which will appear during the follow-up of these patients, and also suggested that ultrasound should be employed more frequently in these particular patients. Although screening programs have demonstrated that HCC can be detected relatively early, these trials have not proven that screening symptomatic patients at higher risk for HCC is cost effective and more importantly significantly influences mortality rates.

The most promising area in HCC research is that of disease prevention. In 1984, in Taiwan, neonatal vaccination for HBV began for children of HbsAg-positive mothers and by 1986 vaccination became universal. The rate of HCC in children aged 6 to 9 years decreased from 0.52 per 100,000 to 0.13 in the first vaccinated cohort (13). The worldwide institution of hepatitis B vaccination will provide even more data on the effectiveness of disease prevention through mass vaccination.

The finding that polyprenoic acid, a retinoid analogue reduces second primaries of HCC after resection raises the possibility that patients at higher risk for HCC may benefit from chemoprophylactic measures (8,14). Further research is underway to develop potent and safe analogues of polyprenoic acid (15). Such compounds may prevent primary hepatomas, since short-term use of polyprenoic acid in low doses inhibited the spontaneous development of mouse hepatomas for 2 years (16).

Cholangiocarcinoma

Bile duct cancer is the second most common primary malignancy of the liver. Approximately 15% to 25% of all primary liver cancers are cholangiocarcinomas. Like gallbladder cancer, the incidence of cholangiocarcinoma increases with increasing age; however, bile duct malignancies have a more even distribution between men and women (17). In temperate countries, the tumor is relatively uncommon. Patients are typically diagnosed in the sixth and seventh decade of life. The incidence in the United States is 1 per 100,000 people per year (18). This is in contrast the incidence of cholangiocarcinoma (CCA) in tropical countries such as Thailand and Southeast Asia, where the tumor accounts for nearly 77% of all primary liver malignancies. The annual frequency per 100,000 population is 7.3 in Israel, 6.5 in American Indians, and 5.5 in Japanese (19).

The majority of bile duct cancers arise from the extrahepatic biliary tree, the hepatic duct bifurcation being the most common site. Recent advances in diagnostic techniques as well as more aggressive surgical approaches to these tumors including liver transplantation, has led to increasing interest in their appropriate management.

Table 1. Etiologic Risk Factors for Cholangiocarcinoma

Hepatolithiasis	Radionuclides
Chlonorchis sinensis	Asbestos
Opisthorchis vivverrini	Dioxin
Choledochal cysts	Nitrosamines
Caroli's disease	Polychlorinated biphenyls
Primary sclerosing cholangitis	Isoniazid
Ulcerative colitis	Methyldopa
Thorium Dioxide (Thorotrast)	Oral contraceptives

Although there are clearly defined risk factors for CCA (Table 1) the mechanism behind its pathogenesis remains unknown. Strong associations have been found between CCA and hepatolithiasis, liver flukes, biliary cystic disease, sclerosing cholangitis and ulcerative colitis, and the radiocontrast agent Thorotrast (17). Weaker associations have been reported between radionucleotides and drugs and the eventual development of CCA.

Hepatolithiasis is a definite risk factor for CCA. In areas where hepatolithiasis is endemic, 5% to 10% of these patients will eventually develop CCA (20-22). Evidence points towards a connection with liver fluke infection and cholangiocarcinoma pathogenesis. There are three bile duct flukes that are acquired in humans who eat raw fish; *Clonorchis sinensis, Opisthorchis viverrini,* and *O. felineus* (23). Infection with the liver fluke *C. sinensis* is common in Asia, where the ingestion of raw fish is common. The parasites enter through the host's duodenum and eventual end up in the intra and extra-hepatic bile ducts. The parasites can become quite long (2.5 cm in length) and can obstruct the flow of bile. This is thought to lead to biliary retention, inflammation, fibrosis, and hyperplasia, which are believed to be the precursors to the eventual development of bile duct cancer (24). The liver fluke *O.viverrini* has also been reported as a risk factor for CCA. *O.viverrini* is endemic to Northeast Thailand where the infection rate is said to approach 90% in some villages (25). The incidence of CCA in this population is estimated at 54 cases per 100,000.

Animal studies indicate that the evolution of CCA may be secondary to specific hepatocarcinogens causing the genetic alteration of pluripotent, periportal stem cells (26). Malignant evolution may be secondary to chronic inflammation and glandular regeneration. Perhaps the most impressive association between a carcinogen and the development of hepatic and bile duct malignancy has been documented with exposure to the radiocontrast agent Thorotrast (17, 27,28). Thorotrast is a 25% colloidal contrast agent used in the 1930's and 1940's that emits energy as alpha particles. It is retained in the reticuloendothelial system for life, with a half-life of 200 to 400 years (29).

Symptoms associated with CCA are those typically associated with biliary obstruction. Painless jaundice occurs in up to 90% of patients. Bacterial overgrowth secondary to biliary obstruction may lead to symptoms of cholangitis. Pruritis, clay colored stools and dark urine are all symptoms associated with hyperbillirubinemia from bile duct obstruction. CCA is a highly malignant tumor with a poor associated prognosis. Patients typically present with late stage disease and it is extremely rare to see survival beyond five years.

Gallbladder Carcinoma

Gallbladder carcinoma is the most common biliary tract cancer and the fifth most common cancer of the gastrointestinal tract. Autopsy studies and data from surgical series reveal an incidence of gallbladder cancer ranging from 0.55% to 1.91% (30). It is typically a disease of the elderly, most commonly diagnosed in the sixth and seventh decades of life. It appears to be more common in women who have a threefold higher incidence than males. Worldwide, gallbladder carcinoma has an unusual geographic and demographic distribution being more common in Israel, Bolivia, and Chile and in the Southwestern United States (31). Very high incidence rates of gallbladder carcinoma have been reported from Israel. The rate of gallbladder cancer in this part of the world is 7.5 per 100,000 men and 13.8 per 100,000 women (17). This in contrast to very low incidence rates in Singapore, India, and Japan. In the United States, 2.5 per 100,000 people will develop gallbladder cancer and the area of highest incidence is in New Mexico where carcinoma of the gallbladder accounts for 8.5% of all cancers (17). Also Japanese-Americans have higher rates of cancer than other populations (32).

Table 2: Risk factors for carcinoma of the gallbladder
Gallstones; chronic cholecystitis
Gallbladder polyps
Peutz-Jeghers syndrome
Choledochal cysts
Anomalous pancreaticobiliary junction
Industrial exposure to carcinogens
Porcelain gallbladder
?High body mass index

Although several risk factors for gallbladder cancer have been identified (Table 2). the cause remains unknown. There appears to be a clear association betweer gallstones, chronic gallbladder inflammation and the eventual development o gallbladder carcinoma. Up to 90% of patients with gallbladder cancer have a histor of gallstones. Chronic typhoid carriers are at six times the risk of developing cance of the gallbladder as compared to the general population (33). Calcification of th gallbladder wall (so called porcelain gallbladder) is associated with longstanding chronic cholecystitis and higher risk of malignancy (34,35). The risk of developing gallbladder cancer increases with increasing gallstone size. Carcinoma is more likely to develop in patients with a single large stone than in those patients with multiple small stones (36).

Several authors have recently raised the concern that an anomalous pancreaticobiliary union may play a role in the pathogenesis of gallbladder cancer (37-39). Most patients with an anomalous ductal union have some congenital dilation of the biliary tree. Whether it is the chronic regurgitation of pancreatic juice itself or the relationship of the abnormal junction to bile stasis and the retention of carcinogens in the biliary tree remains unclear.

There is some evidence to suggest that environmental carcinogens may play a role in the development of gallbladder cancer. Animal studies demonstrate that exposure to nitrosamines and other compounds like o-amino-azotulene causes gallbladder cancer in experimental animals (40-42). A high incidence of gallbladder and biliary tract cancer in individuals working in the rubber industry suggest a link between these cancers and occupational factors (43). Polyps of the gallbladder, particularly those greater than 1 cm in size are associated with higher risk for malignancy and are therefore an indication for cholecystectomy (44,45). Adenomatous polyps of the gallbladder associated with Peutz-Jegher's syndrome are also associated with gallbladder cancer (46).

Carcinoma of the gallbladder produces symptoms that include in decreasing order of frequency, pain, nausea, vomiting, weight loss, and jaundice (47). Physical exam may demonstrate tenderness in the epigastrium or right upper quadrant, mass, jaundice, ascites and hepatomegaly (48). Typically, patients have non-specific laboratory abnormalities and in advanced cases may reflect compromised liver function.

SECONDARY HEPATIC MALIGNANCY

The liver is the first destination of venous blood drainage from multiple intraabdominal organs. As a result of its dual blood supply (75% from the portal vein, 25% from the hepatic artery) and histologic filtering structure, the liver is a common site of metastatic deposits. It has been estimated that 50% of patients in whom the primary tumor drains into the portal vein will develop hepatic metastases.

Colorectal, lung, breast, pancreatic and other visceral adenocarcinomas and carcinoid tumors frequently metastasize to the liver (49). There has been little enthusiasm for resection of nonportal hepatic metastasis (i.e. breast, lung, and melanoma) mainly because of the high probability of extrahepatic metastases. For the most part, only colorectal, pancreatic-neuroendocrine, and carcinoid tumors have a reasonable chance of having liver only metastases. Colorectal cancer metastasis to the liver is by far the most extensively studied and its management continues to evolve. Increasing experience with multi-modality approaches for neuroendocrine liver metastases justifies a review of liver-directed therapies in their management.

Hepatic Colorectal Metastasis

Approximately 160,000 new cases of colorectal cancer are diagnosed each year in the United States, of which 72,000 will eventually develop recurrent disease (50). The majority of these patients will develop some type of liver involvement. Surgeons need to be familiar with the evaluation of patients with colorectal liver metastasis and be able to identify the subgroups of patients who are most likely to benefit from resectional therapies.

The natural history of untreated hepatic metastasis offers little long-term hope for this group of patients. The median survival of patients with untreated metastasis is 3 to 10 months and few patients survive beyond one year (51-56). Even patients with limited metastatic burden, when left untreated, have a dismal prognosis with 5-year survival rates of 2% to 8% (57,58).

Metastases are characteristically asymptomatic and are usually diagnosed by radiographic or biochemical means. When present, symptoms include malaise, fever, weight loss, right upper quadrant abdominal pain, a palpable mass, and occasionally ascites or splenomegaly (59). Jaundice is infrequently present and may be the result of metastatic biliary tract obstruction, or it may occur late in the course of the disease, as a result of loss of functional parenchymal mass and cholestasis.

There is no doubt that appropriately selected patients can benefit from hepatic resection for colorectal metastasis (59). A review of the larger series to date confirms the favorable results of hepatectomy for colorectal metastasis (60-67). Approximately one-third of the patients are 5-year survivors and up to 20% are alive after ten years. The data from these series has also supported the increasing safety with which major hepatic resectional surgery can be performed with operative mortality rates ranging from 2% to 4%. This is likely the result of improved preoperative evaluation and the increasing enthusiasm for aggressive treatment of hepatic tumors based on their favorable prognosis with surgical resection.

In a recent review of 1001 consecutive liver resections at Memorial Sloan Kettering, five factors (listed in Table 3) were found to be predictive of subsequent recurrence (59). The presence of any one of these factors is not an absolute contraindication to surgery, although increasing numbers of negative prognostic indicators is associated with increasing risk of recurrence (59).

Table 3-Clinical Risk Score*
1. Lymph node-positive primary
2. Disease free interval between colon and liver disease <12 months
3. Size of liver tumors >5cm
4. Number of liver tumors greater than one
5. Preoperative CEA level greater than 200 ng/ml
*Each of the 5 unfavorable characteristics above is assigned 1 point. The sum of the positive characteristics is the clinical risk score.

Reprinted with permission from *Advances in Surgery* Vol.34 2000

The calculated clinical risk score shows promise of identifying patients most likely to benefit from an aggressive surgical approach and also helps define those patients at high risk for recurrence. Those patients at risk for recurrence may be further stratified for placement into clinical adjuvant trials.

Hepatic Neuroendocrine Metastasis

Islet cell neoplasms arising from the pancreas and carcinoid tumors are rare neuroendocrine tumors, representing less than 5% of all gastrointestinal malignancies (68-70). Liver neuroendocrine endocrine tumors (NET) represent a heterogeneous group of rare neoplasms with varying patterns of growth and clinical presentation. Liver metastases develop in 46% to 93% of patients with NET and can involve large portions of the liver before becoming symptomatic (71). Although no treatment may be the best treatment for many patients, up to 80% of patients with advanced NET die within 5 years of diagnosis, implying that despite the indolent course of these neoplasms, effective early intervention may be able to impact the natural history of the disease (71-73).

The decision to treat a patient with hepatic NET metastasis should take into consideration the natural history of the disease process and the severity of presenting symptoms (71). Unlike colorectal metastasis, patients with metastatic NET typically follow a protracted and variable time course from the onset of symptoms to death. Even in the setting of advanced disease, a mean survival up to 8.1 years has been reported with a range of up to 41 years (68). Surgeons need to familiarize themselves with the natural history of these tumors when recommending treatment.

The phenotypic manifestations of NET are heterogeneous and symptoms may vary from atypical endocrinopathies, from small isolated metastases, to patients who have near complete replacement of their liver with tumor who are asymptomatic. Advances in the treatment of functional NET have been made through the use of H_2-blockers, proton pump inhibitors, somatostatin, and somatostatin analogue and are considered standard medical therapies. However, most patients become resistant to these types of therapies despite favorable initial response (74,75). These treatments should be used to control symptoms until more definite therapies can be undertaken with an acceptable risk.

The aims of aggressive treatment include the alleviation of hormonal syndromes or pain symptoms refractory to medical management and control of progressive tumor growth. The experience at our institution demonstrates that in selected patients, aggressive liver directed therapy which includes curative surgical resection (CSR) and hepatic artery chemoebolization (HAE) can provide effective improvement in clinical symptoms and may result in sustained tumor control and extend survival.

In our review, patients who underwent a CSR had a 70% 5-year survival. Those patients whose tumors were not amenable to surgical treatment were considered for combination HAE and medical treatment of symptoms. Approximately 90% of our patients achieve palliation of symptoms using this approach. Others have advocated palliative surgical debulking, and in selected patients orthotopic liver transplantation for prolongation of survival and relief of symptoms from metastatic NET (76,77).

CONCLUSION

The appropriate management of both primary and secondary hepatic malignancy remains a formidable challenge to most physicans. The subsequent chapters underscore the importance of a multi-modality approach to the management of tumors of the liver. We attempt to provide the reader with a comprehensive approach to the treatment of these cancers.

A thorough pre-operative assessment of the patient with hepatic malignancy with a personal history and physical examination, along with appropriate radiologic staging, may help identify factors that will predict long-term survival. For the most part, surgical resection remains the primary treatment modality and provides the best chance for prolonged survival and sustained tumor control. Critical components to the treatment of patients with liver tumors are the availability of interstitial therapies and chemoembolization and each will be discussed in detail

When surgery is not possible, endoscopic and percutaneous stenting are affective means for palliation of obstructive jaundice. In selected instances, orthotopic liver transplantation may play a role in the management of nonresectable primary liver cancers.

REFERENCES

1. Greenlee RT, Hill-Harmon MB, Murray T, Thun M. Cancer Statistics, 2001. *CA Cancer J. Clin* 2001 51: 15-36.
2. Parkin D, Pisani P, Ferlay J. Global Cancer Statistics. *CA Cancer J. Clin* 1999: 49(1) 33-64.
3. Sitzmann JV. Malignant Liver Tumors. *Current Surgical Therapy*. St. Louis, Missouri: Mosby, Inc, Cameron JL. (6th edition) 1998: 343-346.
4. El-Serag HB, Mason AC. Rising Incidence of Hepatocellular Carcinoma in the United States. *N Engl J Med 1999;* 340:10 pp 745-750.

5. Cortes-Espinosa T, Mondragon-Sanchez R, Hurtado-Andrade H, et al. Hepatocellular Carcinoma and Hepatic Cirrhosis in Mexico. A 25-year Necroscopy Review. *Hepto Gastroenterology*1997; 44:1401-1403.
6. Reynolds T. Global Cancer Burden Difficult to Assess, Rising Rates Likely. *Journal of the Nat'l Cancer Inst* 1998; 90(10):734-746.
7. Di Bisceglie A, Carithers R, Gores G. Hepatocellular Carcinoma. *Hepatology* 1998; 28(4) 1161-1165.
8. Schafer DF, Sorrell MF. Hepatocellular carcinoma. *Lancet* 1999; 353:1253-57.
9. Beasley RP, Hwang LY, Lin CC, Chein CS. Hepatocellular carcinoma and hepatitis B virus: a prospective study of 22 707 men in Taiwan. *Lancet* 1981; ii: 1129-33.
10. Beebe GW, Norman JE. Study of the likelihood of hepatocellular carcinoma following the 1942 Army epidemic of hepatitis B. In: Tabor E, Di Bisceglie AM, Purcell RH,eds. Etiology, pathology, and treatment of hepatocellular carcinoma in North America. Houston:Gulf Publishing, 1991:3-13.
11. Lasky T, Magder L. Hepatocellular carcinoma p53 G→T transversions at codon 249: the fingerprint of aflatoxin exposure? *Environ Health Perspect* 1997; 105:392-97.
12. Cottone M, Turri M, Caltagirone M, et al. Screening for hepatocellular carcinoma in patients with Child's A cirrhosis: an 8 year prospective study by ultrasound and alfafetoprotein. *J Hepatol*1994; 21:1029-34.
13. Chang MH, Chen CJ, Lai MS, et al. Universal hepatitis B vaccination in Taiwan and the incidence of hepatocellular carcinoma in children. *N Engl J Med* 1997; 336:1855-59.
14. Muto Y, Moriwaki H, Niomiya M, et al. Prevention of second primary tumors by an acyclic retinoid, polyprenoic acid, in patients with hepatocellular carcinoma. *N Engl J Med* 1996; 334: 1561-67.
15. Araki H, Shidoji M, Yamada Y, Moriwaki H, Muto Y. Retinoid agonist activities of synthetic geranyl geranoic acid derivatives. *Biochem Biophys Res Commun* 1995; 209:66-72.
16. Hatekeyama H, Shidoji Y, Omori M, et al. Retardation effect of acyclic retinoid on spontaneous hepatocarcinogenesis without changes in incidence of c-Ha-ras mutations in C3H/HeNCrj mice. *Center Detect Prev* (in press).
17. Pitt HA, Dooley WC, Yeo CJ et al. Malignancies of the biliary tract. *Curr Probl Surg* 1995:32:1.
18. Miller BA, Ries LAG, Hankey BF, et al. SEER Cancer statistics review: 1973-1990. (NIH Publication No. 93-2789). Bethesda, Md: National Cancer Institute, 1993.
19. Waterhouse JC, Muir P, Correa S. Cancer incidence in five countries. Lyon (France): VO3 TARC Scientific Publishers, International Agency for Research in Cancer, 1976.
20. Sheen-Chen SM, Chou FF, Eng HL. Intrahepatic cholangiocarcinoma in hepatolithiasis: a frequently overlooked disease. *J Surg Oncol* 1991; 47:131-5.

21. Fan ST, Lai EC, Wong J. Hepatic resection for hepatolithiasis. *Arch Surg* 1993; 128:1070-4.
22. Chijiiwa K, Ichimiya H, Kuroki S, et al. Late development of cholangiocarcinoma after treatment of hepatolithiasis: immunohistochemical study of mucin carbohydrates and core proteins in hepatolithiasis and cholangiocarcinoma. *Int J Cancer* 1993; 55:82-91.
23. Chapman RW. Risk factors for biliary tract carcinogenesis. *Annals of Oncology* 1999; 10 *Suppl. 4:*s308-311.
24. Schwartz DA: Cholangiocarcinoma associated with liver fluke infection: a preventable source of morbidity in Asian immigrants. *Am J Gastroeneterol* 81:76, 1986.
25. Kurathong S, Lerdverasirikul P, Wonkpaitoon V, et al: *Opisthorchis viverrini* infection and cholangiocarcinoma. A prospective, case-controlled study. *Gastroenterology* 89: 151, 1985.
26. Sell S, Dunsford HA: Evidence for the stem cell origin of hepatocellular carcinoma and cholangiocarcinoma. *Am J Pathol* 134:1347,1989.
27. Baserga R, Yokoo H, Henengar GC. Thorotrast-induced cancer in man. *Cancer* 1960; 13:1021-6.
28. Ito Y, Kojiro M, Nakashima T, et al. Pathomorphologic characteristics of 102 cases of Thorotrast-related hepatocellular carcinoma, cholangiocarcinoma, and hepatic angiosarcoma. *Cancer* 1988; 62:1153-8.
29. Janower ML, Miettinen OS, Flynn MJ. Effects of long-term Thorotrast exposure. *Radiology* 1972; 103:13-20.
30. Piehler JM, Crichlow RW. Primary carcinoma of the gallbladder. *Surg Gynecol Obstet* 1978: 147: 929.
31. Levin B. Gallbladder carcinoma. *Annals of Oncology* 10 *Suppl. 4:* S129-S130, 1999.
32. Krain LS: Carcinoma of the gallbladder in California, 1955-1969. *J Chronic Dis* 25:65, 1972.
33. Maibenco DC, Smith JL, Nava HR, Petrelli NJ, Douglass HO. Carcinoma of the Gallbladder. *Cancer Investigation* 16(1), 33-39 (1998).
34. Polk HC: Carcinoma and the calcified gallbladder. *Gastroenterology* 50:582-585, 1966.
35. Berk RN, Armbuster TG, Salzstein SL: Carcinoma in the porcelain gallbladder. *Radiology* 106:29-31, 1973.
36. Black WC. The morphogenesis of gallbladder carcinoma. In Progress in Surgical Pathology. Masson, New York: Fonoglio CM, Wolff M (eds), 1980:207.
37. Kimura K, Ohto M, Saisho H, Unozawa T, Tsuchiya Y, Morita M, Ebara M, Matsutani S, Okuda K: Association of gallbladder carcinoma and anomalous pancreaticobiliary ductal union. *Gastroenterology* 89: 1258-1265, 1985.
38. Suda K, Miyano T, Konuma I, et al. An abnormal pancreatico-choledocho-ductal junction in cases of biliary tract carcinoma. *Cancer* 1983;52:2086-8.

39. Yamauchi S, Koga A, Matsumoto S, et al. Anomalous junction of pancreaticobiliary duct without congenital choledochal cyst: a possible risk factor for gallbladder cancer. *Am J Gastroenterol* 1987; 82:20-6.

40. Fortner JG: Carcinoma of the gallbladder: The experimental induction of primary cancer. Cancer 8:689, 1955.

41. Fortner JG, Leffall LD: Carcinoma of the gallbladder in dogs. *Cancer* 14:1127, 1961.

42. Kowalewski K, Todd EF: Carcinoma of the gallbladder induced in hamsters by insertion of cholesterol pellets and feeding dimethylnitrosamine. *Pros Soc Exp Biol Med* 136:482, 1971.

43. Mancuso TF, Brennan MJ: Epidemiological consideration of cancer of the gallbladder, bile ducts and salivary glands in the rubber industry. *J Occup Med* 12:333, 1970.

44. Kozuka S, Tsubone M, Yasui A, et al. Relation of adenoma to carcinoma in the gallbladder. *Cancer* 1982; 50:226-34.

45. Yamagiwa H. Mucosal dysplasia of gallbladder: isolated and adjacent lesions to carcinoma. *Jpn J Cancer Res* 1989; 80:238-45.

46. Koichi W, Masao T, Koji Y, et al. Carcinoma and polyps of the gallbladder associated with Peutz-Jeghers syndrome. *Dig Dis Sci* 1987; 32:943-6.

47. Jones RS. Carcinoma of the Gallbladder. *Surg Clin of North Am* 1990:70(6) 1419-28.

48. Piehler JM, Crichlow: Primary carcinoma of the gallbladder. *Surg Gynecol Obstet* 147:929, 1978.

49. Hanks JB, Arnold WS. Hepatic Neoplasms. *Surgery.Scientific Principles and Practice.* Philadelphia, PA:Lippincott-Raven, Greenfield, et al. (2nd edition) 1997: 1008-1022.

50. Roh M. Colorectal Cancer Metastasis to the Liver. *Current Surgical Therapy.* St. Louis, Missouri: Mosby, Inc, Cameron JL. (6th edition) 1998: 352-354.

51. Jaffe BM, Donegan WL, Watson F, et al: Factors influencing survival in patients with untreated hepatic metastases. *Surg Gynecol Obstet* 127:1-11, 1968.

52. Bengmark S, Hafstrom L: The natural history of primary and secondary malignant tumors of the liver: I. The prognosis for patients with hepatic metastases from colonic and rectal carcinoma by laparotomy. *Cancer* 23:198-202, 1969.

53. Goslin R, Steele G, Zamcheck N, et al: Factors influencing survival in patients with hepatic metastases from adenocarcinoma of the colon and rectum. *Dis Colon Rectum* 25:749-754, 1982.

54. Bengtsson G, Carlsson G, Hafstrom L: Natural history of patients with untreated liver metastases from colorectal cancer. *Am J Surg* 141:586-589, 1981.

55. Finan PJ, Marshall RJ, Cooper EH, et al: Factors affecting survival in patients presenting with synchronous hepatic metastases from colorectal cancer: A clinical and computer analysis. *Br J Surg* 72:373-377, 1985.

56. De Brauw LM, De Velde CJH, Bouwhuis-Hoogerwerf ML: Diagnostic evaluation and survival analysis of colorectal cancer patients with liver metastases. *J Surg Oncol* 34:81-86, 1987.
57. Wood CB, Gillis CR, Blumgart LH: A retrospective study of the natural history of patients with liver metastases from colorectal cancer. *Clin Oncol* 2:285-288, 1976.
58. Wagner JS, Adson MA, Van Heerde JA, et al: The natural history of hepatic metastases from colorectal cancer: A comparison with resective treatment. *Ann Surg* 199:502-508, 1984.
59. Fong Y: Hepatic Colorectal Metastasis: Current Surgical Therapy, Selection Criteria for Hepatectomy, and Role for Adjuvant Therapy. *Advances in Surgery* 34:351-373, 2000.
60. Scheele J: Liver resection for colorectal metastases. *World J Surg* 19:59-71, 1995.
61. Fong Y, Fortner JG, Sun R, et al: Clinical score for predicting recurrence after hepatic resection for metastatic colorectal cancer: Analysis of 1001 consecutive case. *Ann Surg* 230:309-321, 1999.
62. Hughes KS, Simon R, Songhorabodi S, et al: Resection of the liver for colorectal carcinoma metastases: A multi-institutional study of patterns of recurrence. *Surgery* 100:278-284, 1986.
63. Scheele J, Stangl R, Altendorf-Hofman A, et al: Indicators of prognosis after hepatic resection for colorectal secondaires. *Surgery* 110:13-29, 1991.
64. Rosen CB, Nagorney DM, Taswell HF, et al: Perioperative blood transfusion and determinants of survival after liver resection for metastatic colorectal carcinoma. *Ann Surg* 216:492-505, 1992.
65. Gayowski TJ, Iwatsuki S, Madariaga JR, et al: Experince in hepatic resection for metastasic colorectal cancer: Analysis of clinical and pathological risk factors. *Surgery* 116:703-711, 1994.
66. Fong Y, Cohen AM, Fortner JG, et al: Liver resection for colorectal metasrases. *J Clin Oncol* 15:938-946, 1997.
67. Nordlinger B, Jeack D, Gulget M, et al: in Nordlinger B (ed): Surgical Resection of Hepatic Metastases: Multicentric Retrospective Study by the French Association Surgery. Paris, Springer, 1992, pp 129-146.
68. Moertel CG. Karnofsky Memorial Lecture: an odyssey in the land of small tumors. *J Clin Onc* 1987; 5:1503-1522.
69. Shebani KO, Souba WW, Finkelstein, et al. Prognosis and survival in patients with gastrointestinal tract carcinoid tumors. *Ann Surg* 1999:229:815-823.
70. Norheim I, Oberg K, Eheodorsson-Norheim E, et al. Malignant carcinoid tumors. *Ann Surg* 1987; 206:115-125.
71. Chamberlain RS, Canes D, Brown KT, Saltz L, Jarnigan W, Fong Y and Blumgart L. Hepatic neuroendocrine metastases: does intervention alter outcomes? *J Am Coll Surg* 2000: 432-445.
72. McEntee Gp, Nagorney Dm, Kvoils LK, et al. Cytoreductive hepatic surgery for neuroendocrine tumors. *Surgery* 1990; 108:1091-1096.

73. Martin JK, Moertel CG, Adson MA, et al. Surgical treatment of functioning metastatic carcinoid tumors. *Arch Surg* 1983; 118: 537-542.
74. Moertel CG, Johnson M, McKusick MA, et al. The Management of Patients with Advanced Carcinoid Tumors and Islet Cell Carcinomas. *Ann Intern Med.* 1994; 120:302-309.
75. Que FG, Nagorney DM, Batts KP, Linz LJ, Kvols LK. Hepatic resection for neuroendocrine carcinomas. *Am J Surg* 1995; 169:36-42.
76. Dousset B, Saint-Marc O, Pitre J, Soubrane O, Houssin D, Chapuis Y. Metastatic endocrine tumors: medical treatment, surgical resection, or liver transplantation. *World J Surg.* 20, 908-915, 1996.
77. Söreide O, Berstad T, Bakka A, et al. Surgical treatment as a principle in patients with advanced abdominal carcinoid tumors. *Surgery* 1992;111:48-54.

2
PATHOLOGIC FEATURES OF PRIMARY AND METASTATIC HEPATIC MALIGNANCIES

Mark Li-Cheng Wu, M.D., Adaora M. Okonkwo, M.D., Jacqueline S. Jeruss, M.D. and M. Sambasiva Rao, M.D.
Northwestern University Medical School, Chicago, IL

INTRODUCTION

In the mammalian liver, 60% of the cells are hepatocytes while the remainder (35%) include biliary epithelium, Kupffer cells, endothelial cells, fat storing cells and connective tissue cells. Although, neoplasms of hepatocytes are the most common liver tumors in humans, a significant number of other neoplasms including tumors of bile duct epithelium can develop. Not too long ago, liver tumors were left untreated because liver was considered as a complex and mysterious organ inaccessible to surgery. Advances in imaging procedures and surgical techniques over the past 30 years have revolutionized the approaches to the treatment of benign and malignant liver tumors. Subsegmentectomy, segmentectomy, lobectomy and transplantation are routinely performed for treatment of primary and metastatic liver tumors with minimal morbidity and mortality rates. Since accurate diagnosis remains the key to sound management, the emphasis of this article is on classification, morphological features and differential diagnosis of malignant neoplasms of liver.

PRIMARY LIVER TUMORS

Classification of primary liver tumors

	Benign tumors	**Malignant tumors**
Epithelial tumors	Hepatic adenoma	Hepatocellular carcinoma
		Hepatoblastoma
	Bile duct adenoma	Cholangiocarcinoma
	Bile duct cystadenoma (mucinous & serous types)	Billiary cystadeno-carcinoma
		Combined hepatocellular-Cholangiocarcinoma
	Billiary papillomatosis	
Non-epithelial tumors	Hemangioma	Epithelioid hemangio-Endothelioma
	Infantile hemangio-Endothelioma	Angiosarcoma

Classification of primary liver tumors (cont'd)

Non-epithelial tumors	Solitary fibrous tumor	Embryonal sarcoma
	Inflammatory myofibro-Blastic tumor	Rhabdomyosarcoma
	Angiomyolipoma	Leiomyosarcoma
		Carcinoid
Tumor-like lesions	Cysts	
	Focal nodular hyperplasia	
	Mesenchymal hamartoma	
	Fatty nodule	

Hepatocellular carcinoma

Hepatocellular carcinoma (HCC) is one of the most common tumors in the world with an estimated 1 million new cases each year. Although, the incidence is much less in western countries, a progressive increase has been seen over the last 20 years. The increased incidence of HCC noted in the U.S. has been attributed to high incidence of hepatitis C virus infection in patients with alcoholic liver disease (1). Other etiologic and risk factors have been identified as being responsible for the high incidence of HCC and possibly explain uneven geographic distribution throughout the world (Table 1).   Although, HCC may develop in non-cirrhotic livers, the majority of patients (about 80%) with HCC have cirrhosis. The pathogenesis of HCC development in cirrhosis is not known. The possible mechanism includes increased susceptibility of dividing hepatocytes associated with cirrhosis to oxidative stress resulting from infections, alcohol and metabolic diseases and exposure to environmental carcinogens leading to initiation phase of neoplastic process. In addition, in the cirrhotic liver there are metabolic and circulatory perturbations that may contribute to promotional and progression phase of tumor development.

Pathology of hepatocellular carcinoma

Although all HCC arise from hepatocytes, their biological behavior is quite variable and unpredictable. In spite of tremendous advances in molecular biology that have revolutionized our understanding of hepatocarcinogenesis there are no reliable molecular clues to predict the behavior of HCC. Features such as size, encapsulation, invasion, differentiation and cytological features are still used for prognostication of these tumors. Here we present a practical scheme for gross and microscopic classification of HCC (Table 2).

Table 1. Risk factors associated with HCC

Factor	Possible Mechanism of Tumor Induction
Dietary contamination by Mycotoxins	Direct DNA damage.
Alcoholic liver damage	Hepatitis, free radical generation, oxidative DNA Damage, cirrhosis.
Hepatitis C virus infection	Chronic necroinflammatory changes, free radical generation, oxidative DNA damage, cirrhosis.
Synergistic effects of HCV Infection + alcoholic Hepatitis	Inflammation, free radical generation, oxidative DNA damage, cirrhosis
Hepatitis B virus infection	Chronic necroinflammatory changes, cell proliferation, free radical generation oxidative DNA damage, cirrhosis, activation of oncogenes by adjacent viral insertion.
Iron overload (Hemochromatosis hemosiderosis)	Hydroxyl radical generation, oxidative DNA damage, cirrhosis.
Copper overload (Wilson's disease, Indian childhood cirrhosis)	Chronic hepatitis, free radical generation, cirrhosis.
Other inherited disorders (α1 -antitrypsin deficiency, porphyria cutanea tarda tyrosinemia)	Chronic inflammation, hepatocyte regeneration, cirrhosis.
Cirrhosis (secondary to any cause)	Increased hepatocyte proliferation, circulatory disturbances, (other factors as mentioned above).

Table 2. Classification of HCC

GROSS	MICROSCOPIC
Encapsulated (Expanding)	Conventional type of HCC
Infiltrating (spreading)	**Morphological variants of HCC**
Multifocal (diffuse)	Fibrolamellar type
Pedunculated	Spindle cell type
	Small cell type
	Sclerosing type
	HCC with osteoclastic giant cells
	Combined hepatocholangiocellular-carcinoma

CONVENTIONAL TYPE OF HCC

Gross pathology

Growth pattern of HCC, irrespective of the size, can provide useful information on the prognosis (2). Approximately 50% of HCC grow by expansion and separated from the adjacent parenchyma by a well-formed capsule. These encapsulated tumors can be large or small and can be seen in both cirrhotic (Figure 1) and non-cirrhotic livers. Encapsulated tumors often lack invasion beyond their capsule, or vascular permeation and are associated with better survival in patients after surgery (3). Formation of capsule around the tumors is considered to be a host defense mechanism rather than compression and collagenization of adjacent stroma. In contrast infiltrating (spreading) HCC's are poorly delineated with invasion into the adjacent parenchyma. These tumors also show frequent vascular invasion. Multifocal (diffuse) type of HCC invariably develops in cirrhotic liver and tumors of various sizes are scattered throughout the liver (Figure 2). Small HCC may be difficult to distinguish from macro-regenerative nodules seen in cirrhosis (4). Multifocality probably represents a combination of multicentric tumor development and intrahepatic metastasis. Pedunculated HCC are rare polyoid tumors connected to the hepatic surface by a stalk. Some pedunculated HCC may represent tumors arising in accessory lobes, or ectopic hepatic tissue or periadrenal metastasis that fuse with the liver. Irrespective of growth pattern, HCC's are soft, tan-white with areas of yellow and green depending on bile production. Cut surface of small tumors is usually homogeneous and fleshy, whereas, large tumors show hemorrhage and necrosis.

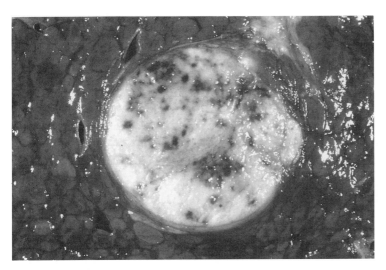

Figure 1. Small encapsulated HCC in a cirrhotic liver.

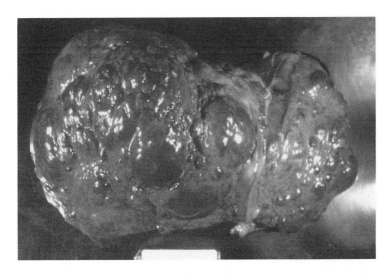

Figure 2. Multifocal HCC in a cirrhotic liver.

Microscopic pathology of conventional type of HCC

This is the most frequent type of HCC displaying cytoarchitectural features of hepatocytes. Tumor cells are usually arrayed in trabecular pattern of variable cell thickness. Plates of 2 to 8 cells and more than 8-cell thickness are referred to as microtrabecular and macrotrabecular patterrns respectively. Trabeculae are separated by sinusoids lined by endothelial cells and Kupffer cells (Figure 3). In some areas, there may be acinar or gland-like spaces containing altered bile resulting from dilatation of canaliculi. The tumor cells are polygonal with eosinophilic, basophilic or amphophilic cytoplasm. In addition, the cytoplasm may contain a variety of inclusions such as fat droplets, Mallory bodies and protein globules normally synthesized by hepatocytes (α-1 antitrypsin, α-1 chymotrypsin, α-fetoprotein, fibrinogen, albumin, ferritin). In some tumors there may be excessive accumulation of glycogen in the cytoplasm imparting clear cell features. Between the tumor cells, well-formed bile canaliculi are present that may not be readily identifiable by light microscope, but can be clearly demonstrated by immunoperoxidase technique using polyclonal carcinoembryonic antigen or electron microscope. Depending on functional differentiation of tumor cells bile may be present in the cytoplasm and canaliculi. The nuclear features vary with degree of tumor differentiation (see below) and they contain prominent eosinophilic nucleoli. Mitotic activity is variable. Some HCC may be associated with marked lymphocyte infiltration that reflects host response to tumor and better prognosis. Vascular invasion of HCC is not uncommon and should be always critically evaluated (Figure 4).

In conventional HCC, the stromal component is minimal and reticulin framework is delicate and sparse. In high grade HCC, the diagnostic trabecular architectural feature is usually lost and these tumors may be difficult to differentiate from metastatic tumors and other primary liver tumors. In such cases, immunohistochemical stains using antibodies to liver specific proteins or other proteins such as α-fetoprotein, α-1 antitrypsin, α-1 microglobulin, albumin, erythropoeitin associated antigen, des-γ-carboxy prothrombin, ferritin, fibrinogen, hepPar-1, cytokeratins and carcinoembryonic antigen are helpful for correct identification of tumors (5-7). Although, positive reaction for liver specific proteins in tumors is specific for the diagnosis of HCC, unfortunately sensitivity is not high.

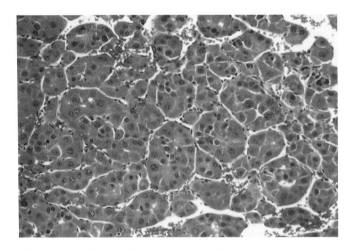

Figure 3. HCC showing trabecular architecture.

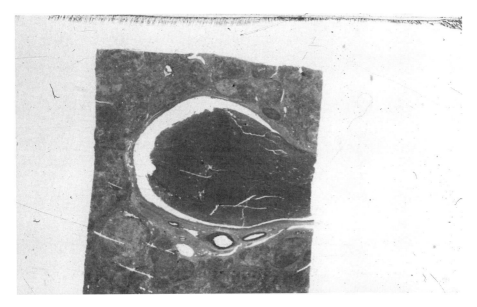

Figure 4. HCC with vascular invasion.

Grading of HCC

Four tier grading system proposed by Edmondson and Steiner (8) based on cytological and architectural features are generally used. (Table 3) Grade 1 HCC, now generally referred to as small early HCC, is characterized by nuclear crowding, cytoplasmic basophilia, microacinar formation and normotrabecular pattern (4,9). Fatty change is a frequent finding in small HCC. With the advent of sophisticated imaging techniques small hepatocellular lesions are readily identified and biopsied. Differentiation of small HCC from precursor lesions is important to avoid unnecessary surgery or over treatment (see below). In grade II HCC, increased nuclear pleomorphism and well-formed trabeculae are present. Grade III HCC show marked cellular pleomorphism with tumor giant cells, frequent mitoses and focal loss of trabecular pattern. Grade IV tumors are usually large, highly anaplastic, lose architectural and cytological resemblance to hepatocytes and may resemble other anaplastic tumors. Okuda et al. (10) have proposed that the degree of tumor differentiation is inversely proportional to the size of the tumor.

It is generally believed that development of HCC in humans, like in experimental animals, develops in a stepwise fashion and is preceded by the formation of precursor lesions (1,4,11). This phenomenon is well documented in livers with cirrhosis (12,13). These precursor lesions include adenomatous hyperplasia (macroregenerative nodule type 1) and atypical adenomatous hyperplasia (macroregenerative nodule type 11). In adenomatous hyperplasia nodules measure around 1 cm in diameter and histologically characterized by slight increase in cell density, lack of cytological atypia and the presence of portal areas with in the nodules. Nodules of atypical adenomatous hyperplasia are slightly larger (1 to 1.5

cm in diameter), and histologically show irregularly distributed portal areas, increased cell density, areas of small cell dysplasia and varying degrees of fatty change. Development of HCC in nodules of atypical adenomatous hyperplasia (nodule in nodule) is well documented.

Table 3. Grading of HCC

Grade	Microscopic features
Grade I	Normotrabecular, microaci, nuclear crowding and cytoplasmic basophilia
Grade II	Well-formed trabeculae, increased pleomorphisim
Grade III	Loss of trabeculae, marked pleomorphisim, tumor giant cells, frequent mitosis
Grade IV	Highly anaplastic

Predictors of prognosis

The survival and prognosis of patients with HCC depends on several factors. Traditionally used pathological criteria for evaluating prognosis in HCC are size, encapsulation, infiltration into the adjacent parenchyma and portal vein infiltration. Of these small size and tumor encapsulation are associated with better prognosis after surgical treatment. In patients with cirrhosis imaging procedures and serum tumor markers like α-fetoprotein and des-γ-carboxy prothrombin and ferritin levels are routinely used for screening to identify small HCC. In addition, a multitude of biological factors such as DNA ploidy, cell proliferation markers, expression of p-53, HSP72, telomerase, P-glycoprotein, E-cadherin are being evaluated in tumors to predict behavior and chemoresponse (14).

VARIANTS OF HCC

Although the incidence of variants of HCC are infrequent, recognition of these variants is important not only because they pose diagnostic problems but also their natural behavior and clinical manifestations can be quite different from conventional HCC.

Fibrolamellar HCC

This variant of HCC is a slow growing tumor, often develops under the age of 25 years in non-cirrhotic livers and is associated with excellent prognosis (15,16). The etiology of these tumors is unknown and no association with viral infections or alcohol consumption has been identified. Underlying chronic liver disease was observed in only 20% of the patients with fibrolamellar carcinomas. For unknown reasons the left lobe is frequently involved than the right lobe.

Pathologic features

Grossly, most of the tumors are large, solitary and well circumscribed with partial or complete encapsulation. However, in some tumors satellite nodules may be present. The cut surface is brown, fleshy with a central scar and connecting fibrous septa resembling focal nodular hyperplasia. (Figure 5A)   Necrosis and hemorrhage are present in large tumors.

These tumors show unique features that include distinct epithelial cells and stroma. The epithelial cells are polygonal with abundant granular eosinophilic cytoplasm and vesicular nuclei containing prominent nucleoli. (Figure 5B) Mitoses are infrequent. Granularity of tumor cells is due to abundant number of mitochondria (oncocytic features) (17). The tumor cells may contain bile, copper, copper associated protein and express both hepatic (cytokeratins 8 & 18) and biliary (cytokeratins 7 & 19) (18,19). In addition 50 % of tumors may contain cytoplasmic eosinophilic globules and pale bodies (clear area of cytoplasm resembling ground glass cells) that represent accumulated α-antitrypsin and fibrinogen respectively (15,18). Positive staining with neuron-specific enolase and serotonin and the presence of neuroendocrine granules also have been reported (20). The stromal component is abundant and is composed of thin multilayered strands of collagenous fibers separating the epithelial cells into trabeculae and nodules. Occasionally, fibrolamellar carcinomas may contain areas of conventional HCC. Fibrolamellar carcinomas may be associated with increased serum levels of vitamin B_{12}-binding protein and neurotensin and normal levels of α-fetoprotein.

Spindle cell type

These tumors are also referred to as sarcomatoid HCC and HCC with sarcomatous change (21,22). The clinical findings and gross morphology are similar to conventional type of HCC. Histologically, these tumors contain spindle cell (sarcomatoid) component and areas of conventional HCC. Sarcomatoid areas contained spindle cells arranged in fascicles and storiform pattern with variable amounts fibrous stroma and can resemble fibrosarcoma, leiomyosarcoma or malignant fibrous histiocytoma. Spindle cells are often stained positively for epithelial and spindle cell markers (21,23). Spindle cell HCC is associated with aggressive behavior characterized by frequent intra and extrahepatic metastasis and significant poor prognosis after resection.

Small cell type

This variant is extremely rare and only 3 cases have been reported. All 3 tumors developed in noncirrhotic livers and exhibited aggressive behavior. Tumor cells were small, polygonal to oval with scant cytoplasm, arranged in nests and trabeculae. Tumor cells stained positively with low molecular weight keratin and α-fetoprotein (24).

Sclerosing type

The sclerosing type of HCC often develops in patients without coexisting cirrhosis and often associated with hypercalcemia (25,26). As the name indicates the tumor is associated with abundant fibrotic stroma containing tumor cells arranged in cords and tubules resembling cholangiocarcinoma. Phenotypically, in 63% of tumors the cells showed hepatocytic features, in 20% ductal features and in the remainder mixed features. Mallory bodies were frequently present in tumor cells. Recurrence of tumor after surgery is rare.

HCC with osteoclastic giant cells

This variant of HCC is very rare and only a few cases have been reported. Histologically, these tumors contain scattered areas of malignant epithelial component with variable degree of differentiation and extensive areas of benign appearing osteoclast-like giant cells. In one giant cell tumor of the liver studied by the authors no evidence of hepatocyte differentiation was seen. HCC with osteoclast-like giant cells should be differentiated from HCC with pleomorphic tumor giant cells (27,28,29).

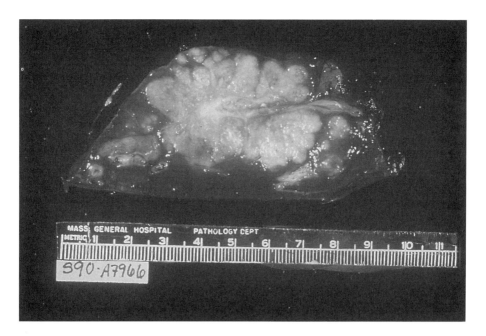

Figure 5A. Gross photograph of fibrolamellar HCC. Cut surface is brown and fleshy with a central scar.

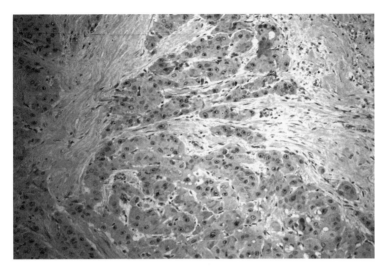

Figure 5B. Photomicrograph showing tumor cells with abundant granular eosinophilic cytoplasm and vesicular nuclei containing a prominent nucleoli.

HEPATOBLASTOMA

Although hepatoblastomas are most common in children under the age of 3 years but are occasionally seen in older children and adults (30-32). In young children, hepatoblastomas are more common in males than in females (2:1 ratio) while in older children there is no sex difference. The etiology of hepatoblastoma is not known and these tumors arise in livers without any preceding chronic liver disease. One third of the patients have various congenital anomalies. In addition, increased incidence of hepatoblastoma in children of familial adenomatous polyposis syndrome has been reported.

The histogenesis of hepatoblastoma is controversial. It is generally believed that both the epithelial and mesenchymal elements are neoplastic and are possibly derived from a common precursor (stem) cell (34). Using cultured chemically transformed rat epithelial cells Tsao and Grisham (35) have produced tumors with features of hepatoblastoma in rats. These findings clearly demonstrated multidirectional differentiation potential of hepatic epithelial cells.

Pathological features

Grossly, these tumors can be solitary and encapsulated or multinodular. The cut surface of the tumor has variegated appearance depending on the microscopic type. Tumors with pure epithelial component are homogeneous with a brown to green surface whereas, tumors with epithelial and mesenchymal components show areas of hemorrhage and necrosis.

Histologically, hepatoblastomas are subdivided into fetal, embryonal, epithelial-mesenchymal, small cell undifferentiated and macrotrabecular types (30,36,37). In fetal subtype, as in the fetal liver, small hepatocytes with prominent nucleoli and eosinophilic cytoplasm are arranged in 2 to 3 cell thick cords. Extramedullary hematopoiesis is seen in the sinusoids.

In the embryonal subtype, the tumor cells are less differentiated than fetal type and may not resemble hepatocytes. The cells are small with high nuclear cytoplasmic ratio, nuclear pleomorphism and increased mitoses. Tumor cells are arranged in cords, sheets and acini and may show areas of squamous differentiation (figure 6). Foci of hematopoiesis can be seen. Mixed epithelial and mesenchymal hepatoblastomas consists of epithelial cells admixed with mesenchymal elements. The mesenchymal components include immature spindle cells, rhabdomyoblasts of varying maturity, osteoid and cartilagenous tissue. Areas of metaplastic squamous epithelium and mucinous epithelium may also be found. Small cell undifferentiated type contain small anaplastic cells arranged in sheets and may mimic neuroblastomas. These tumors are associated with poor prognosis. The macrotrabecular type consists of epithelial cells arranged in thick trabeculae and resembles conventional HCC.

Irrespective of histological subtype, hepatoblastomas are associated with high levels of serum α-fetoprotein and this protein is readily demonstrable in fetal and embryonal cells by immunoperoxidase technique. Patients with hepatoblastomas, except for the small cell and macrotrabecular variants, have excellent prognosis after surgical resection.

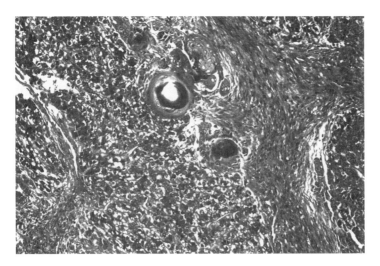

Figure 6. Tumor cells arranged in cords, sheets and acini with areas of squamous differentiation in embryonal subtype of hepatoblastoma.

CHOLANGIOCARCINOMA

Cholangiocarcinoma is an adenocarcinoma arising from biliary epithelium anywhere in the biliary tract. Depending on the site of origin, these tumors are classified as peripheral cholangiocarcinoma (arising in small peripheral intrahepatic bile ducts), hilar type cholangiocarcinoma (arising in right and left hepatic ducts and the area of their junction, also referred to as Klatskin's tumor) and bile duct carcinoma (arising in extrahepatic bile duct) (38,39). The incidence of cholangiocarcinoma is much less common than HCC, and usually affects both the sexes equally over the age of 50. Unlike HCC, no association with alcoholic hepatitis, viral hepatitis or cirrhosis has been found. Exposure to thorotrast and infestation with liver flukes has been causally linked to cholangiocarcinoma (40,41). In addition, several predisposing factors such as Caroli's disease, choledochal cyst, polycystic liver disease, sclerosing cholangitis, inflammatory bowel disease and hepatolithiasis have been identified.

Pathologic features

Grossly, peripheral cholangiocarcinomas are grey-white, firm, unencapsulated tumors that present as a large solitary mass or multiple nodules. Whereas, hilar and bile duct carcinomas present as strictures or diffusely infiltrative lesions.

Microscopically, irrespective of location, cholangiocarcinomas show features of mucin producing adenocarcinomas with abundant desmoplastic stroma. Based on the architectural and cytological differentiation these tumors are classified as well differentiated (grade I), moderately differentiated (grade II), and poorly differentiated (grade III). Well-differentiated cholangiocarcinomas reveal tubular, papillary or tubulo-papillary architecture. The lining epithelium is cuboidal to low columnar with basally located uniform nuclei. (Figure 7) Mitotic activity is infrequent. In poorly differentiated carcinomas gland formation is infrequent, and tumor cells are arranged in clusters or cords. Tumor cells show marked nuclear pleomorphism and frequent mitoses. Moderately differentiated cholangiocarcinomas have features ranging from well differentiated to poorly differentiated tumors. Occasionally, cholangiocarcinomas can show uncommon histological types that include signet ring cells, clear cells, undifferentiated small cells, mucinous carcinoma and adenosquamous features. Poorly differentiated cholangiocarcinomas are difficult to differentiate from metastatic carcinomas and HCC. Proper identification of these tumors is possible with immunohistochemical stains using antibodies to different types of cytokeratins, carcinoembryonic antigen, epithelial membrane antigen, and α-fetoprotein (42-44). In cholangiocarcinomas serum levels of carcinoembryonic antigen and carbohdrate antigen CA 19-9 are increased (45). The incidence of distant and lymph node metastasis in peripheral cholangiocarcinomas is very high than in the hilar type, which may reflect on the advanced stage of the disease at the time of presentation. Hilar tumors are often diagnosed in early stages because of obstructive symptoms.

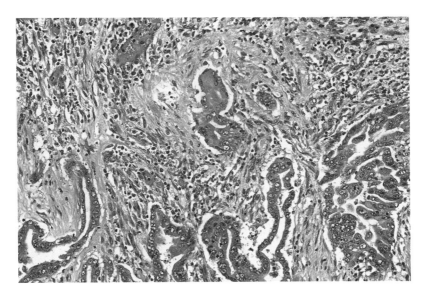

Figure 7. Microscopic view of a well-differentiated cholangiocarcinoma showing cuboidal to columnar lining epithelium with basally located uniform nuclei.

BILIARY CYSTADENOCARCINOMA

This rare cystic malignant neoplasm develops in biliary cystadenoma and choledochal cyst and accounts for 20 to 40% of the reported cases of hepatobiliary cystic tumors (42,46).

Pathologic features

These tumors are well-circumscribed, large multiloculated cysts separated from the adjacent liver by fibrous tissue capsule. The cysts contain clear mucinous or hemorrhagic fluid. Microscopically, the tumors show benign, borderline and malignant areas. In benign areas the lining epithelium is cuboidal to columnar with nuclei that are basally oriented. No cellular atypia is present. In borderline areas there is cellular and nuclear pleomorphism, stratification of nuclei and increased mitosis. In malignant areas, in addition to atypical cellular features, the epithelium is multilayered and may form papillary folds and show invasion into underlying stroma and adjacent liver. Biliary cystadenocarcinoma has much better prognosis after surgical excision compared to cholangiocarcinoma.

PAPILLARY CYSTIC TUMOR

Papillary cystic tumor of the liver is very rare and only a single case has been described (47). The pathological features of this tumor are strikingly similar to papillary cystic tumor of the pancreas. Papillary cystic tumor in the pancreas is now referred to as papillary pseudocystic neoplasm (48). Histologically the tumor contained cuboidal to columnar cells arranged in a papillary pattern and solid sheets. Under electron microscopy, the tumor cells showed features of pancreatic acinar and ductular cells. The diagnosis of papillary cystic tumor of the liver should be made only after exclusion of pancratic primary.

COMBINED HEPATOCELLULAR-CHOLANGIO CARCINOMA

Only the tumors that show features of conventional HCC and cholangiocarcinoma with transitional areas should be included in this category (49). HCC with pseudoglandular features secondary to dilatation of bile canaliculi may be easily confused with this variant. In the combined tumor hepatocellular areas show keratin profile consistent with hepatocytes and in the glandular areas the cells show bile duct epithelium pattern and positive staining for mucin (50). In a case report by Fischer et al., (51) cells in transitional areas showed keratin profile similar to that of bile duct epithelium. Bidirectional differentiation of combined tumors support the hypothesis of existence of bipotential stem cells in the human liver and possible origin of these tumors from those cells.

MALIGNANT VASCULAR TUMORS

Although benign vascular tumors (hemangioma) are very common in the liver, malignant vascular tumors are very rare. Epithelioid hemangioendothelioma and angiosarcoma, two distinct histological types of malignant vascular tumors of endothelial origin, that strongly stain for factor VIII-related antigen, CD31 and CD34, with different biological behavior develop in the liver.

Epithelioid hemangioendothelioma (EH)

These tumors are more common in females (ratio of females to males of 2:1) and occur over a wide age range (2nd to 8th decade). No associated chronic liver disease is present. Role of oral contraceptives in the etiology of EH has been suggested (52,53).

Pathologic features

The tumors often present as multiple, white, firm nodules of varying sizes involving both the lobes. Cut surface is homogeneous with infiltrative margins. Microscopically, the tumor consists of epithelioid to spindle shaped cells occurring singly or arranged in nests or short cords (Figure 8). The epithelioid cells contain abundant eosinophilic cytoplasm and prominent nuclei. In some cells intracytoplasmic vacuoles containing red blood cells can be seen. Mitotic activity is variable. The tumor contains abundant stroma with areas of dense fibrosis, myxoid change and calcification. Areas of necrosis and inflammatory infiltrate can be seen. Extension of tumor cells into large veins and intraluminal growth is frequent. Differentiation of EH from angiosarcoma and epithelial tumors with sclerosis is important because of better prognosis associated with these tumors after lobectomy or transplantation (54).

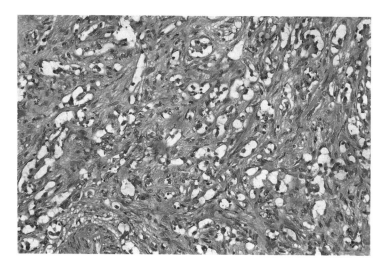

Figure 8. Photomicrograph showing epithelioid homogenous cut surface with infiltrative margins and prominent nucleoli characteristic of hemangioendothelioma.

Angiosarcoma

This tumor affects men more often than women (M: F ratio of 4:1), mostly in the 6th and 7th decades. There is good correlation between exposure to thorotrast, vinyl chloride, and arsenic and the development of angiosarcoma (40,55). In addition, there is also some evidence that radium, inorganic copper, and anabolic steroids may play some role in the pathogenesis of angiosarcoma. However, in many patients no risk factors can be identified.

Pathologic features

Angiosarcoma is often a multifocal disease involving both the lobes and appear as nodules of variable sizes. The cut section shows poorly delineated lesions with gray-white to hemorrhagic areas. Histologically, these tumors consist of predominantly spindle cells arranged in a combination of three basic patterns: sinusoidal, cavernous and solid. In sinusoidal pattern the tumor cells proliferate along sinusoids and there is varying degree of sinusoidal dilatation and atrophy of liver cell cords. In the cavernous pattern the sinusoids become markedly dilated with loss of hepatocytes. The tumor cells are pleomorphic, multilayered and may form papillary folds. In the solid pattern cells grow in sheets without forming vascular spaces and display marked cellular atypia and increased mitoses. Extramedullary hematopoiesis may be present. Infiltration of tumor cells into portal and hepatic veins is common.

Endothelial cells in the liver adjacent to the tumor usually shows hyperplastic and dysplastic changes. The prognosis in angiosarcoma is extremely poor (32).

Embryonal sarcoma

Embryonal sarcoma is also referred to as mesenchymal sarcoma, malignant mesenchymoma and undifferentiated sarcoma, is a rare tumor that commonly afflicts children between the ages of 6 and 10 years and occasionally adults (56). No precursor lesions or predisposing factors have been identified.

Pathologic features

Grossly, these tumors are large, soft, well circumscribed and usually single. On cut section the tumor has variegated appearance with gelatinous, myxoid, cystic, hemorrhagic and necrotic areas (figure 9A). Microscopically, the tumor is composed of primitive anaplastic mesenchymal cells arranged in fascicles, sheets or without any pattern (figure 9B). Typical and atypical mitoses are very common. The matrix is myxoid, rich in acid mucopolysaccharides. PAS-positive, diastase resistant eosinophilic globules, considered to be α-1 antitrypsin, can be seen in the cytoplasm and in the stroma. With in the tumor trapped dilated bile ducts and islands of extramedullary hematopoiesis may be present. In tumors amenable to surgery the prognosis is considered good (32,56,57).

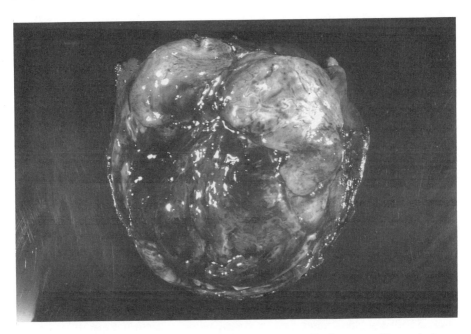

Figure 9A. Gross photograph showing a large circumscribed tumor with a gelatinous cut surface characteristic of embryonal sarcoma.

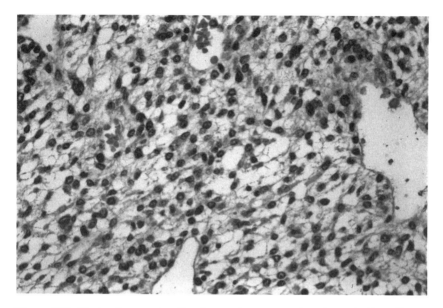

Figure 9B. Photomicrograph of embryonal sarcoma showing spindle cells arranged in fascicles.

OTHER MALIGNANT PRIMARY TUMORS

Various other tumors such as rhabdomyosarcoma, leiomyosarcoma, germ cell tumors, lymphoma and carcinod listed in table 1 occurs very rarely as primary tumors in the liver and shows morphological features similar to those occurring elsewhere in the body. When these tumors are seen in the liver the possibility of metastasis should be considered and ruled out.

METASTATIC TUMORS

In the United States and Europe metastatic tumors of the liver are far more common than primary tumors. Liver is considered as a fertile soil for metastasis from any tumor, although tumors from some organs such as colon, rectum, stomach, pancreas (ductal and islet cell tumors), lung, breast, occular melanomas and gastrointestinal stromal tumors metastasize frequently (58). Liver specific metastasis from these tumors is dependent on several factors such as portal venous drainage, microenvironment, cell adhesion molecules and hepatocyte-derived growth factors (58,59). Because of liver specific factors circulating tumor cells are likely to seed in the liver and grow, thus resulting in liver only metastasis. Under these circumstances surgical therapy, local ablation, regional chemotherapy or chemoembolization may result in palliation, local tumor growth control or even potential cure (60).

With recent advances in imaging techniques liver lesions of smaller size that represent both the primary tumors and metastatic tumors from known and unknown primaries are increasingly identified. Because of significant difference in the treatment of these various tumors proper pathological diagnosis and classification are very important. For differentiation of primary tumors from metastatic tumors and proper identification of metastatic tumors is possible based on characteristic morphological features, and special procedures such as histochemical, immunochemical, ultrastructural studies. In surgical pathology practice a myriad immunohistochemical markers are available that helps in proper identification of tumors (Table 4&5).

Table 4. Immunohistochemical stains for identifying common liver tumors

Tumor	Marker
Hepatocellular carcinoma	CK 8 & 18, polyclonal carcinoembryonic antigen, fibrinogen, α-1 antitrypsin, α-fetoprotein, albumin
Cholangiocarcinoma	CK 7,19 & 20; carcinoembryonic antigen, CA 19-9
Vascular tumors	Factor VIII-related antigen, CD 31 & 34
Metastatic adenocarcinoma	CK 7,19 & 20; carcinoembryonic antigen, CA 19-9, Leu-Leu-M1
Neuroendocrine tumors	Neuron specific enolase, chromogranin, synaptophysin
Lymphoma	Leucocyte common antigen, CD 3 & 20

Table 5. Immunohistochemical stains for identifying specific tumors of the liver

Breast carcinoma	Gross cystic disease fluid protein, estrogen and progesterone receptors
Prostate carcinoma	Prostate specific antigen, prostate specific acid phosphatase
Melanoma	S-100, HMB-45, vimentin

Pathology of metastatic tumors

Grossly, metastatic tumor may be single and circumscribed or multiple with poorly defined margins. Cut surface of the tumor is variable depending on the type of tumor. Melanomas are usually black, choriocarcinomas are hemorrhagic, and undifferentiated tumors and lymphomas display fish-flesh appearance. Microscopically, well and moderately differentiated tumors retain morphologic features of primary tumors. Metastatic tumors from breast and pancreas usually incite a desmoplastic reaction and may be difficult to differentiate from cholangiocarcinoma. Sinusoidal growth pattern is commonly seen with small cell carcinoma of lung and occasionally with other tumors. Liver adjacent to metastatic tumors may show cholestasis, sinusoidal dilatation and atrophy of liver cell cords.

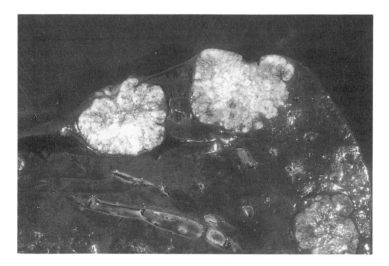

Figure 10A. Gross photograph depicting metastatic colon carcinoma to the liver in a multinodular confluent fashion.

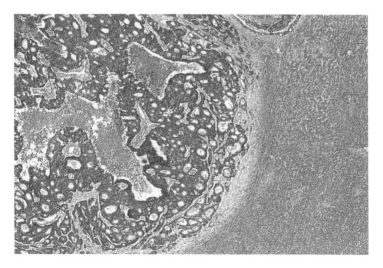

Figure 10B. Corresponding photomicrograph showing metastatic colon cancer with adjacent normal liver.

REFERENCES

1. Okuda K: Hepatocellular carcinoma. J Hepatol 32(Suppl 1): 225-237, 2000.
2. Okuda K, Peters RL and Simson IW: Gross anatomic features of hepatocellular carcinoma from three disparate geographic areas. Proposal of new classification. Cancer 54:2165-2173, 1984.
3. Ng IOL, Lai ECS, Ng MMT and Fan ST: Tumor encapsulation in hepatocellular carcinoma. Cancer 70:45-49, 1992.
4. Kojiro M and Nakashima O: Histopathologic evaluation of hepatocellular carcinoma with special reference to small early stage tumors. Sem Liver Dis 29:287-296, 1999.
5. Fernandez-Izquierdo A and Llombart-Bosch A: Immunohistochemical characterization of 130 cases of primary hepatic carcinomas. Path Res Pract 182: 783-191, 1987.
6. Ganjei P, Nadji M, Albores-Saavedia J, Morales AR: Histologic markers in primary and metastatic tumors of the liver. Cancer 62L1996-1998, 1998.
7. Derrico A, Baccarini P, Florentino M. Ceccarelli C, Bonanzzi C, Ponzetto A, Sccazec JY, Mancini AM and Grigioni WF: Histogenesis of primary liver carcinomas: strengths and weaknesses of cytokeratin profile and albumin mRNA detection. Hum Path 27:599-604, 1996.
8. Edmondson HA and Steiner PE: Primary carcinoma of the liver: a study of 100 cases among 48,900 necropsies. Cancer 7:462-503, 1954.
9. Kondo F, Firooka N, Wada K and Kondo Y: Morphological clues for the diagnosis of small hepatocellular carcinoma. Virch Arch 411:15-21, 1987.
10. Okuda K, Nakashima T, Obata H and Kubo Y: Clinicopathological studies of minute hepatocellular carcinoma: Analysis of 20 cases including 4 with resection. Gastroenterology 73:109-115, 1977.
11. Farber E and Sarma DSR: Hepatocarcinogenesis: a dynamic cellular perspective. Lab Invest 56:4-22, 1987.
12. Theise ND: Macroregenerative (dysplastic) nodules and hepatocarcinogenesis theoretical and clinical considerations. Sem Liver Dis 15:360-371, 1995.
13. Hytiroglou P, Theise ND, Schwartz M, Mor E, Miller C and Thung SN: Macroregenerative nodules in a series of adult cirrhotic liver explants: issues of classification and nomenclature. Hepatology 21:703-708, 1995.
14. Okuda K and Nishioka M: Review of the Japanese literature. Cur Hepatology 17:315-337, 1997.
15. Craig JR, Peters RL, Edmondson HA and Omata M: Fibrolamellar carcinoma of the liver: a tumor of adolescents and young adults with distinctive clincopathologic features. Cancer 46:372-379, 1980.
16. Berman MM, Libbey NP and Foster JH: Hepatocellular carcinoma, polygonal cell type with fibrous stroma- an atypical variant with a favourable prognosis. Cancer 46:1448-1455, 1980.
17. Fachi DC, Shikes RH and Silverberg SA: Ultrastructure of fibrolamellar oncocytic hepatoma. Cancer 50:702-709, 1982.

18. Lefkowitch JH, Muschel R, Price JB, Manbou C and Braunhut S: Copper and Copper-binding protein in fibrolammelar liver cell carcinoma. Cancer 51:97-100, 1983.

19. Berman MA, Burnham JA, Shehan DU: Fibrolamellar carcinoma of the liver: an immunohistochemical study of nineteen cases and a review of the literature. Hum Pathol 19:784-794, 1988.

20. Payne CM, Nagle RB, Paplanus SH and Graham AR: Fibrolamellar carcinoma of liver: a primary malignant oncocytic carcinoid? Ultrastruct Pathol 10:539-552, 1986.

21. Maeda T, Adachi E, Kajiyama K, Takenaka K, Sugimachi K and Tsuneyoshi M: Spindle cell hepatocellular carcinoma. A clinicopathologic and immunohistochemical analysis of 15 cases. Cancer 77:51-57, 1996.

22. Ishak KG, Anthony PP and Sobin LH: Histological typing of tumors of the liver. 2nd Ed. Geneva: World Health Organization, 1994.

23. Haratake J and Horie A: An immunohistochemical study of sarcomatoid liver carcinomas. Cancer 68:93-97, 1991.

24. Zanconati F, Falconieri A, Lamovec JL and Zidar A: Small cell carcinoma of the liver: a hitherto unreported variant of hepatocellular carcinoma. Histopathol 29:449-453, 1996.

25. Omata M, Peters RL and Tatter D: Sclerosing hepatic carcinoma: relationship to hypercalcemia. Liver 1:33-49, 1981.

26. Okuda K and Okuda H: Primary liver cell carcinoma. In: Oxford text book of clinical hepatology, Ed: Bircher J, Benhamon J, Mcintyre N, Rizzetto M and Rodes J. Oxford Medical Publication, Vol 2, pp 1491-1530,1999.

27. Munoz PA, Rao MS and Reddy JK: Osteoclastoma-like giant cell tumor of the liver. Cancer 46:771-779, 1980.

28. Kuwano H, Sonada T, Hashimoto H and Enjoji M: Hepatocellular carcinoma with osteoclast-like giant cells. Cancer 54:837-842,1984.

29. Hood DL, Bauer TW, Leibel SA and Recmahon JT: Hepatic giant cell carcinoma: an ultrastructural and immunohistochemical study. Am J Clin Path 93:111-116,1990.

30. Stocker JT: Hepatoblastoma. Sem Diag Pathol 1994.

31. Reynolds M: Pediatric liver tumors. Sem Surg Oncol 16:159-172,1999.

32. Klatskin A and Conn HO: Neoplasms of the liver and intrahepatic bile ducts. In Histopathology of the liver, Oxford University Press, Oxford Vol 1, pp367-395,1993.

33. Altman HW: Epithelial and mixed hepatoblastoma in the adult. Histological observations and general considerations. Path Res Pract 188:16-22,1988.

34. Ruck P, Xiao JC and Kaiseling E: Small epithelial cells and histogenesis of hepatoblastoma. Electron-microscopic, immuno-electronmiroscopic and immunohistochemical findings. Am J Pathol 148:321,1996.

35. Tsao M and Grisham JW: Hepatocarcinomas, cholangiocarcinomas and hepatoblastomas produced by chemically transformed cultured rat liver epithelial cells. A light and electron-microscopic analysis. Am J Pathol 127:168-181,1987.

36. Lack EE, Neave C and Vawter GF: Hepatoblastoma, a clinical and pathologic study of 54 cases. Am J Surg Pathol 6:693-705,1982.
37. Gonzalez-Crussi F, upton MP and Maurer HS: Hepatoblastoma: attempt at characterization of histologic subtypes. Am J Surg Pathol 6:599,1982.
38. Nakajima T, Kondo Y, Miyazaki M and Okai K: a histopathologic study of 102 cases of intrahepatic cholangiocarcinoma: histologic classification and modes of spreading. Hum Pathol 19:1228-1234, 1988.
39. Yeo CT, Pitt HA and Cameron JL: Cholangiocarcinoma. Surg Clin North Am 70:1429-1447,1990.
40. Ho Y, Kojiro M, Nakashima Ta and Mori T: Pathomorphologic characteristics of 102 cases of thorotrast-related hepatocellular carcinoma, cholangiocarcinoma and hepatic angiosarcoma. Cancer 62:1153-1162,1998.
41. Schwartz DA: Cholangiocarcinoma associated with liver fluke infection: a preventable source of morbidity in Asian immigrants. Am J Gastroenterol 81:76-79,1986.
42. Colombani R and Tsui WMS: Biliary tumors of the liver. Sm Liver Dis 15:402-413,1995.
43. Rullier A, Le Baid B, Fawaz R, Blanc J, Sanic J and Bioulac-Sage P: Cytokeratin 7 and 20 expression in cholangiocarcinoma varies along the biliary tract but still differs from that in colorectal carcinoma metastatsis. Am J Surg Pathol 24:870-876,2000.
44. D'erricoA, Baccarini P, Florentino M, Ceccarelli C, Bonazzi C, Ponzetto A, Scoazec JY, Mancini AY and Grigioni WF: Histogenesis of primary liver carcinomas: strengths and weaknesses of cytokeratin profile and albumin mRNA. Hum Pathol 27:599-604,1996.
45. Jalanko H, Kunsela P, Roberts S, Sippone P, Haghung F and Makela O: Comparison of a new marker CA-19-9T, with α-fetoprotein and carcinoembryonic antigen in patients with upper gastrointestinal disease. J Clin Pathol 37:218-222,1984.
46. Rivaney K, Goodman ZD and Ishak KG: Hepatobiliary cystadenoma and cystadenocarcinoma. A light microscopic and immunohistochemical study of 70 patients. Am J Surg Pathol 18:1078-1091,1994.
47. Kim YI, Kim ST, Lei AK and Choi BI: Papillary cystic tumor of the liver. A case report with ultrastructural observation. Cancer 65:2740-2746,1990.
48. Klimstra DS, Wenig BM and Hefess CS: Solid-pseudopapillary tumor of the pancreas: a typically cystic carcinoma of low malignant potential. Sem Dia Path 17:66-80,2000.
49. Ng IO, Shek TW, Nicholls J and Rea LT: Combined hepatocellular-cholangiocarcinoma: a clinicopathologic study. J Gastroenterol Hepatol 13:34,1998.
50. Kondo Y and Wakajima T: Psuedoglandular hepatocellular carcinoma. A morphologic study. Cancer 60:1032-1037,1987.
51. Fischer HP, Doppl W, Osborn M and Altmannsbuger M:Evidence for a hepatocellular lineage in a combined hepatocellular-cholangiocarcinoma of transitional type. Virch Arch 56:71-76,1988.

52. Ishak KA, Sesterhenn IA, Goodman ZD, Rabin L and Stromeyer FW: Epitheloid hemangioendothelioma of the liver: a clinicopathologic and follow-up study of 32 cases. Hum Pathol 25:839-852,1984.

53. Dean PJ, Haggitt RC and O'hara CJ: Malignant epithelioid hemangioendothelioma of the liver in young women. Relationship to oral contraceptive use. Am J Surg Pathol 9:695-704,1989.

54. Kelleher MB, Inatsuki S and Sheahau DG: Epithelioid hemangioendothelioma of liver. Histopathology 13:999-1008,1989.

55. Popper H, Thomas LB, Teller NC, Flak H and Selikoff IJ: Development of hepatic angiosarcoma induced by vinyl chloride, thorotrast and arsenic. Comparison with cases of unkown etiology. Am J Pathol 92:349-376,1978.

56. Stocker JT and Ishak KG: Undifferentiated (embryonal) sarcoma of the liver. Report of 31 cases. Cancer 42:336-348,1978.

57. Anthony PP: Tumors and tumor-like lesions of the liver and biliary tract. In: Pathology of the liver, Eds: MacSween RMM, Anthony PP, Scheuer PJ, 2nd Edition, Churchhil Livingstone, Edinburgh, pp 574-665,1987.

58. Cody B: Natural history of primary and secondary tumors of the liver. Sem Oncology 10:127-134,1983.

59. Kawamoto K, Onodera H, Kan S and Imamuar M: Possible paracrine mechanism of insulin-like growth factor-2 in the development of liver metastases from colorectal carcinoma. Cancer 85:18-25,1999.

60. Sussman JJ and Ellis LM: Current therapy for hepatic mutations. Cur Hepatol 17:195-215,1997.

3
RADIOLOGIC IMAGING AND STAGING OF PRIMARY AND METASTATIC LIVER TUMORS

Jonathan W. Berlin, M.D., Richard M. Gore, M.D., and Vahid Yaghmai, M.D.
Northwestern University, Evanston, IL
F. Scott Pereles, M.D. and Frank H. Miller, M.D.
Northwestern University Medical School, Chicago, IL

INTRODUCTION

The radiologic imaging and staging of primary and metastatic liver tumors has been revolutionized by advances in ultrasonographic (US) imaging, computed tomography (CT), and magnetic resonance imaging (MRI). In spite of the improved sensitivity in the detection of hepatic malignancies, the ability to differentiate benign from malignant intrahepatic lesions often remains problematic due to extensive overlap in imaging appearances. Additionally, only several liver lesions have a pathognomonic appearance on cross-sectional imaging. As a result, tissue sampling performed with CT or ultrasound guidance is often required to better characterize a hepatic lesion (1-5).

Radiologic staging of hepatic malignancies involves precise localization of the tumor mass using the Couinaud nomenclature (Couinaud) (6), as well as detection of extrahepatic disease that often precludes surgical resection. This requires accurate depiction of extrahepatic lymphadenopathy, ascites, and vascular encasement. Cross-sectional imaging studies of the chest or central nervous system are often required to adequately stage hepatic lesions (7-11). Occasionally, nuclear medicine studies can detect occult skeletal metastases.

Because metastatic disease is the most common malignant tumor of the liver, the first section of this chapter addresses the detection and characterization of hepatic metastasis (2). Subsequent sections discuss the two most common and clinically significant primary hepatic tumors, hepatocellular carcinoma and cholangiocarcinoma (12). The chapter concludes with a brief discussion of the common benign primary hepatic tumors that can simulate malignant lesions on imaging studies.

HEPATIC METASTASES

Effective staging of metastatic disease requires accurate detection of the number, size, and location of intrahepatic metastases, as well as accurate detection of metastatic disease to surrounding lymph nodes and extrahepatic organs. Imaging protocols are designed to maximize detection of small hepatic metastases by utilizing two main strategies: tumor-to-liver contrast differences and increasing spatial resolution. Spatial resolution can be increased on CT and MR scans by using thin sections and contrast differences can be maximized through the use of intravenous contrast material. Most hepatic metastatic lesions greater than one cm in size are detected with modern imaging techniques (7). However, most intrahepatic lesions less than 5mm are not currently detected (2).

Hepatic metastases have a variable appearance on cross-sectional imaging studies that depend upon several factors: the use and timing of intravenous contrast material, the vascularity of the lesion, the degree of hemorrhage and necrosis. Tumors supplied primarily by the hepatic artery are radiographically termed "hypervascular", and those with a greater percentage of vascularity from the portal system are referred to as "hypovascular". Classically hypervascular lesions include primary hepatocellular carcinoma as well as hepatic metastasis from carcinoid, islet cell tumors, pheochromocytoma, renal cell carcinoma, and breast carcinoma.

Metastatic Disease: Ultrasound Appearance

Because of its lesser cost and greater availability, transabdominal ultrasound is the most common primary screening technique used for detection of hepatic metastases worldwide (13-18). The sensitivity of ultrasound approach is that of a noncontrast CT scan (2). Standard transabdominal sonography is limited in patients with heavy body habitus as well as patients who cannot follow respiratory instructions. Additionally, it is highly operator dependent. Intraoperative ultrasound, however, has been shown to have a much higher sensitivity for detection of intrahepatic metastases, with some authors claiming that it is more sensitive than CT or MRI (7).

Recent work with color Doppler sonography has shown that metastatic liver lesions have increased flow within the hepatic artery (8) or an elevated Doppler perfusion index (the ratio of hepatic artery to portal venous flow) (9). Several investigators have advocated the use of intravenous sonographic contrast agents that employ microbubbles to increase lesion conspicuity.

On gray scale sonography, hepatic metastases have a variety of appearances. The most common presentation is a uniformly hypoechoic mass compared to normal hepatic parenchyma (13-14). In general, hypoechoic masses tend to be hypovascular or avascular. Intrahepatic metastases also commonly appear as masses of mixed echogenicity. Occasionally, they can also appear as uniformly hyperechoic lesions. This occurs most often with hypervascular lesions (15-16) but can also be related to intratumoral calcification, which most often occurs in metastases from gastrointestinal primary tumors (Fig. 1), but also can occur with metastatic lesions from ovarian, pancreatic, thyroid, or breast carcinoma. Intrametastatic calcification can produce acoustic shadowing.

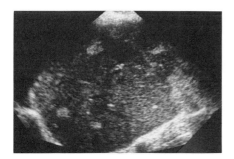 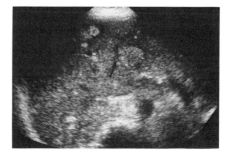

Figure 1. A. *(Left panel)* sagittal sonogram discloses multiple fairly well marginated echogenic metastases from adenocarcinoma of the colon. B. *(Right panel)* several of these metastases (arrows) show a hypoechoic rim. This patient had a colonic primary.

Another sonographic appearance of intrahepatic metastases is that of a "target" or "bulls-eye" lesion, with a hypoechoic halo surrounding a more hyperechoic mass centrally. This is due to compression of normal hepatic parenchyma around the metastatic lesion in some cases (16) and tumor proliferation in other cases (17). Rare sonographic appearances of hepatic metastatic disease include predominantly cystic lesions, usually with mural nodules or septations. This has been described with mucinous tumors of the pancreas, ovary, or colon, as well as with choriocarcinoma and sarcomas.

Metastatic disease can also produce a diffusely infiltrative pattern, without any discreetly definable lesions. Often, this is associated with an irregular hepatic contour, loss of sonographic definition of the intrahepatic vasculature, or with perihepatic fluid. In spite of these sonographic signs, diffusely infiltrative hepatic metastatic disease can often be quite difficult to detect.

Metastatic Disease: CT Appearance

In the United States, CT is the most common cross-sectional imaging modality used to screen for metastatic lesions, largely because of its short examination time, greater ability to detect extrahepatic disease, lesser cost and greater availability compared to MRI.   The most sensitive noninvasive CT technique for detection of metastatic disease utilizes a "triphasic" protocol, designed to maximize differences in conspicuity between the normal liver and tumor.   This imaging protocol requires three separate scanning sets through the liver (pre-contrast, hepatic arterial phase, and portal venous phase).   The arterial and portal venous phases differ in how much time has elapsed between contrast administration and commencement of scanning. Because contrast from the hepatic artery reaches the liver before that from the portal vein, in the arterial phase hypervascular metastases enhance preferentially to the normal liver, and therefore appear hyperdense to surrounding hepatic parenchyma. This difference in conspicuity is lost during the portal venous phase. Because of its limited value detecting hypovascular metastasis as well as practical concerns over radiation dose, triphasic CT is primarily reserved for patients with suspected hypervascular lesions.   Even greater sensitivity for detection of intrahepatic metastases can be achieved with CT arterial portography or CT arteriography (19). However these techniques require catheterization of the splenic, superior mesenteric, or hepatic artery, thus requiring a greater degree of invasiveness and increased cost. Additionally, these imaging modifications require extensive experience with a myriad of artifacts, related to differences in vascular flow within the liver, which can confound interpretation.   With the advent of multi-detector helical CT, the need for this invasive procedure is diminishing.

On non-contrast CT, hepatic metastases most commonly appear hypodense (Fig. 2) relative to normal liver. Occasionally metastases can appear hyperdense on non-contrast CT scans due to hemorrhage, calcification (Fig 3), or extensive fatty infiltration of the liver.

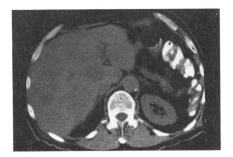 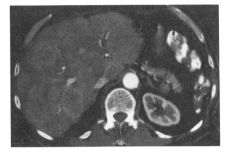

Figure 2. Hypervascular metastases from renal cell carcinoma: CT findings. A.*(Left panel)* non-contrast CT scans shows several poorly defined hypodense regions. B. *(Right panel)* scan obtained during the arterial phase discloses multiple hypervascular metastases.

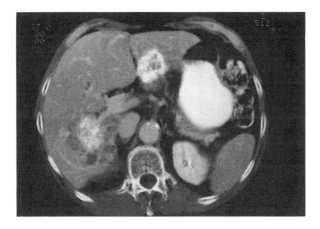

Figure 3. Calcified metastases from this mucinous adenocarcinoma of the colon are demonstrated in both lobes of the liver on this CT scan.

After the intravenous administration of contrast, the appearance of metastatic lesions (see Fig. 2) is dependent on the intrinsic vascularity of the lesion (hypovascular versus hypervascular) and the timing of scanning following contrast administration. During the hepatic arterial phase, hypervascular metastatic lesions appear uniformly hyperdense or contain a hyperdense rim relative to the surrounding liver. Hypovascular lesions most commonly appear hypodense when compared to adjacent hepatic parenchyma during the arterial phase. During the portal venous phase of contrast enhancement, most metastatic lesions (both hypovascular and hypervascular metastases) will appear hypodense compared to normal renal and hepatic parenchyma. They may demonstrate ring enhancement (Fig. 4).

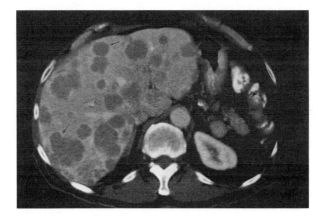

Figure 4. CT scan showing multiple hypodense metastases with a peripheral ring of enhancement identified in this patient with metastatic breast carcinoma.

Scans obtained following the portal venous phase or in patients with a poor contrast bolus (usually secondary to poor intravenous access or scanning delay caused by contrast reaction), differences in lesion-liver conspicuity will decrease, causing some metastatic lesions to appear isodense, obscuring their detection. Occasionally hepatic metastases can appear cystic on CT with a density < 15 HU. This appearance is quite rare, and is usually associated with sarcomas or choriocarcinomas.   Diffuse, infiltrative metastatic disease produces a nodular hepatic contour with non-uniform contrast enhancement. This appearance is commonly associated with perihepatic fluid.

Metastatic Disease: MRI Appearance

Because of higher cost, longer examination time, and probable underestimation of extrahepatic disease, MRI is less commonly used than CT in the detection of hepatic metastases. Intrinsic advantages of MRI include lack of ionizing radiation and inherent multi-planar capability.   Additionally, there is greater contrast difference between the liver and metastatic lesions with MRI compared to CT or ultrasound (4). Hepatobiliary specific MR contrast agents containing manganese have been developed increase the signal of the normal hepatic parenchyma on T1 weighted images, causing metastasis to appear as areas of lower signal intensity. These agents, however, are not yet widely used.   Currently, most abdominal MRI protocols used for detection of liver metastases rely on T1- and T2-weighted images. Following these sequences, T1-weighted images after the intravenous administration gadolinium are obtained.   These post-contrast images may include fat suppression techniques (20).   SPIO (superparamagnetic oxide) particles is another contrast agent taken up by the reticuloendothelial system that, due to its strong paramagnetic effect, renders normal liver and spleen dark (low signal intensity) while metastases, which do not contain Kupfer cells, appear bright (high signal intensity) (21).

Most commonly, hepatic metastases are hypointense (Fig. 5A) compared to normal liver parenchyma on T1-weighted images, and hyperintense (Fig. 5B) relative to normal liver on T2 weighted images. Diffuse metastatic disease can appear as large areas of altered signal (either increased or decreased) compared to normal liver. There are exceptions to these generalizations.   Hemorrhagic metastases or metastatic lesions with excessive mucin content can appear hyperintense on T1-weighted sequences.   Additionally, metastatic melanoma can appear hyperintense on T1-weighted sequences due to the paramagnetic effect of melanin.

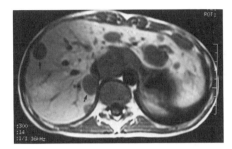 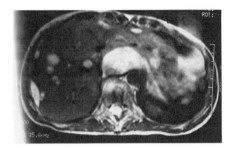

Figure 5. MR appearance of hepatic colorectal metastases. A. *(Left panel)* On T1-weighted images multiple low signal masses (arrows) are identified. B. *(Right panel)* These masses become hyperdense on T2-weighted images.

HEPATOCELLULAR CARCINOMA

Hepatocellular carcinoma (HCC) is the most common primary liver malignancy and the most common type of cancer worldwide. Exclusively the hepatic artery supplies this tumor, so that using the triphasic technique, particularly the arterial phase images, optimizes CT detection. In fact, one study found up to 11% of HCC were only seen with arterial phase imaging (22). Since nearly 90% of these tumors occur in patients with underlying cirrhosis or chronic viral infection (23) detection by imaging is often difficult due to superimposed cirrhotic changes in hepatic morphology. These include distortion of normal hepatic architecture by fibrosis and multiple regenerating nodules, enlargement of the caudate lobe, atrophy of the right hepatic lobe, and diffusely heterogeneous enhancement due to arterial-portal shunting and porto-systemic collaterals. Other factors that decrease the sensitivity of CT in the detection of HCC include the often-multifocal nature of this tumor as well as its variable appearance depending on the size of the lesion. Large lesions often appear slightly heterogeneous with a mosaic pattern of contrast enhancement, whereas smaller lesions appear more homogeneous. Finally, HCC detection is hampered by the non-uniform appearance of lesions, which can occasionally undergo fatty metamorphosis and/or develop an encapsulated rim. These changes develop most commonly in patients from the Eastern Hemisphere (23-24). On non-contrast CT scans, HCC presents as a single or as multiple hypodense or isodense hepatic masses. In patients with extensive fatty infiltration of the liver, however, the lesions can appear hyperdense. Calcification occurs in up to 7% of lesions (24). HCC is most commonly hyperdense during the arterial phase (Fig. 6), and it becomes hypodense (Figs. 7 & 8) on portal venous phase. Encapsulated HCC will demonstrate a hypodense rim on contrast enhanced CT, often demonstrating delayed contrast fill-in (25).

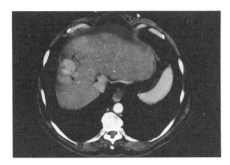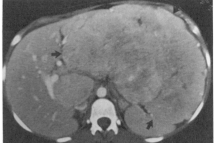

Figure 6. Hepatocellular carcinoma: CT findings in two different patients. A. *(Left panel)* There is a hypervascular lesion seen adjacent to the diaphragm in the right lobe of the liver. B. *(Right panel)* A large vascular lesion replaces the left lobe of the liver.

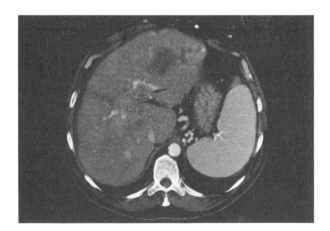

Figure 7. Hepatocellular carcinoma with portal vein thrombosis: CT findings. There is a large hypodense mass within the left lobe of the liver. This is associated with thrombus (arrow) within the left portal vein.

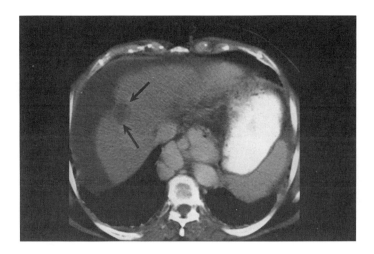

Figure 8. Hepatocellular carcinoma: CT findings. There is a hypodense mass (arrows) within this psoroptic liver. Note the ascites and large varices.

On MRI, most HCC lesions are hypointense relative to liver on T1 weighted images, and slightly hyperintense on T2 weighted sequences. However, lesions with extensive hemorrhage (Fig. 9) or fatty metamorphosis can appear hyperintense on T1 weighted sequences (26). Occasionally, this fatty metamorphosis can be helpful in differentiating of HCC from metastasis through the use of fat-suppression imaging (metastatic lesions do not ordinarily contain fat) (Fig. 10). However, this technique is of limited utility, since other hepatic lesions can also contain fat: focal fatty infiltration, adenoma, intrahepatic lipoma, and angiomyolipoma (12). It is often difficult to distinguish non-siderotic dysplastic cirrhotic nodules from HCC (27) due to the extensive signal variability in HCC. The capsule of a hepatoma often appears hypointense on T1-weighted images and either purely hypointense or layered on T2-weighted images, with an outer hypointense and inner hyperintense ring (28).

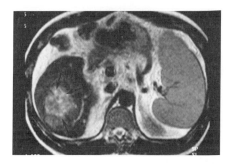
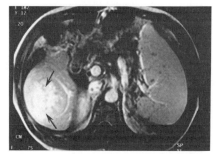

Figure 9 *(previous page)*. Hepatocellular carcinoma: MR findings. A. *(Right panel)* C1 axial MRI demonstrates a large mass in the posterior segment of the right hepatic lobe with heterogeneous signal intensity. The areas of increased signal intensity centrally *(arrows)* represent hemorrhages. B. *(Left panel)* Gradient echo sequence at the same level demonstrates greater prominence of the hemorrhagic area *(arrows)*.

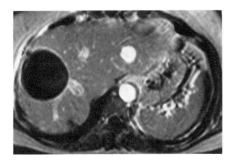 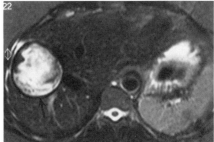

Figure 10. MR of cystic hepatoma. A. *(Left panel)* T1 post gadolinium sequence demonstrates large hypointense mass in the posterior right hepatic lobe with a rim of increased signal intensity due to gadolinium enhancement. B. *(Right panel)* Axial T2 image at the same level again demonstrates large right hepatic mass with a rim of hypointensity, representing the capsule. Note the increased signal intensity essentially likely due to proteinaceous fluid.

The presence of vascular invasion has important staging, prognostic and therapeutic implications in terms of potential liver transplantation and lesion resectability. HCC invades the portal vein in over 40% of cases (29). Arterial-phase CT imaging and dynamically enhanced gadolinium MR imaging can help to differentiate bland thrombus from tumor thrombus by occasionally demonstrating small tumor vessel enhancement of the vascular clot. Extensive portal venous invasion can also be inferred on CT and MR by delayed enhancement of the hepatic segment supplied by the involved portal vein.

Only 50% of HCC lesions present in patients with end stage liver disease are discovered on pre-operative ultrasound. The shrunken, echogenic appearance of the liver often interferes with lesion detection (30). Most HCC lesions less than 3 cm will appear as hypoechoic, relatively homogeneous, well-defined masses. Larger lesions can be more heterogeneous, with hyperechogenicity areas resulting from regions of necrosis, hemorrhage, or fatty metamorphosis. Vascular tumor invasion can be detected by demonstrating arterial Doppler signal or color within echogenic thrombus.

FIBROLAMELLAR CARCINOMA

Fibrolamellar carcinoma is a relatively rare type of HCC that affects younger patients without the traditional risk factors of cirrhosis or hepatitis (31). Characteristically it has a central fibrous scar. These lesions are contained within a single, lobular mass that is hypodense on noncontrast CT scans (Fig. 11) ranging in size from 4 -17 cm in diameter (12) in an otherwise normal-appearing liver. With the exception of the central scar (Fig. 12), fibrolamellar carcinoma enhances rapidly on both CT and MRI, with the mass appearing hyperdense on arterial phase CT imaging. The lack of enhancement of the central scar in fibrolamellar carcinoma helps differentiate this entity from focal nodular hyperplasia, in which the scar enhances with contrast. In one report, however, up to 25% of fibrolamellar carcinoma scars exhibited delayed contrast enhancement.

Sonographically, fibrolamellar carcinoma most often appears as a solitary mass of mixed echogenicity (32). The scar is detected in approximately 33%-60% of cases and appears hyperechoic (33-34). On MR, the central scar in fibrolamellar carcinoma tends to be hypointense on all sequences, whereas the remainder of the mass appears nonspecific, most commonly hypointense on T1 weighted images and hyperintense on T2 weighted sequences. As with contrast enhanced CT, gadolinium enhanced MRI shows rapid heterogeneous enhancement, with delayed imaging demonstrating more homogeneous enhancement of the lesion.

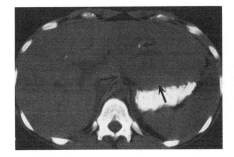 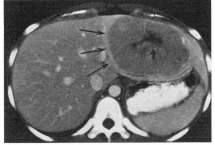

Figure 11. Fibrolamellar carcinoma: CT findings. A. This non-contrast scan demonstrates a hypodense mass *(large arrows)* replacing the lateral segment of the left lobe of the liver. Notice the small region of calcification *(small arrow)*. B. CT obtained following intravenous contrast administration demonstrates a large hypodense hepatic mass in the lateral left hepatic lobe *(arrows)*. Note the peripheral rim of enhancement with a central non-enhancing low-density component representing the central scar (small arrows).

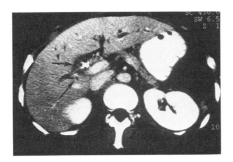 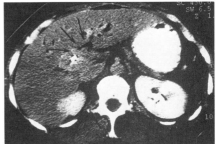

Figure 12. Cholangiocarcinoma: CT findings. A. *(Left panel)* a scan obtained early following the administration of contrast shows a hypodense region in the central portion of the liver *(arrows)*. B. *(Right panel)* Scan obtained 10 minutes later shows delayed enhancement of this central mass *(arrows)*.

CHOLANGIOCARCINOMA

Cholangiocarcinoma is the second most common primary malignant liver tumor after HCC, accounting for approximately 8% of primary intrahepatic neoplasms (12). It most commonly occurs at the confluence of the left and right hepatic ducts (hilar or Klatskin tumor). Hilar cholangiocarcinoma is subclassified into nodular, infiltrating, and papillary types, (35) and is often initially suspected on ultrasound studies performed in patients with jaundice. Sonographic evaluation characteristically reveals intrahepatic biliary dilatation with ducts that rapidly narrow at the confluence due to the tumor mass. Another classic appearance is the presence of intrahepatic ductal dilatation without dilatation of the extrahepatic biliary tract (35). While older studies reported sonographic visualization of a discrete tumor mass in less than fifty percent of cases, (36) more recent investigations with newer sonographic equipment have claimed sensitivity rates of over 90% (37). When a tumor mass is seen, its appearance often is dependent on its subtype: papillary tumors appear as polypoid intraluminal masses; nodular tumors present as a smooth echogenic masses; and infiltrative tumors often do not show a discrete mass, their presence being inferred by an isoechoic "mass effect" displacing adjacent biliary radicals (35). When a mass is identified or when biliary dilatation with an abrupt cutoff is seen, a CT, MR, endoscopic retrograde cholangiopancreatography (ERCP), or magnetic resonance cholangiopancreatogram (MRCP) should then be obtained.

On noncontrast CT, cholangiocarcinoma most commonly appears as an irregular round or oval hypodense mass (Fig. 12A). Initial contrast enhancement is variable and may be central, peripheral, or septated (12) Greater than 50% of intrahepatic cholangiocarcinomas demonstrate homogeneous delayed contrast enhancement (Fig. 12B) on scans performed 6-36 minutes following contrast administration (38). Therefore, in patients with suspected cholangiocarcinoma, delayed scans following contrast administration should be obtained.

Peripheral cholangiocarcinomas can mimic the imaging appearance of intrahepatic metastasis or HCC. Sonographically, peripheral cholangiocarcinomas most commonly appear homogeneously hyperechoic (39). Some lesions, however, are inhomogeneous with hypo or isoechoic region (40-41). These tumors may become quite large due to their late clinical presentation.

The CT and MRI appearance of peripheral cholangiocarcinoma is similar to that of hilar cholangiocarcinoma. As with many other hepatic lesions, the MRI appearance is nonspecific, with most lesions appearing hypointense to surrounding hepatic parenchyma on T1 imaging and hyperintense on T2 imaging (42). On CT, peripheral choangiocarcinomas commonly appear hypodense with slight contrast enhancement peripherally and little enhancement centrally. Ancillary cross-sectional imaging findings can occasionally the correct diagnosis: these include adjacent adenopathy or high-attenuation areas within the mass due to the presence of mucinous material within the bile ducts or tumor cells (43).

BENIGN PRIMARY HEPATIC TUMORS

Hemangioma
Hemangiomas are the most common benign liver tumor, and usually are less than 5cm in diameter. They characteristically appear as uniformly hyperechoic masses (Fig. 13) on ultrasound, making them indistinguishable from hyperechoic metastases (44). Often, they lack detectable flow on color Doppler sonography. On CT, hemangiomas are typically well defined and uniformly hypodense on precontrast scans. After the administration of contrast, hemangiomas typically display nodular peripheral enhancement initially, with "fill in" of the lesion over time (45-46).

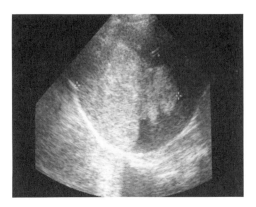

Figure 13. Hemangioma: sonographic features. This large hemangioma demonstrates smooth margins and is uniformly hypoechoic.

On MRI, hemangiomas usually are well defined and hypointense on T1-weighted images, and hyperintense on T2-images. Intravenous gadolinium administration produces initial peripheral enhancement followed by delayed central fill-in (Fig. 14). This pattern of contrast enhancement is so characteristic of a hemangioma that a biopsy is not required. Unfortunately, larger hemangiomas often do not display these unique imaging characteristics, due to the presence of hemorrhage, calcification, and central scars.

Focal Nodular Hyperplasia
Focal nodular hyperplasia is the second most common benign hepatic tumor. It affects a demographically similar group of patients as fibrolamellar HCC and is characteristically subcapsular in location. FNH often is less than 5cm in size, and, like fibrolamellar carcinoma, contains a central scar. On noncontrast CT, FNH is usually a well-defined lesion that is isodense or hypodense compared to normal hepatic parenchyma. After contrast administration, FNH characteristically enhances quickly and washes out quickly, with the central scar occasionally retaining contrast. On MRI the lesions show brisk enhancement during the early arterial phase (Fig. 15).   The central scar of FNH is hypointense on T1-weighted sequences and hyperintense on T2-weighted sequences, in contrast to the central scar of fibrolamellar carcinoma, which is usually hypointense on both imaging sequences.

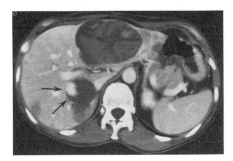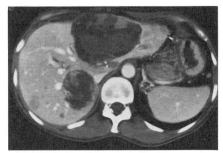

Figure 14 *Previous page.* Hemangioma and adenoma: CT findings. A. *(Left panel)* Peripheral globular enhancement is seen in the adenoma present within the right lobe of the liver *(arrows)*. Note also the hemorrhagic adenoma within the lateral segment of the left lobe of the liver. B. Scan obtained slightly later shows centripetal dissemination of the contrast. A – adenoma; H = hemangioma. *(Right panel)*

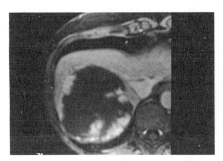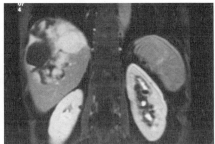

Figure 15. Hemangioma: MR features. A. *(Left panel)* Transverse gradient echo image following the intravenous administration of gadolinium shows peripheral, globular enhancement. B. *(Right panel)* Coronal MR scan in the same patient shows centripetal "filling in" of the lesion.

Hepatic Adenoma

This tumor has very specific demographics, occurring most often in young women taking oral contraceptives, but also affecting patients with glycogen storage disease and athletes abusing anabolic steroids. Adenomas have a propensity to hemorrhage

(Fig. 16) significantly affecting their imaging appearance. These lesions may appear hypodense or hyperdense on non-contrast CT scans depending on the age of hemorrhage. The MRI findings are affected by the age of the hemorrhage as well, with more acute hemorrhage appearing hyperintense on T1 sequences and older hemorrhage appearing darker due to hemosiderin deposition. These lesions enhance rapidly on CT and MR following contrast administration due to the predominantly hepatic arterial supply of the tumor (Fig. 17). Hepatic adenomas tend to appear well defined due to the presence of a tumor capsule.

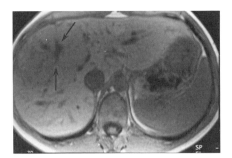 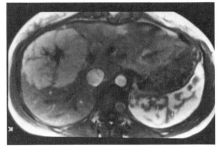

Figure 16.   Focal Nodular hyperplasia.   A. *(Left panel)* Noncontrast MR demonstrates a minimally hypointense mass with a central scar *(arrows)*. B. *(Right panel)* Following the administration of gadolinium there is a brisk enhancement of this lesion with the exception of the central scar.

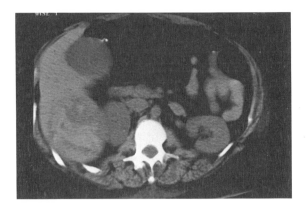

Figure 17.   Adenoma with hemorrhage: CT findings. This non-contrast CT demonstrates hyperdense region within dependent portion of the mass.

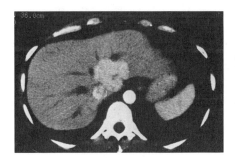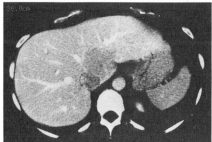

Figure 18. Adenoma: CT features. A. (*Left panel*) during the arterial phase there is dense enhancement of this central lesion. B. *(Right panel)* Notice the prompt "wash out" on slightly later images.

CONCLUSION

Recent developments in CT, MR, and ultrasound enable the radiologist to detect, characterize, and stage a wide variety of malignant tumors. Although MR imaging may be somewhat better at characterizing lesions than CT, the later remains the primary imaging examination for the detection and staging of hepatic lesions at most institutions due to its speed of acquisition and good inherent contrast. Future developments in multi-detector helical CT will further improve the sensitivity and specificity of their technique.

REFERENCES

1. Baker, ME, Pelley R. Hepatic metastases: basic principles and implications for radiologists. Radiology 1995;197:329-337.
2. Meyers, MA (editor). Neoplasms of the Digestive Tract: Imaging, Staging and Management, Lippincott-Raven, 1998; pp361-395.
3. Mahfouz AE, Hamm B, Mathieu D. Imaging of metastases to the liver. Eur Radiol 1996;6:607- 614.
4. Stark DD, Wittenberg J, Butch RJ et al. Hepatic metastases: randomized controlled comparison of detection with MR imaging and CT Radiology 1987;165:399- 406.
5. Taylor HM, Ros PR, Hepatic Imaging: An Overview. Radiol Clin North Am, 1998;36:237-246.

6. Couinaud C. Le foie:etudes anatomiques et chirurgicales. Paris, France: Masson, 1957.
7. Soyer P, Elias D, Zeitoun G et al. surgical treatment of hepatic metastases: impact of intraoperative sonography. AJR 1993;160:511-514.
8. Leen E, Anderson WJ, Wotherspoon H et al. Detection of colorectal liver metastases: comparison of laparotomy, CT, US, and Doppler perfusion index and evaluation of postoperative follow-up results. Radiology 1995;195:113-116.
9. Shuman WP. Liver metastases from colorectal carcinoma: detection with Doppler US-guided measurements of liver blood flow-past, present, future. Radiology 1995; 195:9-10.
10. Paley MR, Ros PR. Hepatic Metastates. Radiol Clin North Am 1998; 36:349-363.
11. Vauthey JN.Liver Imaging: A Surgeon's Perspective. Radiol Clin North Am 1998;36:445-457.
12. Fernandez M, Redvanly RD. Primary hepatic Malignant Neoplasms, Radiol Clin North Am, 1998;36(2):333-348.
13. Green B, Bree RL, Goldstein HM et al. Grey scale ultrasound evaluation of hepatic neoplasms: patterns and correlations. Radiology 1997;124:203-208.
14. Schieble W., Gosink BB, Leopold, GR.   Gray scale echographic patterns of hepatic metastatic disease. AJR 1977;129:983-987.
15. Marchal G, Tshibwabwa-Tumba E, Oyen R et al. Correlation of sonographic patterns in liver metastases with histology and microangiography.   Invest Radiol 1985;20: 79-84.
16. Marchal GJ, Pylyser K, Tshibwabwa Tumba EA et al. anechoic halo in solid liver tumors: sonographic microangiographic, and histologic   correlation. Radiology 1985;156:479-483.
17. Wernecke K, Henke L Vassallo P, Bick U et al. the distinction between benign and malignant liver tumors on sonography: value of a hypoechoic halo. AJR 1992;159:1005-1009.
18. Jones EC, Chezmar JL, Nelson RC. The frequency and significance of small (<1.5cm)hepatic lesions detected by abdominal CT. AJR 1992;158:535-539.
19. Kemmerer SR, Mortele KJ, Ros PR. CT Scan of the Liver. Radiol Clin North Am. 1998;36:247-261.
20. Seigelman ES, outwater EK. MR Imaging of the Liver. Radiol Clin North Am. 1998;36:263-286.
21. Hahn PF, Saini S. Liver-Specific MR Imaging Contrast Agents. 1998; 36:287-298.
22. Baron R, Oliver JH III, Dodd GD III, et al: Hepatocellular carcinoma: Evaluation with biphasic, contrast-enhanced, helical CT. Radiology 1996;199:505-511.
23. Hodgson HJF. Primary hepatocellular carcinoma.   In : Blumgart LH(ed), Surgery of the liver and biliary tract. Edinburgh: Churchill Livingstone, 1994;1341-1347.

24. Freeny P, Baron RL, Teefey SA: Hepatocellular carcinoma: Reduced frequency of typical findings with dynamic contrast-enhanced CT in a non-Asian population. Radiology 1992;182:143-148.

25. Heiken JP, Brink JA, Vannier, MW: Spiral (helical) CT. Radiology 1993;189:647-656.

26. Rummeny E, Weissleder R, Sironi S, et al. Primary liver tumors: diagnosis by MR imaging. AJR 1989;152:63-72.

27. Earls JP, Theise ND, Weinreb JC, et al: Dysplastic nodules and hepatocellular carcinoma: Thin-section MR imaging of explanted cirrhotic livers with pathologic correlation. Radiology 1996;201: 207-214.

28. Kadoya M, Matsui O, Takashima T, et al. Hepatocellular carcinoma: Correlation of MR imaging and histopathologic findings. Radiology 1992;183:819-825.

29. Mathieu D, Guinet C, Bouklia-Hassane A et al. Hepatic vein involvement in hepatocellular carcinoma. Gastrointest Radiol 1988;13:55-60.

30. Dodd, GD III, Miller WJ, Baron RL et al. Detection of malignant tumors in end-stage cirrhotic livers: Efficacy of sonography as a screening technique AJR1992;159:727-733.

31. McLarney JK, Rucker PT, Bender GN. Fibrolamellar Carcinoma of the Liver: Radiologic-Pathologic Correlation. RadioGraphics 1999; 19:453-471.

32. Friedman AC,Lichtenstein JE, Goodman ZD, et al. Fibrolamellar hepatocellular carcinoma. Radiology 1985;157:583-587.

33. Brandt DJ, Johnson CD, Stephens DH et al. imaging of fibrolamellar hepatocellular carcinoma. AJR 1988; 151:295-299.

34. Orsatti G, Hyritoglou P, Thung SN. Lamellar fibrosis in the fibrolamellar variant of hepatocellular carcinoma: a role for transforming growth factor beta. Liver 1997;12:152-156.

35. Bloom CM, Langer B, Wilson SR. Role of US in the detection, characterization, and staging of Cholangiocarcinoma. RadioGraphics 1999;19:1199-1218.

36. Honickman SP, Mueller PR, Wittenberg J et al. Ultrasound in obstructive jaundice: prospective evaluation of site and cause. Radiology 1983;147:511-515.

37. Robledo R, Avertano M, Prieto M. extrahepatic biliary ductal cancer. Radiology 1996;198:869-879.

38. Lacomis JM, Baron RL, Oliver JH III, et al. Cholangiocarcinoma: Delayed CT contrast enhancement patterns. Radiology 1997; 203:98-104.

39. Ros PR, Buck JL, Goodman ZD et al. Intrahepatic cholangiocarcinoma: radiologic-pathologic correlation. Radiology 1988;167:689-693.

40. Wibulpolprasert B, Dhiensiri T. Peripheral cholangiocarcinoma: sonographic evaluation. J Clin Ultrasound 1992;20:303-314.

41. Soyer P, Bluemke DA, Reichle R et al. Imaging of intrahepatic cholangiocarcinoma, 1: peripheral cholangiocarcinoma. AJR 1995;165:1427-1431.

42. Choi BI, Han JK, Shin YM et al. Peripheral cholangiocarcinoma: Comparison of MRI with CT. Abdom Imaging 1995;20:357-360.

43. Choi BI, Lee JH, Han MC et al. Hilar cholangiocarcinoma: comparative study with sonography and CT. Radiology 1989;172:689-692.

44. McArdle CR. Ultrasonographic appearances of a hepatic hemangioma. J Clin Ultrasound 1978;6:124..
45. Nghiem H, Bogost G, Ryan J, Lund P, et al. Cavernous hemangiomas of the liver: enlargement over time. AJR 1997; 169:137-140.
46. Quinn S, Benjamin G. Hepatic cavernous hemangiomas: simple diagnostic sign with dynamic bolus CT. Radiology 1992; 182:545-548.

4
RESULTS OF SURGICAL RESECTION FOR HEPATOCELLULAR CARCINOMA

Sandra M. Jones, M.D. and Mark S. Roh, M.D.
Allegheny Hospital, Pittsburgh, PA

INTRODUCTION

Hepatocellular cancer (HCC) is one of the most common cancers in the world and the incidence is increasing. There are regional differences in the incidence of the disease, with sub-Saharan Africa and the Far East with the highest incidence (>30/100,000) and Northern Europe and the United States with the lowest incidence (<2/100,000) (1). In general, patients with chronic liver injury are at much higher risk for developing HCC. Ten to twenty percent of cirrhotics will develop HCC and in patients with HCC, 60-92% have cirrhosis (2,3). In Western studies the prevalence of cirrhosis in patients undergoing resection is lower, ranging from 4-24% (4-6).

The natural history of HCC varies depending on the size of the tumor at presentation and the severity of underlying liver disease. In patients who are symptomatic at the time of presentation, median survival is less than three months (3,7,8). Patients who are asymptomatic at the time of presentation with small tumors may be eligible for surgical resection. If resected these patients can expect longer survival with 5-year survival rates of 26-58.8% (9-12).

RISK FACTORS

In patients with cirrhosis, risk factors are associated with a higher incidence of HCC. These include male gender, advanced age, race, and history of chronic active hepatitis and chronic hepatitis carrier states. Smoking will increase the risk for HCC in patients with cirrhosis (13). Males are four times more likely to develop HCC than females (14,15). Age is a risk factor for developing HCC, however it varies by region with incidence in the UK and Africa peaking in the 80's and 40's, respectively. Age has also been found to have prognostic significance in patients undergoing resection, with age < 50 being associated with prolonged survival (4). This is thought to relate to the duration of the underlying disease in the patient. Adults who acquire hepatitis B as infants or children may be at a higher risk of developing HCC at an earlier age (14). Certain races have a higher incidence of HCC. This is seen with blacks in Africa and the Chinese in the East and is thought to be secondary to higher incidence of hepatitis B (HBV) in these regions.

Hepatocellular carcinoma rarely occurs in patients without cirrhosis. The etiology is therefore thought to be associated with the causes of cirrhosis, namely viral hepatitis and alcoholism. This is supported by epidemiological evidence that there is a higher incidence of HCC in areas where HBV is endemic. The association was first seen in the Far East with HBV. Development of HCC is related to the chronic inflammation and progressive liver damage caused by hepatitis (1). Molecular studies have demonstrated that HBV-DNA becomes integrated in the hepatic genome and this may enhance chromosomal instability, resulting in microdeletions and/or rearrangements of the host chromosome (1,16).

In western society, however, HBV positivity is not common in patients with HCC. Instead, these patients are positive for Hepatitis C (HCV). The risk for HCC is lower in patients treated with interferon for hepatitis C who had a sustained response compared to patients who did not receive interferon, had a relapse after treatment, or had no response to treatment (17). Other causes of cirrhosis that lead to a higher risk of HCC include metabolic diseases such as hemochromatosis, alpha-1-antitrypsin deficiency, and Wilson's disease. Liver toxins such as aflatoxin B and Thorotrast exposure are also thought to increase the risk of developing HCC. While HCC has been reported in the milieu of hormonal therapy, the association has not been conclusively proven (18).

CLINICAL PRESENTATION

Clinical signs and symptoms of HCC are usually non-specific and may go unrecognized secondary to the underlying liver disease. Symptoms include abdominal distension, abdominal pain, anorexia, fever, malaise, and weight loss. The most common symptoms are pain, malaise and weight loss (8,19,20). Clinical signs of HCC include hepatomegaly, jaundice, ascites, spider nevi, and palmar erythema. In the patient with cirrhosis, the only sign may be the acute deterioration of their disease with rapid development of ascites and jaundice (20). In some patients, signs and symptoms occur with acute rupture of the tumor with resultant hemoperitoneum. Paraneoplastic syndromes are uncommon in Western countries if present will include polycythemia, hypoglycemia, hypercalcemia, and feminization (20). In general HCC presents in three ways: a right upper quadrant mass, the deterioration of the health of a patient with cirrhosis, or as a result of screening of an asymptomatic patient (21).

HCC SURVEILLANCE

There is much debate in the literature regarding the efficacy of surveillance protocols to identify patients with HCC. The goal of any screening program is to detect tumor at an earlier stage where it is still small would be amenable to effective therapy. In HCC, one would ideally detect the tumor while it was small (<5 cm), unifocal, noninvasive and prior to portal vein invasion (14,15,21-27). Patients eligible for screening should have compensated liver disease so that they would be able to withstand surgery.

There is, however, no one test that is both sensitive, specific, easy to perform and widely available. Most of the studies reviewed proposed a combination of interval hepatic ultrasound and interval serum alpha-fetoprotein (AFP) measurement. Normal values for AFP are less than 20 ng/mL. Some feel more rigorous testing for HCC should begin when AFP levels rise above 20 ng/mL (28 Usefulness as a screening test is limited because of its low sensitivity (20-60%). The high specificity (>90%) for serum levels above 250 ug/L demonstrates its utility as a diagnostic agent (14,24,25). Zoli et al, (15) followed AFP levels in a group of patients with cirrhosis and found that levels were rarely elevated above five times normal when small tumors (<5 cm) were detected. An AFP>20 ng/mL at the time of enrollment in a surveillance program was an independent predictor of developing HCC. Other etiologies can lead to an acute rise in serum AFP levels and include viral hepatitis, chronic active hepatitis and massive hepatic necrosis.

Another option is to look at subsets of AFP, which are more sensitive for detecting HCC. Sato et al, (26) examined the lectin-reactive profile of serum AFP in patients with cirrhosis with AFP levels greater than 30 ng/mL and then followed these patients to see which developed HCC. *L.culinaris* agglutinin A-reactive AFP (AFP L3) and erythroagglutinating phytohemagglutinin-reactive AFP (AFP P4 + P5) were most predictive. Seventy-three percent of patients who developed HCC had increased percentage of AFP L3, AFP P4 + P5, or both at the time of diagnosis. No patient with an elevated AFP and no detectable HCC had elevated percentages of AFP L3 or AFP P4 + P5. This study, however, did not address whether early detection of HCC by this method impacted long- term survival or resectability. Another marker considered as screening tests for HCC is des-gamma-carboxyprothrombin, however, the sensitivity for detecting small HCC is only 44%(14,29).

A more promising marker is soluble interleukin-2 receptor (sIL-2R). As part of the inflammatory response to hepatitis, T-cells produce interleukin-2(IL-2) that in turn stimulates the production of sIL-2R. Serum levels of sIL-2R increase in proportion to the degree of inflammatory activity in patients with hepatitis and Izzo et al, (30) found the highest levels to be in patients with HCC. Three patients developed HCC during the study period. These patients were found to have a significant rise in their sIL-2R levels at the time the HCC was diagnosed. Soluble IL-2 receptor level is a promising test for screening patients with hepatitis for HCC.

Hepatic real-time sonography has been advocated as the screening test of choice because it is relatively inexpensive and non-invasive when compared to computed tomography and angiography. Sensitivity of ultrasound for detecting HCC has been reported to vary from 43% to 90% (23,24,31). In the study by Dodd (23), patients with end-stage cirrhosis who were being evaluated for orthotopic liver transplant underwent hepatic sonograms as part of their preoperative work-up. These results were then correlated with resected total hepatectomy specimens. The sensitivity for detecting patients with tumor, and the sensitivity of detecting multiple tumor nodules in the same patient are 43% and 42% respectively. The specificity was 98%. Takayasu et al, (31) found sonography to be 84% sensitive for detecting tumor nodules <5 cm. There are other differences between the studies, which may account for the difference in sensitivity. The patients in Takayasu's study were referred for resection after HCC had already been discovered at another institution, and therefore, further imaging studies were then performed with the knowledge that the patient had a tumor nodule. In the study by Dodd et al, the results of sonography were confirmed by examining total hepatectomy specimens after transplantation, whereas Takayasu's were confirmed by other radiologic imaging studies, intraoperative ultrasound, or resected specimens. Another reason the sensitivity of sonograms may have been lower in the study by Dodd is because the patients had end-stage cirrhosis with small fibrotic livers and the body habitus of western patients tends to be larger than that found in Asian patients.

Currently, most studies recommend a baseline ultrasound in patients presenting with cirrhosis. The schedule for follow-up ultrasound is then determined based on the severity and duration of the patients liver disease and if there is an increase in the AFP level or deterioration of liver function. In general, most studies recommend ultrasound every 6-12 months.

All of the studies have yet to show a survival benefit, decrease in mortality, (21) or decrease in recurrence after resection in patients who have undergone resection after HCC was detected with routine screening (9). It is widely accepted that when HCC is discovered in a symptomatic patient, the disease is usually rapidly fatal. The natural history of an untreated asymptomatic patient with a tumor that is less than 3 cm, is one, two and three year survival rates of 91%, 55% and 13%, respectively. Fifty-percent of the deaths can be attributed to liver failure or complications of their cirrhosis and half due to the malignancy (3). In patients undergoing resection for small (<5 cm) HCC the one, two and three year survival rates are 66.8%, 53.8%, and 41.9%, respectively (32). Future studies are needed to better define a subset of cirrhotics at very high risk for HCC who are also capable of withstanding hepatic resection and would have a low recurrence rate. Additionally, in this era of cost consciousness, screening has not been found to be cost-effective. Estimates for detecting one patient with resectable HCC are range from $51,000 (best case scenario, high HCC incidence) to $183,000 (intermediate case scenario, low HCC incidence) (25).

An efficient way to manage these patients would be to stratify cirrhotic patients into groups, which are more at risk for developing HCC. Patients with cirrhosis could be stratified initially by the etiology of their cirrhosis with hepatitis B, hepatitis C and alcoholic cirrhosis considered high risk. Then the duration of cirrhosis could be used since longer duration of chronic active hepatitis increases the risk of developing HCC due to prolonged liver injury. However, these patients are also more likely to have end-stage liver disease at the time of diagnosis and, therefore, would be ineligible for resection. Zoli et al, (15) identified several risk factors that they found to be independent predictors of developing HCC. Multivariate analysis identified that the entry concentration of alkaline phosphatase (>280 U/L), albumin (<3.5 g/dL), and male sex were independently and significantly related to the appearance of HCC. Therefore, if these indicators are present aggressive screening should be employed and so as to increase the number of patients found to have resectable HCC.

PRE-OPERATIVE ASSESSMENT

Historically, 80-90% of patients with HCC are not eligible for resection at the time of presentation because their preexisting liver disease limits the regenerative capacity of their liver. Resectability rates have improved somewhat with earlier detection secondary to better imaging studies and the use of screening protocols for high-risk patients. Operative mortality has decreased in studies from the East (7,9,33-35) to <10%, making surgical resection an option for patients with HCC. However, results of resection depend heavily on the proper selection of the patient. Factors important in a favorable outcome include the overall health of the patient, the functional reserve of the liver and certain tumor characteristics.

Classification systems such as the Child-Pugh are helpful for stratifying patients. Child-Pugh class C patients with hepatic encephalopathy, refractory ascites, cholestasis with bilirubin over 3.5mg and a prothrombin time below 50% are considered inoperable (20). Child-Pugh class A patients can usually tolerate anatomic resection with minimal morbidity and mortality from liver failure (35). However, in the Child-Pugh class A patient with significant comorbidities and class B patients determining hepatic functional reserve is difficult and often requires additional tests so as to minimize the risk of postoperative morbidity and mortality.

Major morbidity following liver resection is intractable ascites, intractable pleural effusions, and intraperitoneal infection, hemorrhage requiring reoperation, major bile leak and gastrointestinal bleeding. Pre-operative work-up should be designed to identify patients most at risk for these complications. Work-up of the patient thought to be eligible for resection starts with a complete history and physical with particular attention to comorbid conditions such as diabetes mellitus which has been found to correlate with major postoperative complication (p = 0.0001) (36). The presence of uncontrolled ascites is a contraindication to surgical resection as it reflects uncompensated liver failure (37,38). The presence of varices are not a contraindication, however, some advocate aggressive treatment when there is a history of bleeding esophagogastric varices because postoperative hemorrhage is a major complication of hepatic resection (11,35,39).

Laboratory values found to be important prognostic indicators are bilirubin and albumin. These two values have been incorporated into several clinical staging systems including the Okuda Staging System, which also uses tumor size and presence of ascites. Okuda's clinical staging system has been found to have better prognostic value than the TNM staging system (40) because it incorporates these indicators of hepatic function. When patients were divided into the three stages without considering treatment, the median survival for Stage I, II and III was 11.5, 3.0 and 0.9 months, respectively. For those undergoing surgical treatment, median survival of Stage I and II patients was 25.6 and 12.2 months, respectively. There were no Stage III patients in the surgical treatment group (7).

Table 1: Okuda clinical staging

	Tumor Size		Ascites		Albumin		Bilirubin	
Stage	>50% (+)	<50% (-)	(+)	(-)	<3g/dl (+)	>3g/dl (-)	>3mg/dl (+)	<3mg/dl (-)
I	(-)		(-)		(-)		(-)	
II			1 or 2 (+)					
III			3 or 4 (+)					

+: sign of advanced disease

Techniques to Assess Hepatic Reserve Function

There are many proposed tests and scoring systems which have been developed in an attempt to measure the functional reserve of the liver and thus predict who will tolerate surgery. One of the most commonly used is the indocyanine green(ICG) clearance test .ICG is cleared by the liver, cannot be metabolized and does not interfere with enterohepatic circulation. ICG is injected, then venous samples are collected at 3, 5, 7, 10, 15, 10 and 30 minutes after injection. Blood samples are then checked by spectrophotometry at 800 nm to determine the plasma disappearance curves of ICG. The normal serum 15-minute retention rate (ICG R15) is 10% or less. An ICG R15 of > 20% is suggestive of severe cirrhosis. There is, however, no universal agreement on the value that would preclude resection. Theoretically, patients with an ICG R15 of 10% or less should tolerate an anatomic resection.

In the study by Wu, (40) patients with an ICG R15 of >20% were limited to resections of no more that two segments and every effort was made to limit intraoperative blood loss. They also resected as little functional liver as possible which resulted in tumor margins of <1 cm in many patients. Patients with ICG R15 <10% underwent standard anatomic resections. Five-year disease free survival rates were 29.6% in patients with ICG R15<10% and 30.9% in patients with ICG R15 >20%. The difference in these survival rates was not statistically significant. The operative mortality rates were 0.05% and 0% in the patients with ICG R15 of >20% and <10% respectively. Makuuchi, (38) also favors the use of ICG R15 to evaluate liver function and guide the extent of hepatic resection. He recommends that with ICG R15 of <10% a bisegmentectomy or more can be applied, ICG R15 of 10-19% a left lobectomy or right monosegmentectomy, ICG R15 20-29% a subsegmentectomy, ICG R15 30-39% a limited resection and ICG R15 of 40% or more only enucleation. Utilizing this criteria, in-hospital mortality was 2.0% and survival rates during the first five years after resection were 90.2%, 79.2%, 66.2%, 50.8% and 43.7%. Survival did not differ according to the extent of operative resection. Recently, a fingertip probe, similar to pulse oximetry probes, for detecting ICG has been developed which obviates the need for repeated blood draws and makes obtaining this test much easier (41).

Hepatocytes consume an enormous amount of energy for cellular function and measuring mitochondrial function reflects functional reserve. The arterial ketone body ratio (KBR) (acetoacetate/β-hydroxybutyrate) represents the redox state of liver mitochondria, which correlates with the hepatic charge level. Energy metabolism in hepatic mitochondria changes in proportion to blood glucose levels after oral glucose load. Therefore, the Redox Tolerance Index (RTI) measures the change in arterial KBR divided by the change in blood glucose, in response to an oral glucose tolerance test. After a 12-hour fast, patients are given 75 g of glucose. Arterial blood is collected just before taking the glucose, then at 30, 60, 90 and 120 minutes after ingestion and acetoacetate, β-hydroxybutyrate, and blood glucose levels are determined. The KBR/blood glucose ratio is then plotted against time and this is the RTI. In the study by Mori, (42) patients were stratified into three groups based on their RTI: Class I RTI>1.0, Class II 0.5<RTI<1.0, or Class III RTI<0.5. The post-operative mortality was 0%, 3.9%, and 18.4% for Class I, II, and III, respectively. RTI significantly correlated with thirty-day post-operative mortality and is a way of assessing the risk of resection for patients with HCC.

Technetium 99m diethylenetriamine-pentaacetic acid-galactosyl-human serum albumin liver scintography (Tc-GSA) is another test to assess hepatic reserve. This compound will bind directly to receptors on functional hepatocytes. Patients are given a bolus dose of 3 mg of ^{99m}Tc-GSA and the hepatic uptake ratio (LHL15) of ^{99m}Tc-GSA was calculated by dividing the liver activity at 15 minutes by heart plus liver activity at 15 minutes. The blood disappearance ratio (HH15) is then calculated by dividing the heart activity at 15 minutes by the heart activity at 3 minutes. Kwon et al, (43) then calculated a modified receptor index (MRI) by dividing the LHL15 by HH15. The MRI was then compared with ICG R15 and other parameters of conventional liver function in patients undergoing liver resection for HCC. The MRI was found to correlate with the ICG R15 and other conventional liver function tests such as bilirubin, prothrombin time and transaminase levels. Therefore, the Tc-GSA gives a direct measure of functional hepatocytes. There was a discrepancy between the ICG R15 and MRI in eight patients, however, the MRI was found to correlate with histologic disease and ICG R15 did not. This study did not look out outcome or make recommendations on extent of resection based on this test.

In the classification system utilized by the Paul Brousse Hospital, (44) albumin, billirubin, encephalopathy, clinical ascites and coagulation factors II and V are utilized to predict functional reserve. Each of these criteria is assigned a value (Table 2) and patients are stratified into three groups based on the number of criteria: Group A: 0 criteria; Group B: 1 or 2 criteria; and Group C: 3 or more criteria. Estimates of the feasibility of the resection are then made based on the following formula: the quantity of functional liver removed divided by the total quantity of functional liver (expressed as a percentage)), then multiply by the degree of liver insufficiency. The degree of liver insufficiency was graded as follows: group A, 1; group B, 2; and group C, 3. Resection is deemed feasible when the percentage given by the formula was less than 50%. This means that in group A patients, no more than 50% of the functional parenchyma was removed; in-group B, no more than 24%; and in group C, no more than 17.5%.

Table 2

	Number of Criteria
Albuminemia <3 g/100ml	1
Bilirubinemia >30 mmol/l	1
Encephalopathy (disorientation to time and space and/or asterixis	1
Clinical ascites	1
Coagulation factors II and V between 40% and 60%	1
Coagulation factors II and V <40%	2

Thirty-three patients who underwent resection based on this classification system: group A 25 (71%), group B 8 (23%) and group C 2 (6%). There were 5 early postoperative deaths from liver failure, 4 in-group B and 1 in-group C. In 4 of the 5, liver failure was precipitated by portal thrombosis (1 patient), intra-abdominal sepsis (2 patients) and hemorrhagic ascites (1 patient). Of these four patients, three had less than 5% of functional parenchyma resected. One patient had nearly 20% resected. The patient who died of liver failure without other complications had ~25% resected, however, they were found on necropsy to have a tumor in the remaining left lobe. There were no early postoperative deaths in-group A patients.

Evaluation of the Tumor

The biology of the tumor dictates resectability. Tumor characteristics important in determining resectability include size, anatomic location and proximity or involvement of major hepatic vascular structures, number of tumor nodules and whether they are confined to a single lobe or segment. Tumor size is important when considering the volume of liver parenchyma that must be resected to obtain an adequate tumor free margin. The majority of patients cannot tolerate major anatomic resection secondary to their underlying liver disease.

Infiltration into major hepatic vasculature, hepatic and/or portal vein is a contraindication to resection as it predicts distant metastases. Particularly important is an estimate of the volume of tumor as a percentage of liver parenchyma. This may assist in determining which patients would have adequate remaining liver function after resection. Reviewing computed tomography, ultrasonography and angiography assesses these tumor characteristics.

RESECTION

Resection of HCC is undertaken in the setting of cirrhosis. Since the cirrhotic liver has little regenerative capacity, the resection must be meticulously planned so as to minimize the amount of functional liver tissue that is resected (44,45). Intraoperative blood loss must be minimized (4,12,46) since higher intraoperative blood loss has been found to be associated with higher morbidity and mortality in several studies. Nagorney, (4) found that in patients with early postoperative deaths, the average transfusion requirement was 14.5 units whereas in survivors, transfusion requirement averaged 3.1 units (p = 0.002). Similarly, in patients with significant morbidity the average transfusion requirement was 5.8 versus 3.0 in patients without significant morbidity (p = 0.0001). Sitzman (46) found that blood loss (2529mL versus 3983mL, p = 0.08), red cell transfusion (4.0 units versus 6.9 units, p = 0.07) and operative time (3.8 hours versus 4.6 hours, p = 0.005) were significantly related to increased morbidity following resection.

Major complications of hepatic resection in cirrhotic patients include hemorrhage from esophagogastric varices. Several authors (11,35,39) advocate rigorous work-up of patients with a history of bleeding esophagogastric varices in the preoperative setting. Work-up includes esophagogasto-duodenoscopy (EGD) to assess the extent of esophageal and gastric varices. In patients with varices but no history of bleeding, sclerotherapy is the procedure of choice. However, in patients with a history of bleeding varices or risky varices (large varices and varices with "red color sign" endoscopically) the addition of a portal decompression procedure should be considered, such as a distal splenorenal shunt, to the liver resection. There was no difference in outcome equivalent in patients who underwent combined hepatic resection and portal decompression.

There are several techniques for decreasing blood loss during hepatic resection and is dependent upon the size and location of the tumors. For small, superficial tumors one may apply manual pressure to the cut surface of the liver so as to control hemorrhage. Other larger tumors require more complex maneuvers. Inflow occlusion is important to minimize blood loss. The normal liver can tolerate long periods of warm ischemia and 60 minutes is safe. A cirrhotic liver can tolerate 75 minutes of warm ischemia. Wu et al, (45) used intermittent occlusion of the hepatic inflow vessels for 15 minutes and unclamping for 5 minutes. Utilizing this technique, cirrhotic patients can tolerate warm ischemia times as long as 204 minutes without postoperative liver failure.

Paquet et al, (39) described several techniques for decreasing intraoperative blood loss. The first of these is to use sodium nitroprusside to decrease systolic blood pressure to 70mmHg. This in turn decreases the central venous pressure and will decrease blood loss by decreasing the backflow of blood from the vena cava into the hepatic veins. This is used in combination with the Pringle maneuver so as to minimize hepatic blood loss. Another technique utilized in resecting hepatic tumors is total vascular exclusion, (51,52) which is the combination of the Pringle maneuver with the clamping of the IVC both above and below the liver. The risks include pooling in the lower half of the body, which may result in hemodynamic alterations such as decreased cardiac index and arrhythmia due to decreased blood return to the heart. To counteract hemodynamic alteration of total vascular exclusion, double venovenous bypass has been added to the procedure. This provides a circuit that returns blood from the femoral and portal veins to the axillary vein. This technique has been utilized in patients with large tumors, which occupy most of a hepatic lobe, close proximity to the main hepatic vein and/or inferior vena cava (IVC) or tumor thrombus in the IVC or portal trunk. Yamaoka et al, (53) applied this technique to eight patients with cirrhosis and HCC and to twelve patients without cirrhosis, four with HCC, eight with metastatic tumor to the liver. There was no significant difference in the survival of the two groups. The patients with cirrhosis had more complications with all but one experiencing a pleural effusion, increased bilirubin level or gastrointestinal bleeding.

Makuuchi et al, (54) uses both hemihepatic vascular occlusion and subsegmentectomy as a technique for resecting HCC in cirrhotic patients. Hemihepatic vascular occlusion is the selective, mostly unilobar, control of hilar vessels of the liver. It is thought to decrease the biochemical disturbances due to interruption of blood flow to the liver while still minimizing intraoperative blood loss. Another technique for minimizing both resection of functional liver tissue and blood loss is the Makuuchi subsegmentectomy. Indications for Makuuchi subsegmentectomy include small HCC in patients with severe to moderate cirrhosis who would otherwise not tolerate major anatomic resection. Utilizing intraoperative ultrasound, dye is injected into the portal venous structure supplying the tumor just proximal to portal venous tumor extension. Once tatooing of the parenchyma has occurred, resection is carried out along the line of demarcation while employing hemihepatic occlusion so as to minimize blood loss but still perfuse the non-involved lobe. Post-operative mortality in this series was 0%. Survival for 1, 2 and 3 years were 80.3%, 63.3%, and 52.6%, respectively.

COMBINATION THERAPIES

Reports of combination therapies for HCC are becoming more common in the literature. Interest in this has been stimulated by continued low resectability rates despite improved detection and resection strategies for HCC. The goal of combination therapy is to achieve cytoreduction and then to perform sequential resection. Patients ideally suited for combination therapy are those with large, well-encapsulated, solitary tumors confined to one lobe of the liver with no evidence of extrahepatic disease. Cytoreduction therapies include combinations of both systemic and regional chemotherapy, external beam radiation, hepatic artery ligation or embolization and selective portal vein embolization. Ablative therapies can be used in combination with resection intraoperatively. Utilizing these therapies has increased resection rates as high as 51.5% (55).

Preoperative Transcatheter Arterial Embolization

This technique has been effective in treating unresectable primary HCC. Preoperative transcatheter arterial embolization (TAE) (55-58) demonstrated a 25 - 63% reduction in the size of tumors when compared with patients who did not have preoperative TAE (55-58). No difference in operative mortality was observed and a statistically significant improvement in the time to recurrence in patients undergoing TAE was noted in the TAE group (55). Blood loss and operative time were equivalent. However, resection was more difficult in patients who had undergone preoperative TAE because of thickening or adhesions of the hepatoduodenal ligament, severe subhepatic adhesions, biliary tract damage including bile duct necrosis or gangrenous gallbladder, and intrahepatic abscess or focal infarction. In conclusion, preoperative TAE was not indicated for patients already deemed resectable at the time of initial evaluation. TAE is indicated in patients with borderline resectability secondary to tumor bulk where tumor reduction would then render them resectable. The only other indication is to control hemorrhage in patients with ruptured HCC prior to resection.

Selective Portal Vein Embolization

In patients who are unresectable because resection would leave an inadequate functional hepatic parenchyma, selective right portal vein embolization can be performed. This technique has been used mainly in patients with tumors in the right lobe because the right lobe contains approximately two thirds of hepatic parenchyma (59). Emobilization of the right portal vein induces atrophy in the right lobe and hypertrophy of the left lobe, resulting in an increased functional hepatic tissue. Selective right portal vein embolization has been performed in the noncirrhotic patient with biliary or metastatic tumors with an increase in the left lobe volume of 24-64% (59-63) and followed by right hepatectomy. Lee et al, (64) performed this technique in 19 patients with cirrhosis and HCC and the left lobe increased from 479 ± 224 cm^3 to 591 ± 228 cm^3 (p < 0.01). Eleven patients had right lobectomy, one had segmentectomy, and two had small partial resection. One patient who had undergone right lobectomy died postoperative and the other patients had satisfactory postoperative course. The patients tolerate this therapy well and should be considered as a therapeutic option.

Multi-modality Therapy

Multi-modality therapy employs a combination of techniques including both systemic and regional chemotherapy, external beam radiation hepatic artery ligation and isotopic immunoglobulin therapy (65,66). This is utilized in patients who are not eligible for resection secondary to tumor bulk. Although there was no one chemotherapy regimen utilized and different combinations of the above were used, each was able to show no difference in survival between groups having preoperative multi-modality therapy and those having only resection. Operative time and blood loss did increase in patients undergoing multi-modality therapy, however, this was not significant. In both studies there were no operative deaths.

Ablative Therapies

Ablative techniques include cryosurgical, laser and radiofrequency (RF) thermal ablation. These techniques rely on temperature extremes to cause tumor necrosis and are usually employed intraoperatively, although there are reports of percutaneous applications under computed tomography or ultrasound guidance. The use of these techniques in cirrhotic patients with HCC is attractive because they do not require resection of functional liver parenchyma. Ablative techniques can be applied as the only therapy or in combination with resection. Indications include patients with severe cirrhosis that precludes resection, and patients with residual tumor at the cut surface after resection, or small tumors found distant to a large main tumor being resected. Cryotherapy for HCC demonstrates a 5-year survival of 42.1% after cryotherapy plus resection. Radiofrequency interstitial thermal ablation has been applied to small HCC tumors with success although they sometimes require more than one treatment. Rossi et al, (68) have also performed percutaneous RF ablation in patients with small HCC. Twenty-four patients who were not eligible for surgicalresection for small HCC underwent percutaneous RF ablation. There was no morbidity or mortality related to the procedure and local recurrence at the site of RF ablation occurred in two patients at a mean follow-up of 24.8 months. Three and five year survival rates were 67% and 45%, respectively.

ADJUVANT THERAPIES

The overall prognosis of HCC is very poor. Surgical resection is the only potentially curative treatment for HCC, however, of those undergoing resection, about 50% develop recurrence in the first two years and recurrence rates approach 80% in the third year. Recurrence occurs in metastases that are unrecognized at the time of surgery and new tumor foci in the damaged liver parenchyma. Several strategies for postoperative adjuvant therapy have been attempted, however, few show any survival benefit.

Hormonal Therapy

HCC is thought to be a hormonally dependent tumor based on its occurrence in patients who have been treated with oral contraceptives and androgenic steroids. Several trials utilizing antiandrogenic agents for HCC have been reported. These antiandrogenic agents include Tamoxifen (69,70) and Flutamide (71). To date, however, none of these studies has shown a survival benefit or a decrease in recurrence in patients treated in the postoperative setting.

Chemotherapy and Chemoimmunotherapy

Chemotherapies active against HCC have been actively sought and doxirubicin has been found to be the most active agent against HCC with response rates of 10-24% (72). Epirubicin is a newer member in this class and is thought to have less cardiotoxic effects. These agents along with cisplatin and mitomycin C are utilized alone or in combination during chemoembolization of HCC. They are coupled with iodized oil, a process called lipiodolization, which is the administration of chemotherapeutic agents suspended in lipid contrast medium and given via hepatic arterial infusion to HCC. Advantages of lipiodol are that it selectively accumulates only in tissue of HCC for periods ranging from several weeks to over a year (73,74). Lipiodol has no anticancer effect of its own. It's use as a vehicle to suspend other chemotherapeutic agents and because it stays in the HCC tissue for prolonged periods of time, it is thought that this prolongs the exposure of the HCC to the chemotherapeutic agents. Most studies (10,72-75) utilizing chemotherapeutic agents have failed to show a significant survival benefit in the postoperative setting. However, there are trends toward longer disease free survival when multiple chemotherapeutic agents are used (74). Most agree that these agents must be given within the first year after surgery with some advocating administration as early as 6-8 weeks after surgery (72). This is because most recurrences occur during the first year after surgery.

Other Agents

Octreotide and polyprenoic acid are two other agents that are being investigated for their anticancer effect on HCC. Octreotide was recently given to patients in a randomized controlled study (76) and there was a statistically significant survival benefit for the patients who had received octreotide. The mechanism of action of octreotide on HCC is not known for sure. It is thought to act on somatostatin receptors which have been found on HCC itself. It may also work to modulate other tumor trophic hormones such as insulin, insulin like growth factor 1, cholecystokinin B and Gastrin (77).

Another possible anticancer agent is polyprenoic, an acyclic retinoid which may reduce second primaries after HCC resection. This is thought to work as a chemoprophylactic agent because it mainly inhibits the promotion of carcinogenesis but not conversion and progression of carcinoma. This was recently tested in a randomized blinded study and they found a decrease in the occurrence of second primaries following surgery. At the time of publication there was difference in survival between the groups receiving polyprenoic acid and placebo (78).

SUMMARY

The overall prognosis of HCC is very poor because most patients are unresectable at the time of initial evaluation. Surgical resection is the only potentially curative treatment for HCC, however the recurrence rate after resection remains high as well. Utilizing screening protocols which incorporates the use of hepatic ultrasound and biochemical markers, HCC can be identified earlier and enable the patient to withstand surgical resection. Morbidity and mortality after resection is multifactorial and relates to HCC itself, underlying liver disease and comorbid conditions. Utilizing tests such as ICG R15, Redox Tolerance Index and Tc-GSA to define the functional status of the liver and staging systems helps define who will tolerate hepatic resection.

Morbidity and mortality from hepatic resections has also improved with minimizing intraoperative blood loss and minimizing the amount of functional tissue resected. The use of maneuvers such as total vascular exclusion with or without venovenous bypass has expanded the indications for surgery. Utilizing therapeutic combinations, including TAE, portal vein embolization or ablative therapies widens the indications for resection of HCC. Since there are no chemotherapeutic regimens that have been found to prolong survival, surgical resection remains the procedure of choice for treating HCC.

REFERENCES

1. Benvegnu L and Alberti A. Risk factors and prevention of hepatocellular carcinomain HCV infection. Dig Dis Sci 1996 Suppl;41 49S-55S.
2. Lin DY, Liaw YF, Chu CM, Chang-Chien CS, Wu CS, Chen PC, and Sheen IS. Hepatocellular Carcinoma in Noncirrhotic Patients. Cancer 1984; 54: 1466-1468.
3. MacIntosh EL and Minuk GY. Hepatic resection in patients with cirrhosis and hepatocellular carcinoma. SG & O 1992; 174: 245-54.
4. Nagorney DM, van Heerden JA, Ilstrup DM, and Adson MA. Primary hepatic malignancy: Surgical management and determinants of survival. Surgery 1989;106: 740-9.
5. Sesto ME, Vogt DP, and Hermann RE. Hepatic resection in 128 patients: A 24-year experience. Surgery1987;102:846-851.
6. Thompson HH, Tompkins RK, Longmire WP Jr. Major hepatic resection. A 25-year experience. Ann Surg 1983;197:375-88.
7   Okuda K, Ohtsuki T, Obata H, Tomimatsu M, Okazaki N, Hasegawa H, Nakajima Y, and Ohnishi K. Natural history of hepatocellular carcinoma and prognosis in relation to treatment. Cancer 1985; 56: 918-28.
8. Pawarode A, Voravud N, Sriuranpong V, Kullavanijaya P, and Patt YZ. Natural history of untreated primary hepatocellular carcinoma. Am J Clin Oncol 1998; 21:386-391.
9. Lee CS, Sung JL, Hwang LY, Sheu JC, Chen DS, Lin TY, and Beasley RP. Surgical treatment of 109 patients with symptomatic and asymptomatic hepatocellular carcinoma. Surgery1986; 99: 483-490.
10. Izumi R, Shimizu K, and Miyazaki. Postoperative adjuvant locoregional chemotherapy in patients with hepatocellular carcinoma. Hepato-Gastroenterology 1996;43:1415-1420.

11. Nagasue N, Kohno H, Chang YC, Taniura H, Yamanoi A, Uchida M, Kimoto T, Takemoto Y, Nakamura T, and Yukaya H. Liver Resection for hepatocellualar carcinoma: Results of 229 consecutive patients during 11 years. Ann Surg 1993; 217:375-384.
12. Takenaka K, Kawahara N, Yamamoto K, Kajiyama K, Maeda T, Itasaka H, Shirabe K, Nishizaki T, Yanaga K, and Sugimachi K. Results of 280 liver resections for hepatocellualr carcinoma. Arch Surg 1996; 131: 71-76.
13. Tsukuma H, Hiyama T, Tanaka S, Nakao M, Yabuuchi T, Kitamura T, Nakanishi K, Fujimoto I, Inoue A,Yamazaki H and Kawashima T. Risk factors for hepatocellular carcinoma among patients with chronic liver disease. NEJM 1993;328:1797-1801.
14. Regan LS. Screening for hepatocellular carcinoma in high-risk individuals. Arch Intern Med 1989; 149: 1741-4.
15. Zoli M, Magalotti D, Bianchi G, Gueli C, Marchesini G, and Pisi E. Efficacy of a surveillance program for early detection of hepatocellular carcinoma. Cancer 1996; 78: 977-85.
16. Tsai SL and Liaw YF. Etiology and pathogenesis of hepatocellular carcinoma. Dig Surg 1995, 12:7-15.
17. Imai Y, Kawata S, Tamura S, Yabuuchi I, Noda S, Inada M, Maeda Y, Shirai Y, Fukuzaki T, Kaji I, Ishikawa H, Matsuda Y, Nishikawa M, Seki K, and Matsuzawa Y for the Osaka Hepatocellular Carcinoma Prevention Study Group. Relation of Interferon Therapy and Hepatocellular Carcinoma in Patients with Chronic Hepatitis C. Annals Int Med 1998; 129: 94-9.
18. Malt RA, Galdabini JJ, and Jeppsson BW. Abnormal sex-steriod milieu in young adults with hepatocellular carcinoma. World J Surg 1983;7:247-252.
19. Nagasue N, Yukaya H, Hamada T, Hirose S, Kanashima R, and Inokuchi K. The natural history of hepatocellular carcinoma. Cancer 1984; 54: 1461-65.
20. Huquet C, Stipa A, and Gavelli. Primary hepatocellular cancer: Western experienc. In Blumgart LH, ed. Surgery of the Liver and Biliary Tract. Edinburgh: Churchill Livingstone, 19 :p1365-1469.
21. Schafer DF and Sorrell MF. Hepatocellular carcinoma. Lancet 1999; 353: 1253-57.
22. Colombo M, De Franchis R, Del Ninno E, Sangiovanni A, De Fazio C, Tommasini M, Donato MF, Piva A, Di Carlo V, and Dioguardi N. Hepatocellular carcinoma in Italian patients with cirrhosis. N Engl J Med 1991; 325: 675-80.
23. Dodd GD, Miller WJ, Baron RL, Skolnick ML, Campbell WL. Detection of malignant tumors in end-stage cirrhotic livers: efficacy of sonography as a screening techinque. AJR 1992; 159: 727-33.
24. Maringhini A, Cottone M, Sciarrino E, Marceno MP, La Seta F, Fusco G, Rinaldi F, and Pagliaro L. Ultrasonography and alpha-fetoprotein in diagnosis of hepatocellular carcinoma in cirrhosis. Dig Dis Sci 1988; 33: 47-51.
25. Sarasin FP, Giostra E, and Hadengue A. Cost-effectiveness of screening for detection of small hepatocellular carcinoma in western patients with Child-Pugh class A cirrhosis. Am J Med 1996; 171: 422-434.
26. Sato Y, Nakata K, Kato Y, Shima M, Ishii N, Koji T, Taketa K, Endo Y, and Nagataki S. Early recognition of hepatocellular carcinoma based on altered profiles of alpha-fetoprotein. N Engl J Med 1993; 328: 1802-6.
27. Shinagawa T, Ohto M, Kimura K, Tsunetomi S, Morita M, Saisho H, Tsuchiya Y,

Saotome N, Karasawa E, Miki M, Ueno T, and Okuda K. Diagnosis and clinical features of small hepatocellular carcinoma with emphasis on the utility of real-time ultrasonograph. Gastroenterology 1984; 86: 495-502.

28. Bloomer JR. Serum alpha-fetoprotein in nonneoplastic liver diseases. Dig Dis Sci 1980; 25:241-2.

29. Soga K, Watanabe T, Aikawa K, Toshima M, Shibasaki K and Aoyagi Y. Ser des-gamma-carboxy-prothrombin level by a modified enzyme immunoassay method in hepatocellular carcinoma: clinical significance in small hepatocellular carcinoma. Hepato-Gastroenterology 1998; 45:1737-41.

30. Izzo F, Curley S, Maio P, Leonardi E, Imparato L, Giglio S, Cremona F and Castello G. Correlation of soluble interleukin-2 receptor levels with severity of chronic hepatitis C virus liver injury and development of hepatocellular cancer. Surgery 1996;120:100-5)

31. Takayasu K, Moriyama N, Muramatsu Y, Makuuchi M, Hasegawa H, Okazaki N and Hirohashi S. The diagnosis of small hepatocellular carcinomas: efficacy of various imaging procedures in 100 patients. AJR1990; 155: 49-54.

32. Franco D, Capussotti L, Smadja C, Bouzari H, Meakins J, Kemeny F, Grange D, and Dellepiane M. Resection of hepatocellular carcinomas: Results in 72 european patients with cirrhosis. Gastroenterology 1990;98:733-738.

33. Kanematsu T, Takenaka K, Matsumata T, Furuta T, Sugimachi K, and Inokuchi K. Limited hepatic resection effective for selected cirrhotic patients with primary liver cancer. Ann Surg 1984;199:51-56.

34. Makuuchi M, Hasegawa H, and Yamazaki S. Ultrasonically guided subsegmentectomy. Surg Gynec and Obstet 1985;161: 346-350.

35. Nagasue N, Yukaya H, Ogawa Y, Sasaki Y, Chang YC, and Niimi K. Clinical experience with 118 hepatic resections for hepatocellular carcinoma. Surgery 1986;99: 695-701.

36. Shimada M, Matsumata T, Akazawa K, Kamakura T, Itasaka H, Sugimachi K, and Nose Y. Estimation of risk of major complications after hepatic resection. Am J Surg 1994;167: 399-403.

37. Kawasaki, Dig Surg

38. Makuuchi M, Kosuge T, Takayama T, Yamazaki S, Kakazu T, Miyagawa S, and Kawasaki S. Surgery for Small Liver Cancers. Sem Surg Onc 1993;9:298-304.

39. Paquet KJ, Koussouris P, Mercado MA, Kalk JFr, Muting D, and Rambach W. Limited hepatic resection for selected cirrhotic patients with hepatocellular or cholangiocellular carcinoma: a prospective study. Br J Surg 1991; 78: 459-62.

40. Manual for Staging of Cancer. American Joint Committee on Cancer. Pp. 87-89. Philadelphia: J.B. Lippincott, 1988.

41. Kanda M, Taniguchi K, Awazu K, Ishigami Y, Masuzawa M, and Abe H. Continuous monitoring of cardiogreen removal by a diseased liver using an optical sensor. Society of Photo-Optical Instrumentation Engineers 1988;904:39-46.

42. Mori K, Ozawa K, Yamamoto Y, Maki A, Shimahara Y, Kobayashi, Yamaoka Y and Kumada K. Response of hepatic mitochondrial redox state to oral glucose load. Ann Surg 1990;211:438.

43. Kwon AH, Ha-Kawa SK, Uetsuji S, Kamiyama Y, and TanakaY. Use of technetium 99m diethylenetriamine-pentaacetic acid-galactosyl-human serum albumin liver scintography in the evaluation of preoperative and postoperative hepatic functional reserve for hepatectomy. Surgery 1995;117:429-34.

44. Bismuth H, Houssin D, Ornowski J, and Meriggi F. Liver Resections in Cirrhotic Patients: A Western Experience. World J Surg 1986; 10: 311-317.
45. Wu CC, Hwang CR, Liu TJ, and P'eng FK. Effects and limitations of prolonged intermittent ischaemia for hepatic resection and the cirrhotic liver. Br J Surg 1996;83:121-124.
46. Sitzman JV and Greene PS. Perioperative predictors of morbidity following hepatic resection for neoplasm. Ann Surg 1994;219:13-17.
47. Gozzetti G, Mazziotti A, Bolondi L, Cavallari A, Grigioni W, Casanova P, Bellusci R, Villanacci V, and Labo G. Intraoperative ultrasonography in surgery for liver tumors. Surgery 1986;99: 523-529.
48. Huguet C, Nordlinger B, Bloch P, and Conard J. Tolerance of the human liver to prolonged normothermic ischemia. A biological study of 20 patients submitted to extensive hepatectomy. Surg Gynecol Obstet 1978;147: 689-93.
49. Nagasue N, Yukaya H, Suehiro S, and Ogawa Y. Tolerance of the cirrhotic liver to normothermic ischemia. Am J Surg 1984;147:772-5.
50. Kim YI, Kobayashi M, Aramaki M, Nakashima K, Mitarai Y, and Yoshida T. "Early-Stage" cirrhotic liver can withstand 75 minutes of inflow occlusion during resection. Hepato-Gastroenterol 1994;41:355-358.
51. Bismuth H, Castaing D, and Garden OJ. Major hepatic resection under total vascular exclusion. Ann Surg 1989;210:13-19.
52. Habib N, Zografos G, Dalla Serra G, Greco L and Bean A. Liver resection with total vascular exclusion for malignant tumours. Br J Surg 1994;81:1181-1184.
53. Yamaoka Y, Ozawa K, Kumada K, Shimahara Y, Tanaka K, Mori K, Takayasu T, Okamoto R, Kobayashi N, Konishi Y, and Egawa H. Total vascular exclusion for hepatic resection in cirrhotic patients. Arch Surg 1992;127:276-280.
54. Makuuchi M, Mori T, Gunven P, Yamazaki S, and Hasegawa H. Safety of hemihepatic vascular occlusion during resection of the liver. SG & O 1987;164:155-58
55. Nagasue N, Galizia G, Kohno H, Chang YC, Hayashi T, Yamanoi A, Nakamura T, and Yukaya H. Adverse effects of preoperative hepatic artery chemoembolization for resectable hepatocellular carcinoma: A retrospective comparison of 138 liver resections. Surgery 1989; 106: 81-6.
56. Harada T, Matsuo K, Tamesue S, Inoue T, and Nakamure H. Is preoperative hepatic arterial chemoembolization safe and effective for hepatocellular carcinoma? Ann Surg 1996;224:4-9.
57. Hwang TL, Chen MF, Lee TY, Chen TJ, Lin DY, Liaw YF. Resection of hepatocellular carcinoma after transcatheter arterial embolization. Arch Surg 1987;122:756-759.
58. Yu YQ, Xu DB, Zhou XD, Lu JZ, Tang ZY, and Mack P. Experience with liver resection after hepatic arterial chemoembolization for hepatocellular carcinoma. Cancer 1993; 71: 62-5.
59. Kawasaki S, Makuuchi M, Miyagawa S, and Kakzu T. Radical operation after portal embolization for tumor of hilar bile duct. J Am Coll Surg 1994; 178: 480-486.
60. Azoulay d, Raccuia JS, Castaing D, and Bismuth H. Right portal vein embolization in preparation for major hepatic resection. J Am Coll Surg 1995; 181:267-9.
61. de Baere T, Roche A, Vavasseur D, Therasse E, Indushekar S, Elias D, and Bognel

C. Portal vein embolization: utility for inducing left hepatic lobe hypertrophy before surgery. Radiology 1993; 188: 73-77.

62. Nagino M, Nimura Y, Kamiya J, Kondo S, Uesaka K, Kin Y, Hayakawa N, and Yamamoto H. Changes in hepatic lobe volume in biliary tract cancer patients after right portal vein embolization. Hepatology 1995; 21: 434-439.

63. Kawasaki S, Makuuchi M, Kakazu T, Miyagawa S, Takayama T, Kosuge T, Sugihara K, and Moriya Y. Resection for multiple metastatic liver tumors after portal embolization. Surgery 1994; 115: 674-7.

64. Lee KC, Kinoshita H, Hirohashi K, Kubo S, and Iwasa R. Extension of Surgical indications for hepatocellular carcinoma by portal vein embolizaion. World J Surg 1993; 17: 109-115.

65. Zhou XD, Tang ZY, and Yu YQ. Ablative approach for primary liver cancer. Surg Onc Clinics of North America 1996;5:379-390.

66. Sitzman JV and Abrams R. Improved survival for hepatocellular cancer with combination surgery and multimodality treatment. Ann Surg 1993; 217: 149-154.

67 Zhou XD, Tang ZY, Yu YQ, and Ma ZC. Clinical evaluation of cryosurgery in the treatment of primary liver cancer. Cancer 1988;61:1889-1892.

68. Rossi S, Di Stasi M, buscarini E, Cavanna L, Quaretti P, Squassante E, Garbagnati F, and Buscarini L. Percutaneous radiofrequency interstitial thermal ablation in the treatment of small hepatocellular carcinoma. The Cancer J 1995;1:73-81.

69. Castells A, Bruix J, Ayuso C, Roca M, Boix, Vilana R, and Rodes J. Treatment of hepatocellular carcinoma with Tamoxifen: a double blind placebo-controlled trial in 120 patients. Gastroenterology 1995; 109: 917-22.

70. Engstrom PF, Levin B, Moertel CG, and Schutt A. A phase II trial of Tamoxifen in hepatocellular carcinoma. Cancer 1990;65:2641-43.

71. Chao Y, Chan WK, Huang YS, Teng HC, Wang SS, Lui WY, Whang-Peng J, and Lee SD. Phase II study of Flutamide in the treatment of hepatocellular carcinoma. Cancer 1996;77:635-9.

72. Lai ECS, Lo CM, Fan ST, Liu CL, and Wong J. Postoperative adjuvant chemotherapy after curative resection of hepatocellular carcinoma. Arch Surg 1998;133:183-188.

73. Bhattacharya S, Novell JR, Winslet MC and Hobbs KEF. Iodized oil in the treatment of hepatocellular carcinoma. Br J Surg 1994;81:1563-1571.

74. Takenaka K, Yoshida K, Nishizaki T, Korenaga D, Hiroshige K, Ikeda T and Sugimachi K. Postoperative prophylactic lipiodolization reduces the intrahepatic recurrence of hepatocellular carcinoma. Am J Surg 1995;169;400-405.

75. Kawata A, Une Y, Hosokawa M, Wakizaka Y, Namieno T, Uchino J, and Kobayashi H. Adjuvant chemoimmunotherapy for hepatocellular carcinoma patients. Am J Clin Oncol 1995;18:257-262.

76. Kouroumalis E, Skordilis P, Thermos K, Vasilaki A, Moschandrea J, and Manousos ON. Treatment of hepatocellular carcinoma with octreotide: a randomised controlled study. Gut 1998; 42: 442-47.

77. Caplin. Gut 1996;38(Suppl 1):A16.

78. Muto Y, Moriwaki H, Ninomiya M, Adachi S, Saito A, Takasaki KT, Tanaka T, Tsurumi K, Okuno M, Tomita E, Nakamura T, and Kojima T for the Hepatoma Prevention Study Group. Prevention of second primary tumors by an acyclic retinoid, polyprenoic acid, in patients with hepatocellular carcinoma. N Engl J Med 1996; 334: 1561-7.

5

INDICATIONS AND RESULTS OF LIVER TRANSPLANTATION FOR PRIMARY AND METASTATIC LIVER CANCER

Alan Koffron, M.D., Jonathan P. Fryer, M.D., and Michael Abecassis, M.D.

Northwestern University Medical School, Chicago, IL

INTRODUCTION

Orthotopic liver transplantation (OLT) has become an established treatment for end-stage liver disease (ESLD), acute liver failure, and malignant tumors. Transplantation for hepatic malignancies is indicated in the setting of either unresectible lesion(s), or coexistent cirrhosis resulting in both inadequate hepatic reserve and prohibitive portal hypertension.

Despite the theoretical advantages of total hepatectomy, early efforts at hepatic replacement for primary hepatic malignancies generally met with failure (1). Initial enthusiasm for transplantation in patients with hepatic malignancy faded with early recurrence, typically diagnosed within the first 12 to 24 months after OLT (2). Two-year survival after OLT for hepatocellular carcinoma (HCC) was reported to be as low as 17 to 26% (3). These results, probably due to the presence of micro-metastases at the time of surgery, have led transplant surgeons to question the justification of using this treatment modality in this context (4,5). Thus, the proportion of tumor patients undergoing transplantation decreased in the mid-to-late 1980s.

Despite the disappointing outcome in some patients with primary hepatic malignancies, other patients have achieved excellent survival in excess of 12 to 20 years (2,5-9). These long-term survivors demonstrate the potential for cure of these fatal malignancies, providing a stimulus for further attempts at improving outcomes, by identifying prognostic indicators for recurrence such as the use of reverse transcriptase polymerase chain reaction for the detection of albumin mRNA in peripheral blood with HCC (10).

There is ongoing controversy relating to the indications for OLT in the context of large HCC. In the absence of effective non-surgical therapy there remains a strong incentive to carry out OLT for these malignancies. Clinical investigation has identified certain clinicopathological features of patients and tumors which correlate with improved prognosis after transplantation, suggesting that better results can be obtained by stringent preoperative patient selection.

The advent of more accurate diagnostic techniques and identification of a number of prognostic factors associated with poor outcome provide insight into problems inherent in the application of OLT for primary hepatic malignancy (1,2,5-9,11-20). Multimodal therapeutic strategies have been employed yielding benefit in certain categories of hepatic malignancy (1,5,7-9,21-26). More recently, local ablative techniques such as transarterial chemoembolization (TACE) have been employed in attempts at preoperative control of the disease, in order to enhance outcomes following OLT. Although typically used as palliative treatment, initial experience with preoperative TACE suggests a decrease in post-OLT recurrence, possibly due to abating tumor progression during the pretransplant period. Interventions such as adjuvant chemotherapy and radiation are more complex in the immunosuppressed OLT recipient, but such adjunctive therapy may prove useful in preventing or delaying tumor recurrence.

The purpose of this chapter is to review the experience with transplantation for primary and metastatic hepatic cancer in adults. We will outline a diagnostic and staging approach, identify the factors important in patient selection for transplantation, and suggest a possible role for combined modality therapy

DIAGNOSIS

In the United States, metastatic carcinoma to the liver is much more common than primary hepatic malignancy. In adults, 80 to 90% of primary hepatic cancers are HCC (27,28). Furthermore, the incidence of HCC in the USA is increasing, primarily due to the increased incidence of hepatitis C-related cirrhosis (29). Cholangiocarcinoma accounts for the majority of remaining primary hepatic cancers, whereas other tumors, such as cholangiohepatomas occur rarely (30). Because many factors influence outcome after OLT, especially the type of malignancy, it becomes crucial to delineate the type of malignancy and its extent.

Histology

Patients with metastatic disease to the liver or those with metastatic primary hepatic malignancy are not candidates for OLT. Thus, it is extremely important to interpret histologic findings in the context of clinical and other laboratory data. Percutaneous biopsy of hepatic lesions should be obtained for histological examination if there is uncertainty of the diagnosis.

In those patients with a large hepatic mass and elevated alpha-fetoprotein (AFP), the diagnosis of HCC is relatively simple, even without histological confirmation. In contrast, the patients with one or more lesions and only mild AFP elevations usually require biopsy for diagnosis. The risk of needle track seeding should be weighed against the benefit of confirming the diagnosis, especially when the management strategies require a definitive diagnosis (31).

Radiological Investigations

Radiological investigations may be used in lieu of or as a complement to tissue diagnosis. No imaging method provides 100% accuracy in delineating important tumor characteristics. The presence of underlying cirrhosis is problematic, particularly with regard to the value of computed tomography (CT) and ultrasonography. Thus a combination of studies may be required to fully define tumor size, extent, and metastases.

Ultrasonography: The accuracy of ultrasound (US) in detecting HCC varies between groups and operators. A recent study in 100 cirrhotic patients demonstrated a detection rate of 84% of tumor nodules smaller than 3 cm (32), whereas in a prospective evaluation in 200 liver transplant recipients the sensitivity of ultrasound alone in detecting a tumor within a cirrhotic patient was only 50% (33). In this study, 44 lesions among 17 patients were missed (24 measured less than 1 cm: 12 between 1 and 3 cm: 8 larger than 3 cm), the largest missed lesion being 10 cm in diameter and located in the dome of the right lobe. In this study, the US specificity was 98%.

US is of limited accuracy in showing the extent of tumor involvement both within the liver parenchyma and at extrahepatic sites (34) so that detailed information regarding tumor staging cannot be reliably obtained.

Intraoperative US is now utilized in many medical centers and results in an increased sensitivity of 98% (35). US angiography (US in combination with hepatic artery CO_2 microbubble injection) is now being used to differentiate HCC from other nodules based on tumor vascular patterns (36).

Computed Tomography (CT): Contrast-enhanced CT provides a higher level of accuracy than conventional ultrasound in the detection of intrahepatic lesions. Computed Tomography (CT) has been shown to have a detection rate of 87% in HCC lesions over 2 cm, falling to 25% in those less than 1.5 cm (38). In contrast, CT scanning in conjunction with intra-arterial lipiodol represents an improved method for the detection of lesions measuring less than 2 cm, with 93% sensitivity, and better differentiation is possible between small HCC and regenerating nodules. However, lipiodol does not accumulate in early-stage well-differentiated HCC, leading to decreased accuracy in these lesions. (36).

CT arteriography (CTA), a combination of CT and angiography, is useful in the demonstration of hypovascularity in early-stage well-differentiated HCC.   This modality is also useful in the staging of HCC because of its ability to demonstrate vascular invasion (37).   A study of 100 patients with malignant hepatic tumors showed that conventional CT identified 66% of all intrahepatic lesions, and only 5% of those 1 cm or less in diameter, whereas CTA was the most accurate technique, correctly identifying 94% of all intrahepatic tumors, and 82% of those less than 1 cm. Tumor margins were delineated with an accuracy of 93% by CTA, compared with 80% using conventional CT.   However, both CT and CTA were less effective in detecting tumor invasion of the portal vein and inferior vena cava (38).

Magnetic Resonance Imaging (MRI):   The role of MRI in the evaluation of patients with HCC or other tumors is still being fully evaluated.   In early studies (38), MRI has demonstrated a diagnostic sensitivity of 70% declining to 20% for lesions smaller than 1 cm. In those cases with more than three tumor deposits, MRI missed one or more lesions in 71%.   Tumor margins are accurately delineated in 92% of cases, and vascular invasion is detected in 85% of cases, significantly better than either CT or CTA (8% and 30% of cases, respectively) (38). A diagnosis of HCC can often be made by MRI if fatty degeneration, a tumor capsule or vascular invasion are shown (39) and MRI can be useful in evaluating HCC during its early progression from atypical adenomatous hyperplasia (40).   The principal limitation in the use of MRI to detect intrahepatic tumors is patient-induced, motion artifact.

Staging

The TNM staging system applies to all primary hepatic carcinomas, both HCC and cholangiocarcinoma (41,42).   "T" refers to extent of the primary tumor, "N" to the presence or absence of regional node involvement, and "M" to the presence or absence of distant metastasis. These categories are determined by physical examination, imaging procedures, and surgical exploration (43-48). Tumor size, vascular invasion, and number of lesions are important in the recently revised classification (Table). The lowercase letter "p" is placed before the TNM stage to designate postsurgical histopathological classification and "R" indicates the presence of residual tumor. The T category is based on single versus multiple tumor nodules, size of the largest tumor nodule, and vascular invasion determined by imaging procedures in the surgical specimen. Histopathological grading indicates the degree of tumor cell differentiation (well, moderately, poorly, or undifferentiated); however, such grading is not included in the TNM staging of primary hepatic malignancies.

Some view staging celiotomy as a prerequisite to OLT in order to exclude the presence of disease overlooked by other diagnostic modalities (49,50).   A higher surgical mortality after OLT in patients who had undergone a previous staging celiotomy has been reported (5). Abdominal adhesions from the celiotomy could lead to operative difficulties and bleeding at the time of OLT, particularly in cirrhotic patients with portal hypertension.   Theoretically, liver manipulation during celiotomy could favor extrahepatic tumor dissemination. In addition, significant time may elapse between the celiotomy and OLT, making the operative findings obsolete.

Table 1. TNM Staging System

T1	< 2 cm, no vascular invasion
T2	< 2 cm, vascular invasion <u>or</u> > 2 cm, no vascular invasion
T3	> 2 cm with vascular invasion <u>or</u> multiple
T4	Multiple lobes, macrovascular invasion
Stage I, II	T1, T2, N0
Stage III	T3 or N1
Stage IV	T4, any N, or metastasis

PRIMARY HEPATIC NEOPLASMS

Hepatocellular Carcinoma (HCC)

HCC is one of the most common fatal tumors worldwide with an estimated 1 million cases occurring annually (51,52). In the United States there are approximately 13,000 new cases diagnosed each year, and median survival is generally less than 6 months (15,22,53-55). The prognosis for patients with alpha-fetoprotein-negative HCC is somewhat improved, but median survival in this subgroup remains less than 1 year (56,57). Chronic hepatitis B virus infection (HBV) appears to be a major cause of HCC, although tumor incidence in patients with asymptomatic infection is low (58-60). Hepatitis C virus (HCV) appears to be an independent risk factor for HCC in both eastern nations and the Western hemisphere (61-63). Other etiological factors include aflatoxins (64), cirrhosis (including that with hemochromatosis), and alcohol (52,65). HCC is uncommon in cirrhosis resulting from autoimmune hepatitis, Wilson's disease, and primary biliary cirrhosis.

Unfortunately, only 10 to 30% of patients have surgically resectable lesions, of which 30% are cured (15-22,51,66). In general, short of total hepatectomy (lobectomy or trisegmentectomy), the treatment for HCC is currently disappointing (1,3,4,6-24). Early reports suggested that outcomes following transplantation were not substantially improved. A large study of 365 HCC patients treated by OLT reported 2-year and 5-year tumor-free survivals of 9.3% (34/365) and 2.5% (9/365) respectively (9). A more recent study reported actuarial survival of 49%, 37%, and 30% at 1, 2, and 3 years, respectively, for 97 patients who underwent OLT for HCC (13).

Following transplantation, patients with the fibrolamellar variant of HCC as well as those with incidental HCC (those not diagnosed with malignancy before OLT) appear to have a better prognosis than those for whom the presence of HCC was the major indication for OLT. Patients who harbored 'incidental HCC', where the presence of a small focus of hepatocellular carcinoma (HCC) was discovered within the explanted liver after OLT for end-stage liver disease, had excellent long-term survival. Incidental lesions escape detection during routine preoperative screening for HCC and are therefore small (usually less than 3 cm in diameter) and solitary. Macroregenerative nodules, commonly found in explanted cirrhotic livers, may harbor dysplastic, precancerous lesions (67). Tumor recurrence (after OLT) in cases of incidental HCC was found to be lower compared to those patients where a diagnosis of HCC had been made preoperatively (0-13% versus 37-82%) and most of the cases were cured by the procedure (5,6,9,12,68-72). However, long-term survival is not confined to the cases with incidental HCC, as cures have been reported in other patients, where the tumors tended to be small. Some histological types of tumor, for example the fibrolamellar variant of HCC, have also been found to have lower rates of recurrence or were slower growing and less aggressive.

Overall, experience has shown that patients with non-fibrolamellar HCC showed a strong correlation between tumor size and outcome (9,13,16). For example, one study found that patients receiving transplants for HCC lesions larger than 5 cm had 1-, 3-, and 5-year survivals of 51%, 25%, and 25%, respectively. In contrast, patients with tumors smaller than 5 cm had 1-, 3-, and 5-year survivals of 77%, 68%, and 68%, respectively (16).

These and other studies have shown tumor staging to be of significant prognostic value in assessing the surgical treatment of HCC (19).

In view of the poor results with OLT alone in patients with HCC, one important study evaluated patients treated with a combined modality approach using neoadjuvant (preoperative, intraoperative, and postoperative) chemotherapy and OLT (25,26). All patients were known or suspected to have HCC before OLT. None had evidence of extrahepatic tumor, and none had fibrolamellar HCC. Six patients experienced recurrence between 6 and 25 months after OLT, but only one had an initial tumor recurrence in the allograft. Three patients died of recurrent hepatitis B, resulting in a lower overall survival in hepatitis B surface antigen (HBAg)-positive compared with HBAg-negative patients. These authors reported (median follow-up, 39 months), the overall and tumor-free survival rate for the 20 patients in this trial was 55% at 3 years. For the 17 patients with tumors larger than 5 cm, the overall survival rate was 58% and the tumor-free survival rate was 51 % at 3 years.

In summary, analysis of the early experience in treating HCC with OLT has led to the identification of several important prognostic indicators, pivotal in the identification of surgical candidates.

PROGNOSTIC INDICATORS

Tumor size and number

Low rates of tumor recurrence for incidental HCC were first reported in 12 patients, 11 of who remained tumor free during a median follow-up period of 16 months (70). A subsequent report (12) described 14 cases of incidental HCC. Only one of these had a recurrence which was diagnosed at 17 months and led to death 6 months later. The tumor in this case was multifocal, with a maximum tumor nodule size of 3.5 cm. The remaining 13 had unifocal tumors ranging from 0.5 to 7 cm in diameter. Follow-up periods ranged from 3 to 73 months, and at the time of the report, 6 of the patients had survived for longer than 3 years. This study also showed that better results in those patients with tumors diagnosed before transplantation were obtained when the tumors were unifocal and less than 5 cm in diameter. Tumor recurrence was seen in only 2 (7%) of 28 patients in this group, in contrast with 21 (62%) of 34 patients with lesions larger than 5 cm. Disease-free survival figures at 5 years were 71.4% for those with tumors smaller than 5 cm., and 29.1% in the group with larger tumors. A follow-up analysis (72) showed that 1-, 3- and 5-year survival after OLT was 77%, 68% and 68% for small (less than 5 cm) HCC, the corresponding figures for patients with larger tumors being 51%, 25 % and 25 %. In addition, in 18 cases with tumors measuring less than 5 cm in diameter, a mean survival period of 89.6 months was found, in contrast with only 28.1 months in 11 cases with larger tumors. When the number of gross tumors present in the explanted liver was examined, mean survival of 68.6 months was found in cases with single tumors, contrasting with a mean survival period of only 37.9 months in patients with more than one tumor (6). Thus, not only is the size of the main tumor important, but also the number of tumor nodules present has a bearing on subsequent survival. In another study (56 HCC patients) eventual outcome was also found to depend upon the tumor size and the number of deposits (73). The study was divided into three groups. The one with the most favorable outlook comprised those patients with small unifocal tumors measuring less than 4 cm in diameter, with or without much smaller local satellite lesions. None of the cases in this category developed a recurrence of HCC during a mean period of follow-up of 23 months. Four of the 14 cases in this group had incidental HCC, and taken as a whole the group had a 1-year actuarial survival figure of 85.7%, and 57.1 % at 3 and 5 years respectively. The second patient group was made up of patients with unifocal tumors measuring between 4 and 8 cm in diameter in whom tumor recurrence was seen in 40% at a mean time of 16 months after OLT. Five of the six cases with recurrence died as a result of their tumors during the study duration, with a mean survival of more than 3 years. The 1- and 3-year actuarial survival in this group was 66.7%, which declined to 44.4% at 5 years. The group of patients having the worst prognosis were those with either large unifocal lesions which measured 8 cm or more in diameter, or cases with multifocal disease (three or more tumor masses) regardless of the size of any individual lesion. Recurrence of tumor was seen in 21 of the 27 cases in this group (78%), and occurred at a mean post-transplant interval of only 8 months. Nineteen of the 21 with recurrent tumor died after surviving for only 13 months on average; actuarial survival figures were 44.4% and 11.1% at 1 and 3 years.

Unilobar involvement carries a lower risk of tumor recurrence as evidenced by tumor-free survival figures of 81.6%, 67.6% and 67.6% at 1, 3 and 5 years, in contrast with patients where both lobes were involved (72). This latter group had a disease-free survival percentage at 1, 3 and 5 years of only 28.5%. The mean survival period for those with unilobar tumors was significantly higher at 66 months in 51 patients versus 28 months in the 54 cases with involvement of both lobes (6).

Lymph node involvement

Lymph node metastasis, not surprisingly, has been shown to have a major impact on prognosis. In one series patients without nodal involvement had a median survival of 13 months, compared with only 8 months for cases with positive nodes (17). Six-month and 2-year actuarial survival figures in another series for lymph node-negative HCC without cirrhosis were 83% and 75%, compared to only 33% and 11% in those with tumor-positive nodes (3). Two additional studies reported 1-, 2- and 3-year actuarial survival of 43%, 36% and 24% in patients with negative nodes, contrasting with no survivors beyond 12 months in patients with lymph node involvement at the time of transplantation (69,74). The median survival periods for the two groups were 9.5 and 2 months respectively.

Another group (6,71) reported mean survival times after OLT of 10.5 months in lymph node-positive patients, compared with 49.7 months in cases who did not have nodal involvement at the time of operation. The risk of tumor recurrence was found to be more than doubled by lymph node involvement, with recurrence rates for the two groups of 75% and 34% respectively.

TNM stage

The TNM pathological classification of tumor stage (75) has been retrospectively used in two studies demonstrating a clear correlation between TNM staging and survival.

A study of 52 patients (69) demonstrated median survival time for cases with stage II tumors (pT2 pN0 pM0) was 120 months, and only 12 months in patients with stage III (pT1-3 pN0-1 pM0) disease. Those patients with the more advanced stage IVa lesions (pT4 pN0-1 pM0) had a median survival of only 9 months, and cases with stage IVb tumors (pT1-4 pN0-1 pM1) survived for less than a month. The actuarial survival figure for stage II tumor cases was 100% at 5 years; those with stage III disease had 1- and 3-year actuarial survival of approximately 48% and 25% with corresponding figures for the patients with stage IVa disease of approximately 30% and 9%. Another group (6) analyzed results in 105 OLT recipients with HCC, including 10 with the fibrolamellar variant. One- and 5-year actuarial survival for patients with stage I disease was 75%, compared with 1- and 5-year survival of 81.3% and 75% for stage II. Cases with stage III disease had 1-, 3- and 5-year survival of 79%, 56% and 48% and figures for stage IVa tumors at 1, 2 and 3 years were 43.8%, 26.2% and 0%. A total of 45 cases (42.9%) suffered tumor recurrence, causing death in 42 (93%) during the follow-up period of the study. Tumor recurrence rates, disease stages I-IVa, were 0%, 5.3%, 17.4% and 67.8%, respectively. There were ten 5-year survivors with non-fibrolamellar HCC: two had stage I disease, four had stage II disease, and four had stage III disease. There were no 5-year survivors after transplantation for stage IVa disease.

Vascular invasion

The presence of vascular invasion by tumor is associated with a much higher incidence of tumor recurrence. Tumor recurrence was demonstrated in 73% of patients with gross vascular infiltration, compared with 29% of cases without vascular involvement (71). In a later report (72) when 80 cases were analyzed (of whom all had survived the immediate 3-month postoperative period) highly significant differences in outcome were observed. Complete absence of vascular invasion was found in 22 cases and these patients had the lowest risk of tumor recurrence with a tumor-free survival figure of 95.2% at 5 years. This compared with tumor-free survival of 70% at 1 year and 49.8% at 5 years in 30 patients found to have histological evidence of microscopic vascular invasion. In the third group of 28 cases with gross macroscopic vascular invasion, disease-free survival was only 11.9% at 1 year, with no survivors at 3 years. Mean survival figures in the same three groups of patients were 73.2, 43.3 and 21.6 months, respectively (6).

Tumor morphology

A pseudocapsule surrounding the tumor at the periphery was present in 17 of the 80 cases discussed above (72). These 17 patients had disease-free survival figures at 1, 3 and 5 years of 81.6% compared to 51.1%, 37% and 37% in the 63 patients in whom a pseudocapsule was not identified. Well-circumscribed tumors have also been found to recur less frequently after OLT than those with an infiltrative shape. Circumscribed lesions were associated with disease-free survival figures of 70%, 63.2% and 63.2% at 1, 3 and 5 years (72), compared to 1 % and 0% at 1 and 3 years in the patients whose tumors had a more infiltrative configuration (76). Mean survival for patients with circumscribed lesions was 57.2 months compared with 21.8 months for the infiltrating group (6).

Liver capsule involvement does not seem to have a significant deleterious effect on survival. Eight patients with involvement of the liver capsule had tumor-free survival figures of 43.8% at 1, 3 and 5 years, compared with figures of 57.5%, 47.2% and 47.2% in 72 cases without capsular involvement (72). This difference was not statistically significant, but the number of cases in this study was small.

TREATMENT

Adjuvant Therapy and Perioperative Chemoembolization

Hepatic arterial chemoembolization carried out before transplantation has been shown to be a relatively safe procedure and effective in reducing tumor bulk (77). Lipiodol and doxorubicin followed either by gelatin sponge powder or Gelfoam pellets have also been used. A portal vein block must first be excluded because of the risk of inducing massive hepatic necrosis in such cases. Because of a 60-day mortality rate of 37%, the treatment is no longer offered to patients with Child-Pugh class C cirrhosis. Mortality in Child-Pugh classes A and B is 2.8% and 8%, respectively. Chemoembolization can be followed by mild fever and leucocytosis, nausea and anorexia, and hepatic tenderness. Transaminase levels are elevated for a few days. The patient is usually able to be discharged home after 5 days. The treatment can be repeated as necessary, and up to eight (median 2) serial chemoembolization procedures were performed in each patient. Fifty-five patients treated in this way went on to OLT followed by intravenous chemotherapy (78). Tumor-free 3-year survival was 59% for cases with HCC smaller than 3cm, but only 26% for larger lesions.

In addition, doxorubicin (Adriamycin) produces objective responses in only 15 to 20% of patients with advanced HCC and remains the most active agent (51,53,79). Delayed cardiotoxicity is a potential complication with the use of doxorubicin (80). Additional complications of chemotherapy may occur in HCC patients who have undergone liver transplantation. Reactivation of hepatitis B has been reported in patients receiving cytotoxic agents (81,82). Thus far, there is no indication that any particular drug is responsible.

Embolization with or without chemotherapy drugs or lipiodol (77,83-88), alcohol injection of tumors (89-91), biological response modifiers (92), and antiestrogen therapy (93) are alternative liver-directed palliative measures. Monoclonal antibodies raised to antigens on hepatoma cells and alpha-fetoprotein have been described and used as immunotargeting agents (94-96).

Surgical Options

If there is no evidence of extrahepatic disease, resection should always be considered in noncirrhotic livers with HCC, if anatomically feasible. However, over 85% of HCCs in the U.S.A. are associated with cirrhosis. In cirrhotic livers with favorable HCC tumors (i.e. ≤ 5cm, ≤ 3 tumors, confined to one lobe), transplantation is associated with better disease-free survival than resection (97,98). However, due to the limited number of organs available for transplantation, resection should still be considered in certain circumstances, since resection can be curative in a some patients (99). Curative resections will help some patients by allowing them to avoid lifelong immunosuppression and others by making more donor livers available.

Candidates must be carefully selected to avoid postoperative complications commonly associated with resection such as liver failure, bleeding, bile leaks, ascites, and sepsis. In general, resection of cirrhotic livers is reasonably safe in patients with Child's A cirrhosis with no portal hypertension where a segmental or subsegmental resection are required. Careful attention must be paid to the amount of cirrhotic liver resected. While, there are no fool-proof methods for calculating the requisite functional hepatocyte mass in every cirrhotic patient, some approaches have been reliable and reproducible (100). In some cases non-resectable lesions can be made resectable (101) using preoperative portal vein embolization.

HCC patients with no evidence of extrahepatic disease that are not resection candidates, should be considered for transplantation. Unfortunately, the supply of cadaveric organs falls short of the demand, and these patients must go on a waiting list for a liver transplant. Currently, priority on the waiting list is determined by waiting time and medical urgency. Typically, cirrhotics with HCC are not sick enough from their liver disease to qualify for the highest priority categories, and they can wait over a year for an available liver. To control the growth and spread of the tumor while waiting, preoperative tumor ablative strategies such as transarterial chemoembolization (TACE), ethanol injection, microwave ablation, and resection are typically incorporated into the overall treatment regimen. Other strategies which can potentially decrease a given patient's waiting time include the use of Hepatitis B or C positive donors, respectively, in Hepatitis B or C recipients, and the use of split livers. Finally, the use of right or left lobar segments from living donors may provide another important source of livers for patients with HCC (102).

FIBROLAMELLAR HCC (FLHCC)

Fibrolamellar variant of HCC (FLHCC) usually occurs in a non-cirrhotic liver, has a peak incidence in young adults, and the prognosis after OLT appears to be more favorable than for non-fibrolamellar HCC. It is a slower growing tumor, with metastases appearing later in its clinical course. However, as with other tumors arising in a non-cirrhotic liver, the early natural history of FLHCC is usually silent, most patients only presenting when the tumor is of substantial size. Late presentation is almost certainly the major factor underlying the high rates of tumor recurrence.

In a series of FLHCC treated by liver resection or transplantation (103) eight patients underwent a radical subtotal hepatic resection. Seven had clear surgical resection margins, and none of these suffered recurrent disease. The eighth case developed recurrent intra-abdominal deposits within 8 months, which were removed at laparotomy 3.5 years after the original resection. Six other patients in this series had, tumors which were considered unresectable, and were treated by transplantation, of these, cases with tumor invasion into adjacent organs at the time of OLT resulted in recurrence, whereas in patients without invasive disease no recurrence has occurred.

A multicenter review in 1991 (9) identified only 33 patients who had received a liver graft for FLHCC. Of these, 13 (39%) developed recurrent disease, of which 10 had died. Sixteen (48 %) survived 2 years, and 10 of these had remained tumor-free. The actuarial survival was 60% at 2 years and 55% at 5 years, and an overall rate of tumor recurrence of 39%. Other reports show similar recurrence rates of between 38% and 83%, actuarial survival figures of 80 to 100% (1 year), 60 to 70% (2 years), 46 to 57% (3 years), and 33 to 57% (5 years).

Despite high rates of tumor recurrence in patients with advanced disease, survival after OLT for FLHCC compares favorably with cases of non-fibrolamellar HCC. Tumor recurrence after transplantation for FLHCC seems to occur later compared with other types of primary hepatic malignancies. The fibrolamellar variant of HCC has been shown to be an independent factor of favorable prognosis, tumor recurrence being 16 times less likely than in cases with non-fibrolamellar HCC (6,72).

CHOLANGIOCARCINOMA

Cholangiocarcinoma is a neoplasm of the bile duct epithelium and is divided into two types: peripheral (intrahepatic) and extrahepatic (major hepatic ducts or common bile duct) (26,104). Hilar cholangiocarcinoma is also known as the Klatskin tumor. These tumors usually are mucin-secreting adenocarcinomas and are difficult to distinguish from metastatic adenocarcinomas even with a panel of immunohistochemical stains (105,106). Cholangiocarcinomas are frequently multicentric, indolent, and locally invasive. Extrahepatic metastases occur more frequently with peripheral cholangiocarcinomas (80%) than with the hilar type (40%) (104). Etiological factors include clonorchiasis, ulcerative colitis, sclerosing cholangitis, fibrocystic diseases, and anabolic steroids. Surgical resection for hilar or peripheral cholangiocarcinoma has yielded an average survival of 18 to 24 months, however many patients present with unresectable disease (27,82,107,108).

The diagnosis of cholangiocarcinoma in the context of primary sclerosing cholangitis (PSC) is notoriously difficult. In a series of 126 cases of PSC (109) cholangiocarcinoma was present in 6 (23%) of 26 cases who had a liver transplant. The tumor was diagnosed or suspected before OLT in four, but was an incidental finding in two. These two cases remained tumor free and are now still alive and free of tumor at 5 years 7 months and 6 years post-transplant. These cases emphasize the need for regular screening in PSC and aggressive efforts by cytology or histology to diagnose the tumors at an early stage.

Early reports have suggested that OLT is not curative for cholangiocarcinoma (70,110-112). More recently, improved survival has been noted, but overall the results are discouraging. One large series found that OLT for cholangiocarcinoma resulted in 44% recurrence and 39% mortality from recurrent disease alone. These recurrences occurred within 12 months of OLT in 52%, and within 2 years in 70%.

Survival was 30% at 2 years and 17% at 5 years (9). No difference was found between peripheral and Klatskin lesions.

Another study (5) reports a 3-month survival after OLT of only 54% (14 cases) among 26 cases with either peripheral or central cholangiocarcinoma. Tumor recurrence occurred at a median time of 56 weeks after transplantation. Of the seven with hilar lesions, six died of recurrent disease within a year (median survival 34 weeks).

Another report (71) describes 19 cases of hilar cholangiocarcinoma, and two peripheral cholangiocarcinomas treated by OLT. One of the two patients with peripheral cholangiocarcinoma had recurrence at 20 months. Of the 19 hilar lesions, 17 survived the operation and 11 (65%) developed recurrent disease. Recurrence was diagnosed within 12 months in 10 of the 11.

Accurate preoperative tumor staging is of paramount importance if the results of OLT for cholangiocarcinoma are to be improved upon. Many centers now undertake lymph node sampling either at a separate celiotomy or as a frozen section procedure on the day of transplantation with a back-up case available. When lymph node status (cases with central tumors) is considered, striking differences in survival have been observed, with over 80% survival at 2 years for the patients free of nodal metastasis, contrasting with less than 20% survival for the same periods in those with positive nodes (3).

OTHER PRIMARY HEPATIC NEOPLASMS

Hepatoblastoma: This tumor is the most common malignant primary liver tumor in children under 5 years. Transplantation may play a role in patients with unresectable lesions that show some response to aggressive chemotherapy. Favorable prognostic factors include the presence of fetal epithelium in the tumors, absence of vascular invasion, and absence of extrahepatic extension. A report of 18 cases of OLT for hepatoblastoma demonstrated recurrent tumor in 6 (33%) (9). Recurrence was early, on average 6 months after OLT, and all presented within 18 months. Four of the six died. There were five 2-year survivors who are apparently tumor-free, after periods of follow-up of 25 to 116 months. The actuarial tumor-free survival figure was 50% at 2 and 5 years. Encouraging results have been obtained even following resection of pulmonary lesions.

Epithelioid Hemangioendothelioma (EHE): This rare malignant tumor of endothelial origin that may arise in the liver usually in the absence of pre-existing cirrhosis. The natural history seems to be variable, and an association with oral contraceptive use has been reported (113). Some patients have a lengthy clinical course, while in others, tumor growth rapidly progresses to death within a few months from hepatic failure. The diagnosis is usually made by liver biopsy. The microscopic appearance may suggest other primary liver or metastatic tumors, but the presence of positive immunohistochemical staining for factor VIII-related antigen confirms the diagnosis. Morphological appearance does not correlate well with biological behavior and, therefore, the prognosis is unpredictable. Tumors are commonly multiple, bilobar, subtotal resection is usually not an option, and chemotherapy is also usually ineffective (114). Interestingly, extrahepatic tumor is not a contraindication to OLT and does not correlate with survival (2,115,116). A series of 21 patients transplanted for this malignancy (9) demonstrates recurrent disease in 7 (33%) during a mean follow-up period of 43 months. The actuarial survival was 82% at 2 years and 43% at 5 years, most of the deaths due to recurrence. Recurrence occurred predominantly in patients with extrahepatic extension of disease at the time of OLT.

Sarcoma and Hemangiosarcoma: Hepatic angiosarcoma, a very rare malignant neoplasm, may be induced by exposure to vinyl chloride, thorotrast, arsenic and radium, and only a small number of patients have been treated by OLT. World wide, 14 cases are reported where 9 (64%) developed recurrent cancer and died. Only two patients survived longer than 2 years, both succumbing to metastatic disease at or before 28 months (9).

METASTATIC HEPATIC NEOPLASMS

Liver transplantation has been criticized as therapy for metastatic tumors due to two predominant adverse sequelae: imminent tumor recurrence and the finding that malignant tumor growth is accelerated following immunosuppression (117). Early surgical mortality and recurrence-related mortality is common in reported series.

In a series of 42 recipients undergoing OLT for metastatic malignancy (118), 22 patients had neuroendocrine tumors including carcinoid (5), gastrinoma (3), glucagonoma (2), insulinoma (1), vipoma (1), somatostatinoma (1), and indeterminate (9). Twelve patients had metastatic adenocarcinoma. The remaining patients had malignant stromal tumor (7) and metastatic ocular melanoma (1). The alimentary tract contained the majority of primary lesions (intestine and pancreas, 17 and 16 patients, respectively). The patients were assessed by standard radiologic and endoscopic modalities to define the primary site and tumor extent, and patients with distant metastases were excluded from transplantation. Surgical procedures ranged from total hepatectomy and OLT to aggressive approaches such as upper abdominal exenteration followed by en bloc transplantation of the liver, pancreas, and adjacent gastrointestinal tract (organ cluster transplantation). Early mortality was high (23.8%). The 1-year survival rate was 59.5%, diminishing to 24.2% at five years. Survival rates of patients with neuroendocrine tumor appeared improved compared to patients with gastrointestinal stromal tumor or adenocarcinoma. Tumor recurrence within 1 year was followed by death within 2 years of the transplantation procedure and was the cause of late mortality in all groups.

Occasionally, OLT performed for neuroendocrine metastasis provides excellent relief of symptoms. In one report comprising four cases (2 carcinoid, 1 pancreatic apudoma, and 1 primary liver neuroendocrine-type tumor) peptide hormone levels fell to within the normal range following OLT (119). Two patients (primary apudoma and carcinoid syndrome) remained alive at 38 and 22 months after OLT, respectively. The other two cases remained free of symptoms but died of chronic graft rejection prior to 1-year post-OLT. Follow-up of the two survivors reveals that the patient with apudoma was alive over 8 years, but the other case had recurrent carcinoid symptoms and died from metastasis-related intestinal obstruction at 4 years 7 months post-OLT. Another series (120) described five patients who had OLT for neuroendocrine tumors (carcinoid, glucagonoma, and gastrinoma). The patients with carcinoid died at 2 and 9 months from graft rejection and recurrence of a coexistent incidentally found cholangiocarcinoma, respectively. Two of the patients had their primary pancreatic lesion removed at the time of OLT and remained alive with no evidence of residual disease at 7 and 16 months. The fifth case was alive and symptom free at 34 months, but with a marginally elevated glucagon level. *En bloc* resections of liver, pancreas, distal stomach and duodenum with transplantation of liver, pancreas and duodenum has also been described (121).

The results of transplantation for non-neuroendocrine liver metastases have been extremely poor due to rapid tumor recurrence and death secondary to carcinomatosis. For example, in one series (5), tumor recurrence resulted in death between 22 and 41 weeks following OLT. These cases included carcinoma of the colon and pancreas, leiomyosarcoma of the small intestine, meningiosarcoma and nephroma. The largest review of OLT for hepatic metastasis reported similar results (9). In this report, 41 cases included carcinoma of the colon (10), malignant carcinoid (9), intestinal leiomyosarcoma (5), mammary carcinoma (3), gastrinoma (2), glucagonoma (2), and a case of meningioma, neuroblastoma, renal cell carcinoma, pancreatic cystosarcoma, hemangioperisarcoma, seminoma, vipoma, melanoma, acute myeloid leukemia, and one unknown primary tumour. Twenty-four (59%) patients had developed recurrent disease. Specific recurrence rates were as follows: carcinoma of the colon (70%), carcinoid (67%), mammary carcinoma (100%), and leiomyosarcoma (40%). Only eight cases survived longer than 2 years. The actuarial survival for the whole group was 38% at 2 years and 21% at 5 years, most of the deaths in the intervening 3 years were due to tumor recurrence.

Metastatic malignancy is considered a systemic disease. In this situation, even aggressive surgical extirpation of tumor-bearing organs or regions alone is not curative. In practice, however, one-third of patients with hepatic metastasis from colorectal cancer survive more than 5 years after hepatic resection. Hepatic resection is still considered the treatment of choice for metastatic tumors of the liver.

CONCLUSION

Because of the shortage of donor organs, liver transplantation cannot be justified in the vast majority of patients with advanced malignancy of the liver. However, we cannot conclude that patients with malignant hepatic tumors are to be excluded entirely from liver transplantation. In order to ensure satisfactory outcomes following OLT for hepatic malignancy, several maxims need to be applied. A specific diagnostic approach to these malignancies needs to be utilized, including histologic diagnosis, thorough radiologic assessment. This will identify the important prognostic indicators in the process of selecting patients for OLT such as tumor size, morphology, stage and the presence of vascular invasion. Combined modality treatment, including adjuvant chemotherapy and/or TACE, may improve those lesions which are associated with poorer outcomes.

Continuing efforts to treat specific patients with hepatic tumors with transplantation may be justified. Rational criteria for patient selection promoting acceptable results require an individual approach to patients, and the general assumption that in most cases adjuvant therapy may play a essential role in decreasing the incidence of recurrence.

REFERENCES

1. Starzl TE, Demetris AJ, Van Thiel D. Liver transplantation. *N Engl J Med* 321:1014-1022, 1092-1099, 1989.
2. Klintmalm GB, Stone MJ. Liver transplantation for malignancy. *Transplant Rev* 4:52-8, 1990.
3. Pichlmayr R. Is there a place for liver grafting for malignancy? *Transplant Proc* 20(suppl) 1):478-82, 1988.
4. Olthoff KM, Millis JM, Rosove MH, et al. Is liver transplantation justified for the treatment of hepatic malignancies? *Arch Surg* 125:1261-8, 1990
5. O'Grady JG, Polson RJ, Rolles K, et al. Liver transplantation for malignant disease. *Ann Surg* 207:373-9, 1988
6. Iwatsuki S, Gordon RD, Shaw BW Jr, Starzl TE. Role of liver transplantation in cancer therapy. *Ann Surg* 202:401-7, 1985
7. Pichlmayr R, Ringe B, Bechstein WO, et al. Approach to primary liver cancer. *Recent Results Cancer Research* 110:65-73, 1988
8. Ringe B, Wittekind C, Bechstein, WO, et al. The role of liver transplantation in hepatobiliary malignancy. *Ann Surg* 209:88-98, 1989
9. Penn I. Hepatic transplantation for primary and metastatic cancers of the liver. *Surgery* 110:726-35, 1991
10. Carr BI, Kar S. An assay for hepatoma micrometastases: albumin gene expression in peripheral blood from patients with advanced hepatocellular carcinoma (HCC) (abstr). *Hepatology* 14:108A, 1991
11. Neuhaus P, Broelsch CE, Ringe B, Pichlmayr R. Liver transplantation for liver tumors. *Recent Results Cancer Research*. 100:221-8, 1986.

12. Koneru B, Cassaville A, Bowman J, et al. Liver transplantation for malignant tumors. *Gastroenterology Clin North Amer* 17:177-93, 1988.
13. Jenkins RL, Pinson CW, Stone MD. Experience with transplantation in the treatment of liver cancer. *Cancer Chemother Pharmacol* 23(Suppl):S104-9, 1989.
14. Pichlmayr R. Indications for liver grafting in hepatic tumors. In Bannasch P, Keppler D, Weber G, eds. Liver Cell Carcinoma. Boston, Kluwer Academic, 1989, pp 491-7.
15. Flye MW, McCullough CS. Liver transplantation for malignant disease. *Principles Pract Oncol* 3:1-12,1989.
16. Yokoyama I, Todo S, Iwatsuki S, Starzl TE. Liver transplantation in the treatment of primary liver cancer. *Hepatogastroenterology* 37:188-93, 1990.
17. Ismail T, Angrisani I, Gunson B, et al, Primary hepatic malignancy: the role of liver transplantation. *Br J Surg* 77:983-7, 1990.
18. Ringe B, Pichlmayr R, Wittekind C, Tusch G. Surgical treatment of hepatocellular carcinoma: experience with liver resection and transplantation in 198 patients. *World J Surg* 15:270-85, 1991.
19. Iwatsuki S, Starzl TE, Sheahan DG, et al. Hepatic resection versus transplantation for hepatocellular carcinoma. *Ann Surg* 214:221-9, 1991.
20. Stevens L, Piper J, Emond J, et al. Liver transplantation for controversial indications: alcoholic liver disease, hepatic cancers, and viral hepatitis. *Transplant Proc* 23:1915-6, 1991.
21. Van Thiel DH, Carr B, Iwatsuki S, et al. Liver transplantation for alcoholic liver disease, viral hepatitis, and hepatic neoplasms. *Transplant Proc* 23:1917-21, 1991.
22. Van Thiel DH, Carr BI, Yokoyama I, et al. Liver transplantation as a treatment of hepatocellular carcinoma. In Tabor E, Di Bisceglie AM, Purcell RH, eds. Etiology, Pathology, and Treatment of Hepatocellular Carcinoma in North America. Houston, TX, Gulf, 1991, pp 309-15.
23. Haug CE, Jenkins RL, Rohrer RJ, et al. Liver transplantation for primary hepatic cancer. *Transplantation* 53:376-82, 1992.
24. Ellis LM, Demers MI, Roh MS. Current strategies for the treatment of hepatocellular carcinoma. *Curr Opin Oncol* 4:741-51, 1992.
25. Stone MJ, Klintmalm G, Polter D, et al. Neoadjuvant chemotherapy and orthotopic liver transplantation for hepatocellular carcinoma. *Transplantation* 48:344-7, 1989.
26. Stone MI, Klintmalm GBG, Polter D, et al. Neoadjuvant chemotherapy and liver transplantation for hepatocellular carcinoma: a pilot study in 20 patients. *Gastroenterology* 104:196-202, 1993.
27. Ahlgren JD. Neoplasms of the hepatobiliary system. In Calbresi P, Schein PS, eds. Medical Oncology. New York, McGraw-Hill, 1993, pp 713-39.
28. Craig JR, Peters RI, Edmondson HA. Tumors of the Liver and Intrahepatic Bile Ducts. Washington, DC: Armed Forces Institute of Pathology, 1989.
29. El-Serag HB, Mason AC. Rising incidence of hepatocellular carcinoma in the United States. *N Engl J Med* 340:745-50, 1999.

30. Goodman ZD, Ishak KG, Langloss JM, et al. Combined hepatocellular-cholangiocarcinoma. *Cancer* 55:124-35, 1985.
31. McPeake J, and Williams R. Liver transplantation for malignancy: the current position. In Terblanche J, ed. Hepatobiliary Malignancy, It's Multidisciplinary Management, Edward Arnold, London, 1994, pp 595-618.
32. Takayasu K, Moriyama N, Muramatsu Y, et al. The diagnosis of small hepatocellular carcinomas: efficacy of various imaging procedures in 100 patients. *Am J Roentgenol* 155: 49-54, 1990.
33. Dodd GD, Miller WJ, Baron RL, Skolnick ML, Campbell WL. Detection of malignant tumours in end-stage cirrhotic livers: efficacy of sonography as a screening technique. *Am J Roentgenol* 159: 727-33, 1992.
34. Miller WJ, Federle MP, Campbell WL. Diagnosis and staging of hepatocellular carcinoma: comparison of CT and sonography in 36 liver transplantation patients. *Amer J Roentgenol* 157:303-6, 1991.
35. Parker GA, Lawrence W, Horsley S, et al. Intraoperative ultrasound of the liver affects operative decision making. *Ann Surg* 209:569-77, 1989.
36. Kudo M. Imaging Diagnosis of Hepatocellular Carcinoma. *Seminars in Liver Disease* 19;297-310, 1999.
37. Tsunetomi S, Ohto M, Iino Y, et al. Diagnosis of small hepatocellular carcinoma by computed tomography: correlation of CT findings and histopathology. *J Gastroenterol Hepatol* 4:395-404, 1989.
38. Sitzmann JV, Coleman J, Pitt HA, et al. Preoperative assessment of malignant hepatic tumors. *Am Surg* 159:137-43, 1990.
39. Rummeny E, Weissleder R, Stark DD, et al. Primary liver tumors: diagnosis by MR imaging. *Am J Roentgenol* 159:137-43, 1989.
40. Muramatsu Y, Nawano S, Takayasu K, et al. Early hepatocellular carcinoma: MR imaging. *Radiology* 181:209-13, 1991.
41. Cohen MB, Haber MM, Holly EA, et al. Cytologic criteria to distinguish hepatocellular carcinoma from normoplastic liver. *Am J Clin Pathol* 95:125-30, 1991.
42. Beahrs OH, Henson DE, Hutter RVP, Kennedy W, eds. Manual for Staging of Cancer. Philadelphia, JB Lippincott, 1992, pp 89-91.
43. Foster JH. Evaluation of asymptomatic solitary hepatic lesions. *Ann Rev Med* 39:85-93, 1988.
44. Rummeny E, Weissleder IT, Stark DD, et al. Primary liver tumors: diagnosis by MR imaging. *Am J Roentgenol* 152:63-72, 1989.
45. Ferrucci JT. Liver tumor imaging. *Cancer* 67:1189-95, 1991.
46. Miller WJ, Federle MP, Campbell WL. Diagnosis and staging of hepatocellular carcinoma: comparison of CT and sonography in 36 liver transplantation patients. *Am J Roentgenol* 157:303-6, 1991
47. Johnson CD. Magnetic resonance imaging of the liver. current clinical applications. *Mayo Clin Proc* 68:147-56, 1993.
48. Edelman RR, Warach S. Magnetic resonance imaging. *N Engl J Med* 328:708-16, 785-91, 1993.

49. Calne RY, Williams R, Rolles K. Liver transplantation in the adult. *World J Surg* 10: 422-31, 1986.
50. Krom RA, Gips CH, Houthoff HJ, et al. Orthotopic liver transplantation in Groningen, The Netherlands (1979-1983). *Hepatology* 4(suppl):61S-65S, 1984.
51. Di Bisceglie AM, Rustgi VY, Hoofnagle JH, et al. Hepatocellular carcinoma. *Ann Intern Med* 108:390-401, 1988.
52. Ahlgren JD, Wanebo HJ, Hill MC. Hepatocellular carcinoma. In Ahlgren JD, Macdonald JS, eds. Gastrointestinal Oncology. Philadelphia, JB Lippincott, 1992, pp 417-36.
53. Nerenstone SR, Ihde DC, Friedman MA. Clinical trials in primary hepatocellular carcinoma: current status and future directions. *Cancer Treat Rev* 15:1-31, 1988.
54. Falkson G, Cnaan A, Schutt AJ, et al. Prognostic factors for survival in hepatocellular carcinoma. *Cancer Res* 48:7314-8, 1988.
55. Falkson G. Treatment for patients with hepatocellular carcinoma: state-of-the-art. *Ann Oncol* 3:336-7, 1992.
56. Taketa K. α-fetoprotein: reevaluation in hepatology. *Hepatology* 12:1420-32, 1990.
57. Epstein B, Ettinger D, Leichner P, Order SE. Multimodality cisplatin treatment in nonresectable alpha-fetoprotein-positive hepatoma. *Cancer* 67:896-900, 1991.
58. Beasley RP. Hepatitis B virus. *Cancer* 61:1942-56, 1988.
59. Wands JR, Blum HE. Primary hepatocellular carcinoma. *N Engl J Med* 325:729-31, 1991.
60. de Franchis IT, Meucci G, Vecchi M, et al. The natural history of asymptomatic hepatitis B surface antigen carriers. *Ann Intem Med* 118:191-4, 1993.
61. Simonetti RG, Cammi C, Fiorello F, et al. Hepatitis C virus infection as a risk factor for hepatocellular carcinoma in patients with cirrhosis. *Ann Intern Med* 116:97-103, 1992.
62. Tabor E, Kobayashi K. Hepatitis C virus, a causative infectious agent of non-A, non-B hepatitis: prevalence and structure-Summary of a conference on hepatitis C virus as a cause of hepatocellular carcinoma. *J Natl Cancer Inst* 84:86-90, 1992.
63. Tsukama H, Hiyama T, Tanaka S, et al. Risk factors for hepatocellular carcinoma among patients with chronic liver disease. *N Engl J Med* 328:1797-1801, 1993.
64. Wogan GN. Aflatoxins as risk factors for hepatocellular carcinoma in humans. *Cancer Res* 52(Suppl):2114-8S, 1992.
65. Deugnier YK Guyader D, Crantock L, et al. Primary liver cancer in genetic hemochromatosis: A clinical, pathological, and pathogenetic study of 54 cases. *Gastroenterology* 104:228-34, 1993.
66. Iwatsuki S, Starzl TE. Personal experience with 411 hepatic resections. *Ann Surg* 208:421-434, 1988.

67. Theise ND, Schwartz M, Miller C, Thung SN. Macroregenerative nodules and hepatocellular carcinoma in forty-four sequential adult liver explants with cirrhosis. *Hepatology* 16:949-55, 1993.

68. Olthoff KM, Millis JM, Rosove MH, Goldstein LI, Ramming KP, Busuttil RW. Is liver transplantation justified for the treatment of hepatic malignancies? *Arch Surg* 125:1261-6, 1990.

69. Ringe B, Wittekind C, Bechstein WO, Bunzendahl H, Pichlmayr R. The role of liver transplantation in hepatobiliary malignancy. A retrospective analysis of 95 patients with particular regard to tumor stage and recurrence. *Ann Surg* 209:88-98, 1989.

70. Iwatsuki S, Gordon RD, Shaw BJ, Starzl TE. Role of liver transplantation in cancer therapy. *Ann Surg* 202:401-7, 1985.

71. Yokoyama I, Todo S, Iwatsuki S, Starzl TE. Liver transplantation in the treatment of primary liver cancer. *Hepatogastroenterology* 37:188-93, 1990.

72. Yokoyama I, Sheahan DG, Carr B, et al. Clinicopathologic factors affecting patient survival and tumor recurrence after orthotopic liver transplantation for hepatocellular carcinoma. *Transplant Proc* 23:2194-6, 1991.

73. McPeake JR, O'Grady JG, Zaman S, et al. Liver transplantation for primary hepatocellular carcinoma: tumor size and number determines outcome. *J Hepatol* 18:226-34, 1993.

74. Pichlmayr R, Ringe B, Wittekind C, et al. Liver grafting for malignant liver tumors. *Transplant Proc* 21:2403-5, 1989.

75. Hermanek P, Sobin LH. *TNM Classification of Malignant Tumors.* 4th ed. Berlin: Springer-Verlag, 1987.

76. Stone MJ, Klintmalm GBG, Polter D, et al. Neoadjuvant chemotherapy and liver transplantation for hepatocellular carcinoma: a pilot study in 20 patients. *Gastroenterology* 104:196-202, 1993.

77. Bismuth H, Morino M, Sherlock D, et al. Primary treatment of hepatocellular carcinoma by arterial chemoembolization. *Am J Surg* 63:387-94, 1992.

78. Bismuth H, Chiche L, Adam R, Castaing D. Surgical treatment of hepatocellular carcinoma in cirrhosis: liver resection or transplantation? *Transplant Proc* 25:1066-7, 1993.

79. Friedman MA. Chemotherapy for patients with hepatocellular carcinoma: Prospects and possibilities. In Tabor E, Di Bisceglie AM, Purcell RH, eds. Etiology, Pathology, and Treatment of Hepatocellular Carcinoma in North America. Houston, TX, Gulf, 1991, pp, 287-292.

80. Steinherz U, Steinherz PG. Delayed anthracycline cardiac toxicity. *Principles Pract Oncol* 5:1-15, 1991.

81. Chemotherapy and hepatitis B (editorial). *Lancet* 2:1136-7, 1989.

82. Vogt DP. Current management of cholangiocarcinoma. *Oncology* 2:37-43, 1988.

83. Kanematsu T, Furuta T, Takenaka K, et al. A 5-year experience of lipiodolization: Selective regional chemotherapy for 200 patients with hepatocellular carcinoma. *Hepatology* 10:98-102, 1989.

84. Venook AP, Stagg RJ, Lewis BJ, et al. Chemoembolization for hepatocellular carcinoma. *J Clin Oncol* 8:1108-14, 1990.

85. Yamashita Y, Takahashi M, Koga Y, et al. Prognostic factors in the treatment of hepatocellular carcinoma with transcatheter arterial embolization and arterial infusion. *Cancer* 67:385-91, 1991.

86. Raoul JI, Bretagne JF, Caucanas JP, et al. Internal radiation therapy for hepatocellular carcinoma. *Cancer* 69:346-52, 1992.

87. Yu Y, Xu D, Zhou X, et al. Experience with liver resection after hepatic arterial chemoembolization for hepatocellular carcinoma. *Cancer* 71:62-5, 1993.

88. Kanematsu T, Matsumata T, Shirabe K, et al. A comparative study of hepatic resection and transcatheter arterial embolization for the treatment of primary hepatocellular carcinoma. *Cancer* 71:2181-6, 1993.

89. Livraghi T, Bolondi L, Lazzaroni S, et al. Percutaneous ethanol injection in the treatment of hepatocellular carcinoma in cirrhosis. *Cancer* 69:925-9, 1992.

90. Tanaka K, Nakamura S, Numata. K, et al. Hepatocellular carcinoma: treatment with percutaneous ethanol injection and transcatheter arterial embolization. *Radiology* 185:457-60, 1992.

91. Shiina S, Tagawa K, Niwa Y, et al. Percutaneous ethanol injection therapy for hepatocellular carcinoma: Results in 146 patients. *Am J Roentgenol* 160:1023-8, 1993.

92. Lai CI, Lau JYN, Wu PC, et al. Recombinant interferon-alpha in inoperable hepatocellular carcinoma: a randomized controlled trial. *Hepatology* 17:389-94, 1993.

93. Farinati F, Salvagnini M, de Maria N, et al. Unresectable hepatocellular carcinoma: a prospective controlled trial with tamoxifen. *J Hepatol* 11:297-301, 1990.

94. Carlson RI, Ben-Porath E, Shouval D, et al. Antigenic characterization of human hepatocellular carcinoma. *J Clin Invest* 76:40-51, 1985.

95. Takahashi H, Ozturk M, Vilson B, et al. In vivo expression of two novel tumor-associated antigens and their use in immunolocalization of human hepatocellular carcinoma. *Hepatology* 9:625-34, 1989.

96. Keegan-Rogers V, Wu GY. Immunotargeting in the diagnosis and treatment of liver cancer. *Hepatology* 9:646-8, 1989.

97. Bismuth H, Chiche L, Adam R, et al. Liver resection versus transplantation for hepatocellular carcinoma in cirrhotic patients. *Ann Surg* 218:145-51, 1993.

98. Mazzaferro V, Regalia E, Doci R, et al. Liver transplantation for the treatment of small hepatocellular carcinomas in patients with cirrhosis. *N Engl J Med* 334:693-9, 1996.

99. Llovet JM, Fuster J, Bruix J. Intention-to-treat analysis of surgical treatment for early hepatocellular carcinoma: resection versus transplantation. *Hepatology* 30:1434-40, 1999.

100. Kanematsu T, Takenaka K, Furuta T, et al. Acute portal hypertension associated with liver resection. Analysis of early postoperative death. *Arch Surg* 120:1303-5, 1985.

101. Elias D, Debaere T, Roche A, et al. Preoperative selective portal vein embolizations are an effective means of extending the indications of major hepatectomy in the normal and injured liver. *Hepatogastroenterology* 45:170-7, 1998.
102. Marcos A, Ham JM, Fisher RN, et al. Single-center analysis of the first 40 adult-to-adult living donor liver transplants using the right lobe. *Liver Transpl* 6:296-301, 2000.
103. Starzl TE, Iwatsuki S, Shaw BJ, Nalesnik MA, Farhi DC, Van Thiel D. Treatment of fibrolamellar hepatoma with partial or total hepatectomy and transplantation of the liver. *Surg Gynecol Obstet* 162:145-8, 1986.
104. Nakajima T, Kondo Y, Miyazald M, Okui K. A histopathologic study of 102 cases of intrahepatic cholangiocarcinoma. *Hum Pathol* 19:1228-34, 1988.
105. Ma CK, Zarbo RJ, Frierson HF, Lee MW. Comparative immunohistochemical study of primary and metastatic carcinomas of the liver. *Am J Clin Pathol* 99:551-7, 1993.
106. Swanson PE. Diagnostic immunohistochemistry. *Am J M Pathol* 99:530-2, 1993.
107. Wanebo HJ, AhIgren JD, Macdonald JS, eds. Gastrointestinal Oncology. Philadelphia, JB Lippincott 1992, pp399-416
108. Chen MF, Jan YY, Wang CS, et al. Clinical experience in 20 hepatic resections for peripheral cholangiocarcinoma. *Cancer* 64:2226-32, 1989.
109. Farrant JM, Hayllar KM, Wilkinson ML, et al Natural history and prognostic variables in primary sclerosing cholangitis. *Gastroenterology* 100:1710-7, 1991.
110. Calne RY. Liver transplantation for liver cancer. *World J Surg* 10:76-80, 1986.
111. Iwatsuki S, Klintmalm GBG, StarzI TE. Total hepatectomy and liver replacement (orthotopic liver transplantation) for primary hepatic malignancy. *World J Surg* 6:81-5, 1982.
112. Neuhaus P, Proelsch C, Ringe B, Pichlmayr R. Liver transplantation for liver tumors. In: Herfarth C, Schlag P, Hohenberger P, eds. *Therapeutic Strategy in Primary and Metastatic Liver Cancer.* New York: Springer Verlag, 1986:221-8.
113. Weiss JW, Enzinger FM. Epithelioid haemangioendothelioma: a vascular tumor often mistaken for a carcinoma. *Cancer* 50:970-81, 1982.
114. Forbes A, Portmann B, Johnson P, Williams R. Hepatic sarcomas in adults: a review of 25 cases. *Gut* 28:668-74, 1987.
115. Marino IR, Todo S, Tzakis AG, et al. Treatment of hepatic epithelioid hemangioendothelioma with liver transplantation. *Cancer* 62:2079-84, 1988.
116. Kelleher MB, Iwatsuld S, Sheahan DG. Epithelioid hemangioendothelioma of liver. *Am J Surg Pathol* 13:999-1008, 1989.
117. Yokoyama I, Carr B, Saitsu HL, et al. Accelerated growth rates of recurrent hepatocellular carcinoma after liver transplantation. *Cancer* 68:2095-2100, 1991.
118. Busuttil R, Klintmalm G, eds. *Transplantation of the Liver,* Philadelphia, WB Saunders 1996, pp130-133

119. Arnold JC, O'Grady JG, Bird GL, Caine RY, Williams R. Liver transplantation for primary and secondary hepatic apudomas. *Br J Surg* 76:248-9, 1989.
120. Makowka L, Tzakis AG, Mazzaferro V, et al. Transplantation of the liver for metastatic endocrine tumors of the intestine and pancreas. *Surg Gynecol Obstet* 168:107-11, 1989.
121. Lobe TE, Vera SR, Bowman LC, Fontanesi J, Britt, LG, Gaber AO. Hepaticopancreaticogastroduodenectomy with transplantation for metastatic islet cell carcinoma in childhood. *J Pediatr Surg* 27:227-9, 1992.

6

CHEMOEMBOLIZATION AND INTERSTITIAL THERAPIES FOR HEPATOCELLULAR CARCINOMA

D. Michael Rose, M.D.
John Wayne Cancer Institute, Santa Monica, CA
William C. Chapman, M.D.
Vanderbilt University Medical Center, Nashville, TN

INTRODUCTION

Hepatocellular carcinoma (HCC) remains one of the most common malignancies worldwide, causing approximately 1,250,000 deaths annually (1). In the United States, HCC accounts for 1% of all new cancer diagnoses and 2% of all cancer deaths (2). According to data collected by the Surveillance, Epidemiology, and End Results (SEER) Program of the National Cancer Institute, HCC survival rates in this country are dismal with an overall five-year survival of 3%. Patients with localized disease had an 8% five-year survival compared to <2% in patients with either regional or distant disease (2). Surgical resection is the preferred treatment for HCC; unfortunately, only 20% of all patients with HCC are suitable candidates for resection (3,4). Of those who undergo resection, approximately 30-70% will have a hepatic recurrence (3-5). With the preponderance of patients not eligible for surgical intervention, multiple alternative approaches have been developed including hepatic-directed therapies (transcatheter arterial chemoembolization, hepatic artery ligation) and local tumor ablation (percutaneous ethanol injection, cryosurgical ablation, interstitial laser photocoagulation, microwave tumor coagulation, radiofrequency ablation). This chapter will examine the rationale and results with two of these modalities: transcatheter chemoembolization and percutaneous ethanol injection.

TRANSCATHETER ARTERIAL CHEMOEMBOLIZATION

Transcatheter arterial chemoembolization (TACE) is a hepatic-directed therapy that takes advantage of relatively selective hepatic arterial tumor vascularization. HCC's derive approximately 80-85% of their blood supply from the hepatic artery. Normal hepatic parenchyma is supplied primarily by the portal vein as well as the hepatic artery (1,3,6). Chemotherapeutic agents can be delivered angiographically with concomitant embolization to theoretically increase local chemotherapeutic dwell time and induce tumor ischemia. Multiple regimens have been applied with TACE; however, the majority of which have utilized doxirubicin, cisplatin or a combination of these agents. Embolization is generally achieved through the use of gelatin foam particles or powder. Some investigators have recommended gelatin foam because its degradation occurs in several weeks allowing repeated TACE treatments that may improve prognostic outcomes (3).

Lipiodol is an ethyl ester of the fatty acid of poppyseed oil containing 38% iodine (1). This agent concentrates in neoplastic tissue within the liver, possibly due to abnormal tumor vasculature or lymphatic drainage. The exact mechanism for this deposition is unclear. Lipiodol may increase contact time of chemotherapeutic agents due to its selective deposition and may also cause selective micro-embolization of the tumor (3,6). Multiple TACE techniques have been reported throughout the literature with variable sequences of partial versus complete embolization. The procedure at Vanderbilt University Medical Center consists of a standardized approach by an experienced group of interventional radiologists. Arterial access is achieved via a femoral or brachial approach and hepatic arteriography is performed. A suspension of doxirubicin, lipiodol and gelatin foam particles is produced and selective left or right hepatic artery chemoembolization is performed. Selective lobar chemoembolization is performed at two separate TACE sessions with a third study to confirm, and if required, complete embolization.

Reported Series

The critical analysis of TACE has been hampered by a lack of randomized, prospective data. Median survivals, subgroups and statistical analysis of the predominate Western series is presented in Table 1, divided according to type of study design. Of note, the two reported prospective randomized trials failed to show a significant improvement in overall survival (7,8). However, both of these studies were multi-center collaborations with relatively few patients in each arm. Pelletier et al reported a decreased median survival of 4 months in 21 patients receiving TACE compared to a 6 month median survival in patients receiving supportive care only (7). This is the only study in the Western literature that reports a decreased survival with the utilization of TACE for patients with HCC. The Group d'Etude et de Traitement du Carcinome Hepatocellulaire reported their results with 50 patients undergoing TACE in 24 institutions (8). While no statistically significant difference was noted in survival when compared to supportive care only, median survivals were increased from 8 to 19 months and the estimated relative risk of death was 1.4 in the conservatively managed group compared to the chemoembolization group.

The remainder of the studies presented in Table 1 are retrospective with either historically matched or non-matched controls. Of note, all of these studies demonstrate a significant improvement in overall patient survival when compared to patients receiving supportive care only (9-16). Examination of the median survivals of these studies shows a consistent three-fold improvement in survival in those patients undergoing TACE.

Table 1: WESTERN SERIES OF TACE FOR HCC

Prospective, Randomized

Author	Year	Therapy	n	Med Surv	p
Pelletier (7)	1990	Dox + Gel	21	4	NS
		Supportive Care	21	6	
French Group (8)	1995	Cis + Lip + Gel	50	19	0.13
		Supportive Care	46	8	

Retrospective, Matched Historical Controls

Author	Year	Therapy	n	Med Surv	p
Vetter (9)	1991	Dox + Lip + Gel	30	12	<0.001
		Supportive Care	30	3	
Bronowicki (10)	1994	Dox, Cis, or Epi + Lip + Gel	127	18	<0.0001
		Supportive Care	127	5	
Stefanini (11)	1995	Dox + Lip + Gel	69	21	<0.001
		Supportive Care	64	3	

Retrospective, Non-Matched Controls

Author	Year	Therapy	n	Med Surv	p
Bronowicki (12)	1996	Dox, Cis, or Epi + Lip + Gel	42	36	<0.0001
		Supportive Care	33	11	
Stuart (13)	1996	Dox + Lip + Gel	137	14	<0.01
		Supportive Care	81	2	
Marcos-Alvarez (14)	1996	Dox + Lip + Gel	30	13	<0.05
		Supportive Care	22	5	
Ryder (15)	1996	Dox + Lip + Gel	67	9	NR
		Non-Surgical Therapy	118	3	
Rose (16)	1999	Dox + Lip + Gel	35	9	<0.0001
		Supportive Care	31	3	

Dox=doxirubicin, Cis=cisplatin, Epi=epirubicin, Lip=lipiodol, Gel=gelatin-foam particles or powder, NS=not statistically significant, NR=not reported, Med Surv=median survival (months)

Published studies from Asian series report findings similar to those reported from the Western centers. The majority of large Asian studies show a survival benefit to TACE with actuarial one-year survivals between 24% and 80% (3,4). However, despite multiple reports of the benefit of TACE, no randomized, prospective trials have been reported from Eastern centers. Liu and Fan state that such a controlled trial would be very difficult in Eastern countries as TACE is viewed as an established and effective treatment and has become the standard of care in these centers (3).

Several extensive reviews of the current treatment of HCC point out the relative shortcomings of the available data on TACE. Liu and Fan report that TACE is generally considered an effective treatment for HCC, although improved survival has yet to be shown in a prospective, randomized fashion (3). Trinchet and Beaugrand also question the statistical benefit demonstrated in available studies and call for further investigation (6). Lehnert and Herfarth point out that with the large number of variables in patients with HCC, a number of diligent studies will be required to establish optimal treatment parameters and patient selection (17). Clearly, there is a need for further investigation into the utility and appropriate application of TACE. The use of ^{131}I-labeled lipiodol is one example of the possible further application of TACE (18).

Morbidity
In order to validate TACE as an appropriate palliative procedure for HCC, the procedure itself must be safe. The morbidity of TACE is primarily secondary to the postembolization syndrome (19). This consists of transient and self-limited fever, abdominal pain, nausea, vomiting and anorexia. Previous studies have reported relatively high incidences of major complications following TACE. Bismuth et al reported a series of 291 patients undergoing TACE with 31 episodes of cholecystitis [11%], duodenal ulceration [6 patients], hepatic abscess [4], splenic infarction [3], and pancreatitis [2] (20). Berger et al from the M.D. Anderson Cancer Center reported an experience with a total of 314 TACE treatments or hepatic artery embolizations in 121 patients (21). Hepatic abscess was noted in 6 patients, and hepatic failure in an additional four patients. Overall, major complications occurred after 16 embolization treatments and 5 patients died as a direct result of intervention. This group concluded that the procedure is a safe palliative treatment; yet strongly emphasize the need for close monitoring and aggressive care at the time of

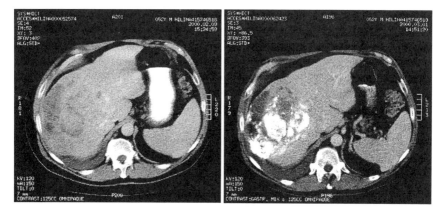

Figure 1. CT scan demonstrating large right lobe hepatocellular carcinoma before (left panel) and after (right panel) chemoembolization with mitomycin, adriamycin, cisplatin, lipiodol, and gelfoam. The early post-chemoembolization CT on the right confirms proper targeting of the tumor (note bright CT signal from lipiodol) and provides contrast enhancement to follow tumor size in future studies.

TACE. Lopez et al reported an experience with TACE in unresectable hepatic malignancies and found only transient adverse side effects associated with the postembolization syndrome (22). Similar results were seen in our series with the exception of one patient who developed ATN requiring hemodialysis following TACE (16). Overall, the Vanderbilt group has found TACE to be a safe procedure in properly selected patients. However, we also encourage close peri-procedural monitoring, intravenous hydration, and specialized care with staff familiar with the potential hazards of the procedure.

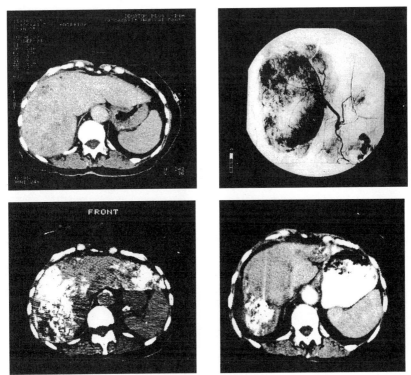

Figure 2. CT scan (upper left panel) demonstrating multifocal hepatocellular carcinoma prior to angiogram (upper right panel) and chemoembolization. The lower left panel shows the early CT result following separate right and left lobe chemoembolization. This was followed by marked tumor involution (lower right panel) on CT scanning 3 years following the initial procedure. The patient ultimately died 3 and ½ years following the initial procedure from multiple lung metastases.

Portal vein obstruction has clinically been considered a contraindication to TACE due to the risk of subsequent hepatic insufficiency. Lee et al reported a series if 31 patients with HCC and main portal vein obstruction who underwent TACE and compared outcomes with 16 untreated controls (23). No difference in degradation of hepatic function was noted in either group. The authors concluded that TACE may be considered in patients with main portal vein obstruction provided they had good hepatic function and collateral portal circulation.

Prognostic Factors

Several Western studies have examined the prognostic factors associated with improved outcomes following TACE. Farinati et al found that Child's class, Okuda staging (24), number of TACE treatments, AFP-responsiveness, and concurrent tamoxifen therapy, correlate with increased survival (25). Mondazzi et al found age, Child's class, serum bilirubin, Okuda stage, tumor size, degree of lipiodol tumor labeling, use of gelatin foam, change in tumor size and change in AFP levels to significantly impact survival by univariate analysis (26). The report of TACE from Vanderbilt did not demonstrate any factors that had a statistically significant impact on survival; however, those patients who responded with a decrease in serum AFP levels following TACE did have an increase in median survival from 7 to 13 months (16). Similarly, cirrhotic patients had a decreased survival of 9 months compared to 13 months in non-cirrhotic patients. Not surprisingly, patients with improved hepatic reserve and evidence of response to therapy had better outcomes.

Neoadjuvant TACE

The overall poor outcomes with the treatment of HCC have led to a number of multi-modality approaches including the use of TACE as a neoadjuvant preoperative treatment. The rationale for this approach includes the treatment of microscopic subclinical disease and the hope of downstaging larger lesions so they can be considered for resection. The data is largely retrospective in nature and overall shows little difference in disease-free or overall survival following resection. Lu et al performed neoadjuvant TACE in 44 patients and compared outcomes to 76 non-matched controls undergoing resection without TACE (27). Overall survival was similar; however, the subgroup of patients with lesions greater than 8 cm had significantly better overall and disease-free survival. Majno et al reported their results with preoperative TACE in 49/76 liver resections and 54/111 transplant recipients (28). Again, no difference was noted in overall survival. This group, however, identified a significant improvement in patients undergoing TACE who also were downstaged or who had total tumor necrosis. This subset improvement was noted in both the resection and transplant patients. The authors also noted that downstaging of previously unresectable lesions allows for a curative resection in 10% of their patient population. Finally, Harada et al reported outcomes with 98 patients undergoing preoperative TACE compared to 35 who underwent resection only (29). Once again, no difference was noted in overall or disease-free survival. A distinct reduction in tumor mass was noted in half the patients and the authors concluded that neoadjuvant TACE should be confined to patients with borderline resectability.

Preoperative TACE may downstage large, bulky lesions and allow resection in some cases. Overall survival from large retrospective series have failed to demonstrate a survival advantage; however, certain subsets of patients may benefit. Similar to the utilization of TACE as a primary treatment for HCC, the neoadjuvant role of this therapeutic modality awaits confirmation by randomized, prospective data.

CONCLUSIONS

TACE can be safely applied to a properly selected group of patients with HCC who are not candidates for surgical resection. Median survival appears to be significantly increased in these patients when compared to non-matched controls receiving only supportive care in the same time period. Unfortunately, little randomized, prospective data is available to absolutely define the long-term outcomes following TACE and to better define a population of patients who would most benefit. Further prospective trials of sufficient number remain necessary in order to answer these critical questions.

PERCUTANEOUS ETHANOL INJECTION

Probably the most common therapy utilized for the treatment of HCC throughout the world is percutaneous ethanol injection (PEI). Sugiura first described this for the treatment of small HCC in 1983 (30). PEI is a local tumor ablative technique whose mechanism of action is dependent on the toxic effects of ethanol. Ethanol diffuses into cells causing protein denaturation, cellular dehydration and subsequent coagulation necrosis (31, 32). Local fibrosis and small vessel thrombosis also occur in the region of injection.

PEI is generally performed by two different techniques (33). The most common is a "multi-session" approach performed in an outpatient setting with local anesthesia. Multi-session treatment is performed under radiologic guidance (usually ultrasound) at which time a single 20 or 22 gauge needle is inserted into the lesion. The total volume of ethanol injected is generally from 8-10 ml per session. The volume can be estimated form the following formula:

$$V = 4/3 \, \pi \, (R + 0.5)^3$$

Where V is the volume of total injectate and R is the radius of the lesion. The 0.5 factor allows for a volume adequate enough for a "margin" of normal tissue to be destroyed with the ablation. Obviously, this represents a guideline only for the total volume of ethanol. Based on these calculations, the approximate volume of ethanol for a 1-cm tumor is 4 ml; 2 cm, 14 ml; 3 cm, 33 ml; and 5 cm, 113 ml. The maximum volume injected in the outpatient setting in most centers is 20 – 30 ml (56). Even with this volume limitation, some patients can develop system effects of alcohol intoxication, and require close observation immediately following the procedure. Livraghi states that the number of sessions required for an adequate ablation is approximately twice the lesion diameter in centimeters (33).

PEI may also be utilized as a "single session" in which large volumes of ethanol are injected into more advanced lesions with the patient under general anesthesia. This technique was first introduced by Livraghi and colleagues in 1993 as an attempt to treat larger or multiple lesions (34). This approach is more aggressive with a somewhat higher complication rate compared to conventional, multi-session PEI.

Reported Series

The majority of the reported series following PEI are retrospective reviews of outcomes with no controls. In these series, mean survival rates at 1, 2 and 3 years are 93%, 80%, and 68%, respectively (31). These series represent a heterogeneous group of patients with single or multiple lesions generally less than 5 cm in size.

Several other authors have made comparisons to non-treated cohorts and have found significant improvements in outcomes in those patients undergoing PEI. The Italian Cooperative HCC Study Group performed a retrospective analysis of 391 patients with Child's A or B cirrhosis and a single HCC less than 5 cm in size (35). Comparable 3-year survival rates were noted in patients undergoing PEI or resection (79% vs. 71% in Child's A patients and 41% vs. 40% in Child's B patients). Untreated patients had statistically significantly lower 3-year survival rates of 26% and 13% in Child's A and B cirrhotics, respectively. A similar comparison between patients with single HCC's less than 4 cm in size has been reported by Castells et al (36). Overall survival rates between patients undergoing resection versus PEI were not significantly different. In a series of comparable patients with HCC, Okuda reported a 45% 5-year survival in Child's A patients treated by PEI versus no patients surviving in a non-treated group (37).

Overall, PEI appears to offer a survival advantage in the studies that have compared treatment to supportive therapy only. Certainly, a degree of selection bias may be introduced in the choice of those patients undergoing PEI. Of interest, several of the discussed series have shown similar outcomes between surgical resection and PEI, again bringing to bear the impact of selection in these series. No randomized, prospective data has been generated regarding the outcomes with PEI versus no treatment, and this is unlikely to be done. Livraghi et al state that due to the efficacy and safety of this modality, a no-treatment control group has been considered unethical (38).

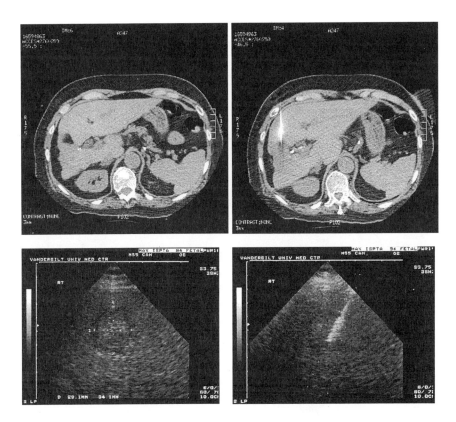

Figure 3. Percutaneous alcohol instillation in a patient with advanced cirrhosis and a small right lobe hepatocellular carcinoma. The upper panels show tumor targeting under CT guidance with corresponding ultrasound views before and during alcohol instillation (lower panels).

Morbidity

Percutaneous ethanol injection appears to be associated with very few adverse outcomes, overall. Conventional, multi-session PEI is particularly safe with transient pain, fever and a feeling of ethanol intoxication being the most common complications (31, 33). Pain is most often localized to the injection site and analgesic requirements appear to be associated with total volume of injectate. Transient increases in serum transaminases are also commonly noted following PEI, generally less than those noted with TACE. Livraghi reports that among 1643 patients, collected by various authors, no deaths were noted and major complications ranged from 1.3 – 2.4% (38). Infrequent major complications include pleural effusion, pneumothorax, ascites, myoglobinuria, hemobilia, liver abscess, splenic abscess, and partial hepatic infarction (31).

Single-session PEI has been associated with higher rates of complications and mortality than the standard low-volume multi-session approach. The mortality rates are between 1.4 – 11% with complication rates up to 58% (38). Deaths have been noted secondary to upper gastrointestinal bleeding, particularly in Child's class C patients (31). Fatal extensive thrombosis of the entire portal tree has also been reported (39). In contrast, Tapani et al have reported their experience with various volumes of injected ethanol and have attempted to correlate complications with increased volume (40). While the incidence of acute pain did increase with increasing volumes from 10 ml to 200 ml, the incidence of serious complications was extremely rare and not associated with total volume.

Needle-track seeding is a potential complication associated with PEI, particularly in the context of a single patient undergoing multiple sessions with multiple needle passes per session. The estimated risk of needle-track implantation with fine-needle aspiration biopsy is approximately 0.0005% (31, 41). The majority of reports of needle-track seeding are anecdotal; however, Sammack et al reported 2 cases of implantation among a total of 32 patients treated between 1993 and 1997 for an incidence of 6.2% (42). Ishii et al reported a 1.1% incidence in 4/348 patients undergoing PEI (43). Risk factors identified for implantation in these patients included lesions $\geq$ 2 cm in size, enhancement on early phase dynamic CT scanning, and moderate tumor cell differentiation. The reasons for these factor remains uncertain, as does the etiology of seeding itself.

Prognostic Factors

Factors influencing survival following PEI are, not surprisingly, related primarily to tumor volume and intrinsic hepatic function. Patients with single lesions less than 3 cm have improved survivals when compared to larger or multiple lesions (31, 32). Child's A patients also have significantly better outcomes compared to B or C patients. The majority of Child's A patients treated with PEI die of progression of their neoplastic disease, while Child's C patients tend to expire secondary to progressive cirrhosis and hepatic failure (38). The prognostic significance of AFP levels is controversial. Lencioni et al noted significantly better survival in patients with initial AFP levels less than 200 µg/L (44). Livraghi et al found AFP levels to be predictive only in patients with multiple lesions and AFP levels > 200 µg/L (38).

Recurrence is extremely common in patients treated by PEI, ranging from 64 – 98% at 5 years (31). Ishii et al examined predictive factors for recurrence after PEI (45). Among nine separate variables examined by univariate analysis in 31 patients, AFP levels $\leq$ 20 ng/ml and absence of cirrhosis were associated with significantly lower recurrence rates. A separate report by the same author examined factors associated with local recurrence only and found size > 3 cm to be the most predictive factor (46).

CONCLUSIONS

Percutaneous ethanol injection appears to be efficacious and safe in the management of selected patients with HCC. Clearly, those individuals with more limited disease and better hepatic function have improved outcomes. Selection (similar to TACE) becomes paramount in the choice of optimal therapy. Larger volume single-session PEI is effective as well; however, this does come at an increased cost in morbidity and mortality. Similar to TACE, little to no randomized, prospective data is available. Overall, PEI is a valuable method of local tumor ablation and remains an important component in the management of patients with HCC.

COMBINED TACE AND PEI

TACE is an effective regional therapy for HCC; however, recurrences are common and are felt to be secondary to portal perfusion at the rim of the tumor. PEI is an excellent local ablative technique but, again, recurrence is the rule and this modality does not address sub-clinical disease within the liver. In an attempt to overcome the limitations of TACE and PEI, several authors have proposed combining each as a multi-modal approach for the treatment of HCC.

Lencioni et al have reported prospectively acquired outcomes in patients with HCC's between 3 and 8 cm in size undergoing TACE and PEI (47). Actuarial survival at 5 years was 59% for Child's A patients and 35% for Child's B cirrhotics. In a similar report, Tanaka et al noted a 35% survival in patients receiving combination therapy (48). Stage of cirrhosis and size of the largest lesion were independently associated with survival in this study.

Several authors have compared combination TACE and PEI to treatment with TACE alone. Yamamoto et al reported a retrospective series of 100 patients equally divided into TACE alone or with PEI (49). Actuarial survival at 3 years was 50% for combination therapy compared to 20% for TACE alone, with number of lesions and tumor embolus within the portal vein being the most significant prognostic factors in the combination therapy group. Tateishi et al reported similar finding in a retrospective analysis of 17 patients receiving both TACE and PEI compared to 18 patients undergoing TACE alone (50). Median survival was 38 months in patients undergoing combined therapy compared to 21 months with TACE alone. Bartolozzi et al performed a randomized, prospective trial comparing these two approaches (51). Fifty-three patients were randomized to TACE and PEI [26 pts] or TACE alone [27 pts]. Median disease-free survival was significantly improved in the combination group (20 vs. 10 months), as was disease-free actuarial survival at three years (52% vs. 30%).

A recent report compared 132 patients with inoperable HCC who received one of four treatments: PEI alone, TACE alone, PEI and TACE, or best supportive care (52). The patients were stratified to treatment groups based on number of lesions, size of largest lesion, and accessibility of the lesions to PEI. Median survival was greatest in patients undergoing combined therapy, followed by PEI alone, TACE alone and best supportive care (25, 18, 8 and 2 months, respectively). Multivariate analysis in this series revealed that combined therapy was a strong independent predictor of survival even though the groups were dissimilar due to initial stratification.

The combination of TACE and PEI is an attractive option on many levels and appears to be supported by the available data. Combination therapy has also been proposed in the treatment of intrahepatic recurrence following resection (53, 54) and as preoperative therapy in patients awaiting liver transplantation (55).

CONCLUSIONS

Chemoembolization and interstitial therapy with percutaneous ethanol injection are critical components in the treatment of patients with hepatocellular carcinoma. Each has advantages and disadvantages and each is best suited for a selective population of patients with HCC. The data suggests that in carefully selected populations, a combination of the two may provide the most benefit in inoperable patients. Clearly, the importance of a multi-modality approach at a center capable of offering all therapies is paramount. Only in this fashion can the best outcomes in these difficult patients be realized.

REFERENCES

1.   Venook AP. Treatment of hepatocellular carcinoma: too many options? *J Clin Oncol*, 1994;12(6):1323.
2.   Carriaga MT, Henson DE. Liver, gallbladder, extrahepatic bile ducts, and pancreas. *Cancer*, 1995;75(1 Suppl):171.
3.   Liu C-L, Fan S-T. Nonresectional therapies for hepatocellular carcinoma. *Am J Surg*, 1997;173:358.
4.   Farmer DG, Rosove MH, Shaked A, Busuttil RW. Current treatment modalities for haepatocellular carcinoma. *Ann Surg*, 1994;219(3):236.
5.   Bruix   J.   Treatment   of   hepatocellular   carcinoma.   *Hepatology*, 1997;25(2):259.
6.   Trinchet J-C, Beaugrand M. Treatment of hepatocellular carcinoma in patients with cirrhosis. *J Hepatol* , 1997;27:756.
7.   Pelletier G, Roche A, Ink O, et al. A randomized trial of hepatic arterial chemoembolization in patients with unresectable hepatocellular carcinoma.. *J Hepatol* 1990;11:181.
8.   Groupe d'Etude et de Traitement du Carcinome Hepatocellulaire. A comparison of lipiodol chemoembolization and conservative treatment for unresectable hepatocellular carcinoma. *N Engl J Med*, 1995;332(19):1256.
9.   Vetter   D,   Wenger   JJ,   Bergier   JM,   et   al.   Transcatheter   oily chemoembolization   in   the   management   of   advanced   hepatocellular

carcinoma in cirrhosis: results of a western comparative study in 60 patients. *Hepatology*, 1991;13(3):427.

10. Bronowicki JP, Vetter D, Dumas F, et al.. Transcatheter oily chemoembolization for hepatocellular carcinoma: a 4-year study of 127 patients. *Cancer,* 1994;74(1):16.

11. Stefanini GF, Amorati P, Biselli M, et al.. Efficacy of transarterial targeted treatments on survival of patients with hepatocellular carcinoma: an italian experience. *Cancer*, 1995; 75(10):2427.

12. Bronowicki J-P, Boudjema K, Chone L, et al. Comparison of resection, liver transplantation and transcatheter oily chemoembolization in the treatment of hepatocellular carcinoma. *J Hepatol*, 1996;24:293.

13. Stuart KE, Anand AJ, Jenkins RL. Hepatocellular carcinoma in the united states: prognostic features, treatment outcome, and survival. *Cancer*, 1996;77(11):2217.

14. Marcos-Alvarez A, Jenkins RL, Washburn WK, et al. Multimodality treatment of hepatocellular carcinoma in a hepatobiliary specialty center. *Arch Surg*, 1996;131:292.

15. Ryder SD, Rizzi PM, Metivier E, et al. Chemoembolisation with lipiodol and doxorubicin: applicability in british patients with hepatocellular carcinoma. *Gut*, 1996; 38:125.

16. Rose DM, Pinson CW, Brokenbrough AT, et al. Transcatheter arterial chemoembolization as primary treatment for hepatocellular carcinoma. *Am J Surg* (in press).

17. Lehnert T, Herfarth C. Chemoembolization for hepatocellular carcinoma: what, when, and for whom? *Ann Surg*, 1996;224(1):1.

18. Raoul J-L, Guyader D, Bretagne J-F, et al. Prospective randomized trial of chemoembolization versus intra-arterial injection of ^{131}I-labeled-iodized oil in the treatment of hepatocellular carcinoma. *Hepatology*, 1997;26(5):1156.

19. Cohen SE, Safadi R, Verstandig A, et al. Liver-spleen infarcts following transcatheter chemoembolization: a case report and review of the literature on adverse effects. *Dig Dis Sci,* 1997;42(5):938.

20. Bismuth H, Morino M, Sherlock D, et al. Primary treatment of hepatocellular carcinoma by arterial chemoembolization. *Am J Surg*, 1992;163:387.

21. Berger DH, Carrasco CH, Hohn DC, Curley SA. Hepatic artery chemoembolization or embolization for primary and metastatic liver tumors: post-treatment management and complications. *J Surg Oncol*, 1995;60:116.

22. Lopez RR, Pan S, Lois JF, et al. Transarterial chemoembolization is a safe treatment for unresectable hepatic malignancies. *Am Surg*, 1997;63:923.

23. Lee H-S, Kim JS, Choi IJ, et al. The safety and eficacy of transcatheter arterial chemoembolization in the treatment of patients with hepatocellular carcinoma and main portal vein obstruction. *Cancer*, 1997; 79(11): 2087.

24. Okuda K, Obata H, Ohtsuki T, et al. Prognosis of primary hepatocellular carcinoma. *Hepatology*, 1984;4(1):3S.

25.   Farinati F, De Maria N, Marafin C, et al. Unresectable hepatocellular carcinoma in cirrhosis: survival, prognostic factors, and unexpected side effects after transcatheter arterial chemoembolization. *Dig Dis Sci*, 1996;41(12):2332.

26.   Mondazzi L, Bottelli R, Brambilla G, et al. Transarterial oily chemoembolization for the treatment of hepatocellular carcinoma: a multivariate analysis of prognostic factors. *Hepatology*, 1994;19(5):1115.

27.   Lu C-D, Peng S-Y, Jiang X-C, Chiba Y, Tanigawa N. Preoperative transcatheter arterial chemoembolization and prognosis of patients with hepatocellular carcinoma: retrospective analysis of 120 cases. *World J Surg*, 1999; 23: 293.

28.   Majno PE, Adam R, Bismuth H, et al. Influence of preoperative transarterial lipiodol chemoembolization on resection and transplantation for hepatocellular carcinoma in patients with cirrhosis. Ann Surg, 1997; 226(6): 688.

29.   Harada T, Matsuo K, Inoue T, et al. Is preoperative hepatic arterial chemoembolization safe and effective for hepatocellular carcinoma? *Ann Surg*, 1996;224(1):4.

30.   Sugiura N, Takara K, Ohto M, Okuda K, Hirooka N. Percutaneous intratumoral injection of ethanol under ultrasound imaging for treatment of small hepatocellular carcinoma. *Acta Hepatol Jpn*, 1983; 24: 920.

31.   De Sanctis JT, Goldberg SN, Mueller PR. Percutaneous treatment of hepatic neoplasms: a review of current techniques. *Cardiovasc Intervent Radiol*, 1998; 21: 273.

32.   Lee MJ, Mueller PR, Dawson SL, et al. Percutaneous ethanol injection for the treatment of hepatic tumors: indications, mechanism of action, technique and efficacy. *Am J Radiol*, 1995; 164: 215.

33.   Livraghi T. Percutaneous ethanol injection in the treatment of hepatocellular carcinoma in cirrhosis. *Hepato-gastroenterol*, 1998; 45: 1248.

34.   Livraghi T, Lazzaroni S, Pellicano S, et al. Percutaneous ethanol injection of hepatic tumors: single-session therapy with general anesthesia. *Am J Radiol*, 1993; 161: 1065.

35.   Livraghi T, Bolondi L, Buscarini L , et al. No treatment, resection, and ethanol injection in hepatocellular carcinoma: a retrospective analysis of survival in 391 patients with cirrhosis. Italian Cooperative HCC Study Group. *J Hepatol*, 1995; 22:522.

36.   Castells A, Bruix J, Bru C, et al. Treatment of small hepatocellular carcinoma in cirrhotic patients: a cohort study comparing surgical resection and percutaneous ethanol injection. *Hepatology*, 1993; 18: 1121.

37.   Okuda K. Intratumoral ethanol injection. *J Surg Oncol Suppl*, 1993; 3:97.

38.   Livraghi T, Giorgio A, Marin G, et al. Hepatocellular carcinoma and cirrhosis in 746 patients: long-term results of percutaneous ethanol injection. *Radiology*, 1995; 197(1): 101.

39.   Lencioni R, Cioni D, Uliana M, Bartolozzi C. Fatal thrombosis of the portal vein following single-session percutaneous injection therapy of hepatocellular carcinoma. *Abdom Imaging*, 1998; 23: 608.

40.   Tapani E, Soiva M, Lavonen J, Ristkari S, Vehmas T. Complications following high-dose percutaneous ethanol injection into hepatic tumors. *Acta Radiologica*, 1996; 37: 655.

41.   Shimada M, Maeda T, Saitoh A, Morotomi I, Kano T. Needle track seeding after percutaneous ethanol injection therapy for small hepatocellular carcinoma. *J Surg Oncol*, 1995; 58: 278.

42.   Sammack B, Yousef B, Abd El Bagi M, et al. Needle track seeding following percutaneous ethanol injection for treatment of hepatocellular carcinoma. *Hepato-gastroenterol*, 1998; 45: 1097.

43.   Ishii H, Okada S, Okusaka T, et al. Needle tract implantation of hepatocellular carcinoma after percutaneous ethanol injection. *Cancer*, 1998; 82: 1638.

44.   Lencioni R, Caramella D, Bartolozzi C. Hepatocellular carcinoma: use of color doppler US to evaluate response to treatment with percutaneous ethanol injection. *Radiology*, 1995; 194: 113.

45.   Ishii H, Okada S, Nose H, et al. Predictive factors for recurrence after percutaneous ethanol injection for solitary hepatocellular carcinoma. *Hepato-gastroenterol*, 1996; 43: 938.

46.   Ishii H, Okada S, Nose H, et al. Local recurrence of hepatocellular carcinoma after percutaneous ethanol injection. *Cancer*, 1996; 77: 1792.

47.   Lencioni R, Paolicchi A, Moretti M, et al. Combined transcatheter arterial chemoembolization and percutaneous ethanol injection for the treatment of large hepatocellular carcinoma: local therapeutic effect and long-term survival rate. *Eur Radiol*, 1998; 8: 439.

48.   Tanaka K, Nakamura S, Numata K, et al. The long term efficacy of combined transcatheter arterial embolization and percutaneous ethanol injection in the treatment of patients with large hepatocellular carcinoma and cirrhosis. *Cancer*, 1998; 82: 78.

49.   Yamamoto K, Masuzawa M, Kato M, et al. Evaluation of combined therapy with chemoembolization and ethanol injection for advanced hepatocellular carcinoma. *Semin Oncol Suppl*, 1997; 24(2): S6-50.

50.   Tateishi H, Kinuta M, Furukawa J, et al. Follow-up study of combined treatment (TAE and PEIT) for unresectable hepatocellular carcinoma. *Cancer Chemother Pharmacol Suppl*, 1994; 33: S 119.

51.   Bartolozzi C, Lencioni R, Caramella D, et al. Treatment of large HCC: transcatheter arterial chemoembolization combined with percutaneous ethanol injection versus repeated transcatheter arterial chemoembolization. *Radiology*, 1995; 197: 812.

52.   Allgaier H-P, Deibert P, Olschewski M, et al. Survival benefit of patients with inoperable hepatocellular carcinoma treated by a combination of transarterial chemoembolization and percutaneous ethanol injection – a single-center analysis including 132 patients. *Int J Cancer*, 1998; 79: 601.

53.   Sato M, Watanabe Y, Iseki N, et al. Chemoembolization and percutaneous ethanol injection for intrahepatic recurrence of hepatocellular carcinoma after hepatic resection. *Hepato-Gastroenterol*, 1996; 43: 1421.

54.   Ishii H, Okada S, Sato T, et al. Effect of percutaneous ethanol injection for postoperative recurrence of hepatocellular carcinoma n combination with transcatheter arterial chemoembolization. *Hepato-Gastroenterol*, 1996; 43: 644.

55.   Veltri A, Grosso M, Martina MC, et al. Effect of preoperative radiological treatment of hepatocellular carcinoma before liver transplantation: a retrospective study. *Cardiovasc Intervent Radiol*, 1998; 21: 393.

56.   Paulson EK. Ethanol injection of treatment of liver tumors. In: Malignant liver tumors: current and emerging therapies. Pierre-Alain Clavian (ed.); Blackwell Science, Malden, Massachusetts, 1999: 181-188.

7

DIAGNOSIS AND MANAGEMENT OF INTRAHEPATIC AND EXTRAHEPATIC CHOLANGIOCARCINOMA

Steven A. Curley, M.D., F.A.C.S.
The University of Texas M.D. Anderson Cancer Center, Houston, TX

INTRODUCTION

Cholangiocarcinomas are malignant tumors that arise from the epithelium of the intrahepatic or extrahepatic bile ducts. Cholangiocarcinomas are rare compared with hepatocellular carcinoma, comprising less than 10% of primary malignancies of the liver (1). In the United States, approximately 3,000 patients are diagnosed with cholangiocarcinoma annually (2). The autopsy incidence of cholangiocarcinoma is low also, being reported in 0.089-0.46% of necropsies (1). Cholangiocarcinomas are diagnosed most frequently in the fifth and sixth decades of life (3). There is only a slight male preponderance of cases of cholangiocarcinoma. Cholangiocarcinomas can arise at any site in the intra- or extrahepatic biliary system, but perihilar tumors comprise two-thirds of the cases of cholangiocarcinoma (3) (Fig. 1).

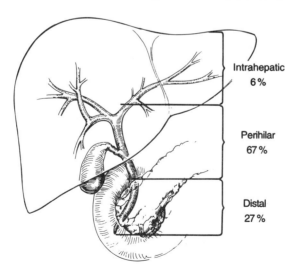

Figure 1. The distribution of 294 cholangiocarcinomas into intrahepatic, perihilar, and distal subgroups. (From Nakeeb et al, with permission, 3).

CAUSATIVE FACTORS

There are distinct differences between the factors associated with cholangiocarcinoma and those associated with hepatocellular carcinoma (Table 1). Cholangiocarcinoma does not appear to be associated with hepatitis B or C virus infection, or mycotoxin exposure (1). Only 10-20% of cholangiocarcinomas occur in cirrhotic patients, compared with the 70-90% of hepatocellular carcinomas that arise in cirrhotic livers (2,4,5). A cohort study in Denmark of 11,605 patients with cirrhosis indicated a 60-fold increased risk for developing hepatocellular cancer and a 10-fold increased risk for cholangiocarcinoma (5). Frequently the cirrhosis associated with cholangiocarcinomas is a subacute secondary biliary type that results from the neoplastic obstruction of the bile ducts, indicating that some cases of cirrhosis in cholangiocarcinoma patients are the result of the tumor rather than their cause.

Table 1. Factors associated with an increased risk to develop cholangiocarcinoma compared with factors associated with hepatocellular carcinoma.

Cholangiocarcinoma	Hepatocellular carcinoma
Liver fluke infection	Cirrhosis
Clonorchis sinensis	Chronic hepatitis B virus infection
Opisthorchis viverrini	Chronic hepatitis C virus infection
Congenital/chronic cystic dilation of the bile ducts	Aflatoxin B_1 ingestion
Choledochal cyst	Chronic ethanol ingestion
Caroli's disease	Primary biliary cirrhosis
Hepatolithiasis	Hemachromatosis
Primary sclerosing cholangitis	Alpha-1-antitrypsin deficiency
Ulcerative colitis	Glycogen storage disease
Thorotrast exposure	Hypercitrullnemia
Cholelithiasis	Porphyrias
Asbestos	Hereditary tyrosinemia
Dioxin (Agent Orange)	Wilson's disease
Polychlorinated diphenyls	Hepatotoxin exposure
Nitrosamines	Thorotrast
Isoniazid	Polyvinyl chloride
Methyldopa	Carbon tetrachloride

Cholangiocarcinoma is more prevalent in Southeast Asia than in other parts of the world. The higher incidence in this geographic region is related to parasitic infection with the liver flukes *Clonorchis sinensis* and *Opisthorchis viverrini* (6,7). Infestation by other biliary parasites, such as *Fasciola hepatica* and *Schistosomiasis japonica*, does not appear to have similar carcinogenic effects (8). Liver flukes induce hyperplasia, fibrosis, and adenomatous proliferation of human biliary epithelium and are associated with hepatolithiasis (9,10). The fluke infestation suggests a direct etiologic role in the subsequent development of cholangiocarcinoma, but this relationship is not established unequivocally. It is interesting to note that in a Syrian Golden hamster model, administration of dimethylnitrosamine alone does not cause neoplasia, but this agent given to animals with liver fluke infection leads to the development of cholangiocarcinomas (11,12).

Several disorders that can produce chronic inflammation of the bile ducts have been associated with an increased risk of developing cholangiocarcinoma. These include polycystic liver disease, choledochal cysts, congenital dilation of the intrahepatic bile ducts (Caroli's syndrome), sclerosing cholangitis (occasionally in association with inflammatory bowel disease), hepatolithiasis, and cholelithiasis (13-22). Hepatolithiasis is not a common disorder, and only 5-7% of patients with documented hepatic stones develop cholangiocarcinoma (21, 22). The reported incidence of cholangiocarcinoma developing in areas of congenital cystic dilation of the bile duct, including choledochal cysts and Caroli's disease, ranges from 3-30% (23, 24). Patients with primary sclerosing cholangitis are also at increased risk to develop cholangiocarcinoma with incidence rates ranging from 9-40% (25-27). Patients with ulcerative colitis may also develop sclerosing cholangitis, but cholangiocarcinoma occurs in only 0.4-1.4% of individuals with ulcerative colitis (25). In patients with sclerosing cholangitis, whether associated with ulcerative colitis or not, radiologic distinction between sclerosing cholangitis and cholangiocarcinoma is often impossible. A recent study showed that the serum tumor marker CA19-9 had 89% sensitivity and 86% specificity in diagnosing cholangiocarcinoma in patients with sclerosing cholangitis (28). Combining serum CA19-9 levels with serum CEA levels may further increase the diagnostic accuracy to detect cholangiocarcinoma in patients with sclerosing cholangitis (29)

Patients who underwent diagnostic radiographs with intravenous injection of Thorotrast (thorium dioxide) are at high risk of developing hepatocellular carcinoma, angiosarcoma, and cholangiocarcinoma (30,31). Cholangiocarcinoma is the most frequent hepatic neoplasm reported in patients who have received Thorotrast. Exposure to several drugs or carcinogens has also been linked to an increased risk to develop cholangiocarcinoma (Table 1). Because cholangiocarcinoma is a relatively rare neoplasm, it has been difficult to prove the pathogenesis of cholangiocarcinoma related to any of these factors, but it is clear that chronic inflammation of the biliary tree by any cause is associated with an increased risk of developing cholangiocarcinoma.

It has been suggested that hepatocellular carcinoma and cholangiocarcinoma arise from a common hepatic progenitor or 'stem' cell in response to chronic injury and subsequent cellular proliferation (32). Evidence supporting this theory occurs in patients who present with combined hepatocellular carcinoma and cholangiocarcinoma (33,34). Approximately 3% of patients with hepatocellular carcinoma have histologic evidence within or adjacent to the cancer of coexistent cholangiocarcinoma (34). Evaluation of a variety of cell surface markers in the cholangiocarcinoma and hepatocellular carcinoma cells of patients with combined tumors indicates a high degree of homology in the expression of cell surface molecules between the two malignant cell types (33,34). Furthermore, the only consistent genetic alterations that have been detected in cholangiocarcinomas are loss of heterozygosity in regions of chromosomes 5 and 17 that are also lost in hepatocellular carcinoma (35). These findings suggest a common origin from a pluripotential cell type in patients with combined hepatocellular carcinoma and cholangiocarcinoma, but definitive proof has not yet been provided.

Chronic inflammation of the biliary system or exposure to genotoxic agents concentrated in bile may produce damage to the DNA of biliary epithelial cells leading to the development of cholangiocarcinoma. Mutations in the p53 tumor suppressor gene and in the K-ras protooncogene have been identified in cholangiocarcinoma patients (36-38). There may be geographic and population-based differences in the mutations rates of these two genes in cholangiocarcinoma, but alterations in p53 and K-ras are observed in significant proportions of patients with any of the identified factors (Table 1) that increase risk to develop cholangiocarcinoma. Overexpression of c-erbB-2, a protooncogene that encodes a transmembrane protein which is highly homologous to epidermal growth factor receptor, has been confirmed in human cholangiocarcinoma cells and in benign proliferative biliary epithelium from patients with hepatolithiasis, primary sclerosing cholangitis, and live fluke infestation (39). Alterations in c-erbB-2 expression may occur early in the chronic inflammation-induced proliferation of biliary epithelium leading to malignant transformation. Chronic inflammation may also produce the overexpression of the Bcl-2 protooncogene observed in cholangiocarcinomas that may promote tumorigenesis by inhibiting normal apoptotic processes (40).

CLINICAL PRESENTATION

The clinical features of cholangiocarcinoma are nonspecific and depend on the location of the tumor. The usual clinical presentation of patients with hilar cholangiocarcinoma is painless jaundice. Patients may also report concomitant onset of fatigue, pruritus, fever, vague abdominal pain, and anorexia. The serum liver function tests in patients with hilar cholangiocarcinoma commonly demonstrate obstructive jaundice, with alkaline phosphatase and total bilirubin levels elevated in greater than 90% of patients (2). Cholangiocarcinomas that arise in peripheral bile ducts within the hepatic parenchyma usually reach a large size before becoming clinically evident. Patients with these large peripheral hepatic tumors usually present with hepatomegaly and an upper abdominal mass, abdominal and back pain, and weight loss (2). Jaundice and ascites are late and usually preterminal sequelae in patients with large intrahepatic cholangiocarcinomas. Jaundice associated with a large hepatic cholangiocarcinoma is caused by a combination of extension of the tumor to the bifurcation of the left and right hepatic ducts and by compression of contralateral bile ducts by the expanding tumor.

Serum alkaline phosphatase levels are elevated in greater than 90% of patients with cholangiocarcinoma (3). Serum bilirubin also is elevated in the majority of cholangiocarcinoma patients, particularly in those with a tumor arising in the central portion of the liver or the extrahepatic hilar bile ducts (41). In contrast to hepatocellular carcinoma, serum alpha-fetoprotein (AFP) levels are abnormal in less than 5% of cholangiocarcinoma patients (3). There is an increase in serum carcinoembryonic antigen (CEA) levels in 40-60% of cholangiocarcinoma patients (3,42). Another tumor marker, CA 19-9, is elevated in over 80% of patients with cholangiocarcinoma (42). Mild anemia occurs occasionally, but other serum laboratory studies are usually normal. However, clinically significant hypercalcemia in the absence of bone metastases has been described in several patients with large hepatic cholangiocarcinomas (43). In one case, the hypercalcemia was caused by release of parathyroid hormone-related protein by the cholangiocarcinoma (44).

PATHOLOGY

Cholangiocarcinomas appear grossly as fine, gray-white tumors. Cholangiocarcinomas originating in the periphery of the hepatic parenchyma usually are solitary and large, but satellite nodules occasionally are present (1,45). Gross tumor invasion of large portal or hepatic veins occurs much less frequently than in hepatocellular carcinoma. The gross and microscopic appearance of intrahepatic cholangiocarcinomas may have prognostic significance because tumors with periductal infiltration have a higher incidence of lymph node and intrahepatic metastasis (46). Metastases to regional lymph nodes, the lungs, and the peritoneal cavity are more common in cholangiocarcinoma than in hepatocellular carcinoma. When the tumor causes longstanding biliary obstruction, the liver may show secondary biliary cirrhosis.

Microscopically, low cuboidal cells that resemble normal biliary epithelium characterize cholangiocarcinoma. Varying degrees of pleomorphism, atypia, mitotic activity, hyperchromatic nuclei, and prominent nucleoli are noted from area to area in the same tumor. In more poorly differentiated tumors, solid cords of cells without lumens may be present. Rarely, a clear cell variant of cholangiocarcinoma occurs which must be distinguished from clear cell renal carcinoma with liver metastasis (47). Cholangiocarcinomas are mucin-secreting adenocarcinomas, and intracellular and intraluminal mucin often can be demonstrated. The presence of mucin is useful in differentiating cholangiocarcinoma from hepatocellular carcinoma. The presence of bile production by cholangiocarcinoma can also be useful in distinguishing this tumor from a hepatocellular carcinoma. Immunohistochemical staining that is positive for epithelial membrane antigen and tissue polypeptide antigen may be useful in confirming a diagnosis of cholangiocarcinoma (48,49). Immunohistochemical staining for cytokeratin subtypes can be helpful in differentiating cholangiocarcinoma from metastatic colorectal carcinoma (50). Cholangiocarcinomas are usually locally invasive with spread along nerves or in subepithelial layers of the bile ducts.

DIAGNOSTIC STUDIES

Peripheral intrahepatic cholangiocarcinoma is often difficult to distinguish pathologically and radiographically from a deposit of metastatic adenocarcinoma within the liver. While transabdominal ultrasonography can detect an intrahepatic malignant tumor greater than 2 cm in diameter, ultrasound findings do not differ between cholangiocarcinomas, liver metastases from extrahepatic adenocarcinomas, and multinodular hepatocellular carcinoma (51). Computed tomography (CT) demonstrates a rounded, low attenuation mass with irregular or lobulated margins (Fig. 2). Satellite lesions may be evident, particularly when using helical CT during the optimal period of hepatic contrast enhancement. Calcification within the tumor is present in 25% of cases, and a central scar is observed in 30% (52). Magnetic resonance imaging (MRI) shows a nonencapsulated mass with irregular margins that is hypointense compared to normal liver on T1-weighted and hyperintense on T2-weighted images. The peripheral rim of the tumor usually enhances following MRI contrast administration. A hyperintense central scar is best seen on T2-weighted images, but the CT and MRI characteristics of intrahepatic cholangiocarcinomas may be present in other types of hepatic tumors (52).

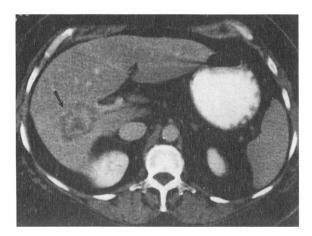

Figure 2. High-resolution, helical CT scan during the late venous contrast phase in a patient with an intrahepatic cholangiocarcinoma. The periphery of the tumor (arrow) has irregular margins and is hypodense relative to the surrounding liver parenchyma. A relatively hypovascular area of scar is evident in the center of the tumor.

The diagnosis of pancreatic cancer is considered frequently in patients presenting with painless jaundice. For this reason, a CT scan of the abdomen may be the first radiologic study obtained. Patients with painless jaundice due to pancreatic cancer may or may not have a mass in the head of the pancreas on a CT scan. They will, however, have dilation of the extrahepatic biliary tree and gallbladder (if the latter has not been removed previously). In contrast, a diagnosis of hilar cholangiocarcinoma should be suspected in the patient with painless jaundice whose CT scan demonstrates dilated intrahepatic bile ducts with a normal gallbladder and extrahepatic biliary tree. High-resolution, helical CT scans can provide information on the location of an obstructing biliary tumor and may suggest the extent of involvement of the liver and porta hepatis structures by the tumor (Figs. 3,4). Multiphasic helical CT can correctly identify the level of biliary obstruction by a hilar cholangiocarcinoma in 63-90% of patients (53-55). Preoperative helical CT is also useful in demonstrating lobar or segmental liver atrophy caused by bile duct obstruction or portal vein occlusion (53) (Fig. 5). However, helical CT is not accurate in assessing the resectability of hilar cholangiocarcinomas because of limited resolution in evaluating intraductal tumor spread and a significant false positive and false negative rate in demonstrating portal vein or hepatic artery involvement by tumor (53-55).

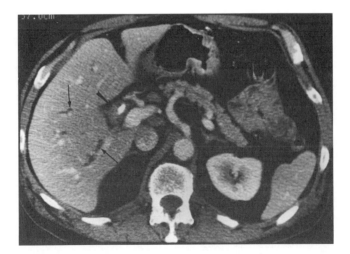

Figure 3. High-resolution, helical CT scan in a patient with obstructive jaundice. The scan demonstrates a tumor (large arrow) anterior to the portal vein with a stent (white area adjacent to large arrow) in place. Dilated intrahepatic bile ducts (small arrows) are evident in the right lobe of the liver.

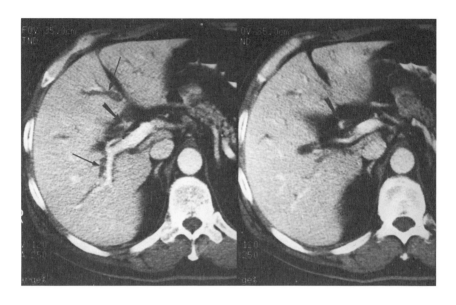

Figure 4.   High-resolution, helical CT scan in another patient presenting with obstructive jaundice.   The small tumor mass (large arrow, left and right panels) is seen as a vascular mass in the bile duct at the hepatic hilum.   Dilated intrahepatic ducts (small arrows) are evident.

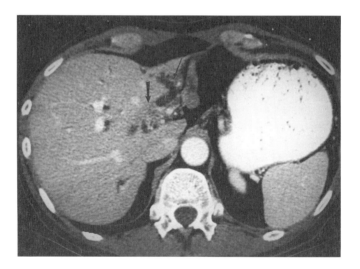

Figure 5. High-resolution, helical CT scan in a patient presenting with several months of increasing pruritus followed by the development of clinically evident jaundice.   The relatively hypodense hilar cholangiocarcinoma (large arrow) is evident.   Marked atrophy of the left hepatic lobe is noted with dilated intrahepatic bile ducts (small arrow) but little remaining hepatic parenchyma is evident.

Ultrasound is the simplest noninvasive study for the jaundiced patient. Like the CT scan, ultrasound can demonstrate a nondilated gallbladder and common bile duct associated with dilated intrahepatic ducts. Additionally, as gray-scale ultrasonography has improved, finding a hilar bile duct mass in 65-90% of patients (56,57) supports the diagnosis of cholangiocarcinoma. Ultrasound and CT scan may be used to demonstrate the presence of intrahepatic tumor due to direct extension or noncontiguous metastases, and enlarged periportal lymph nodes suggesting nodal metastases (57,58). Even intraoperative ultrasonography is suboptimal for detecting intraductal spread by hilar cholangiocarcinoma, correctly demonstrating the extent of tumor spread away from the primary biliary tumor in only 18% of cases (59). Intraoperative ultrasonography can be used to screen for noncontiguous liver metastases from the primary biliary cancer, and can accurately detect direct tumor invasion of the portal vein or hepatic artery in 83.3% and 60% of cases, respectively (59). Recently, endoscopic ultrasonography and intraductal sonography findings have been described in patients with bile duct cancer, but the small number of patients studied precludes determination of the staging accuracy of these techniques (60).

Similar to the intrahepatic variety, hilar cholangiocarcinoma usually shows hypointensity on T1 and hyperintensity on T2-weighted MRI. Dilated intrahepatic bile ducts are evident in patients with obstructing tumors, and lobar atrophy is seen in cases of portal venous occlusion. Fast low-angle shot (FLASH) MR with contrast-enhanced coronal imaging has been used to demonstrate intraluminal extension of tumor and to distinguish between blood vessels and bile ducts (61, 62). Magnetic resonance cholangiopancreatography (MRCP) and MR virtual endoscopy can demonstrate hilar bile duct obstruction by tumor with dilated intrahepatic ducts (61, 63). The advantages of MRCP over direct cholangiography include noninvasiveness and possible visualization of isolated bile ducts. However, MRCP may have limitations relative to direct cholangiography because evaluation of tumor extent is limited by spatial resolution (63).

Cholangiography definitively demonstrates a lesion obstructing the left and right hepatic duct at the hilar confluence (Fig. 6), and percutaneous transhepatic cholangiography (PTC) and endoscopic retrograde cholangiopancreatography (ERCP) are both useful in assessing patients with extrahepatic biliary obstruction. A prospective, randomized comparison of PTC and ERCP in jaundiced patients concluded that both techniques had similar diagnostic accuracy (64). PTC was 100% accurate at demonstrating obstruction at the confluence of the left and right hepatic ducts, while ERCP had an accuracy of 92% in demonstrating these lesions. ERCP has the additional benefit of providing a pancreatogram. A normal pancreatogram helps to exclude a small carcinoma of the head of the pancreas as a cause of biliary obstruction. Some investigators have recommended combined PTC and ERCP to establish the extent of the lesion in the bile ducts; however, such concomitant studies are helpful only in selected patients with complete obstruction of the biliary tree (65). Cytologic specimens can be obtained at the time of PTC and

ERCP. The presence of malignant cells in bile or bile duct brushings is confirmed in
approximately 50% of patients undergoing PTC or ERCP (64,65).

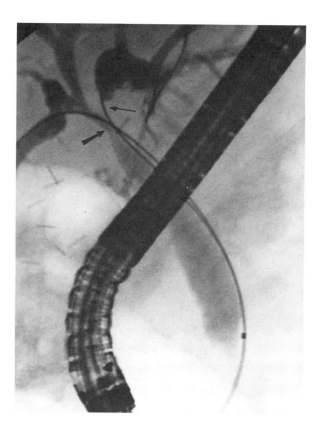

Figure 6.   Endoscopic retrograde cholangiopancreatography (ERCP) showing a
malignant stricture of the right hepatic (large arrow) and left hepatic (small arrow)
bile ducts with marked dilatation of the intrahepatic bile ducts.   This hilar
cholangiocarcinoma was unresectable based on tumor extension into secondary and
tertiary biliary radicals of both lobes of the liver.

Drainage of the obstructed biliary tree with partial or complete relief of jaundice and
associated symptoms can be achieved with PTC.   Improvements in catheter
technology led to the development of endoprostheses that can be placed across the
malignant obstruction into the duodenum to allow internal drainage (66). It must be
emphasized that providing symptomatic relief for patients by decompressing the
biliary tract should not be the primary reason to place these catheters. Prospective,
randomized studies have failed to demonstrate a benefit in terms of a decrease in
hospital morbidity or mortality by preoperative decompression of biliary obstruction

(67,68). However, the catheters are useful in identifying and dissecting the hepatic duct bifurcation at the time of operation and aid in the reconstruction of the biliary tract following extirpation of the tumor (69,70). Although ERCP can be employed to place an internal stent across a malignant hilar obstruction, the success rate with this procedure is much lower than with PTC (71).

Positron emission tomography (PET) is being evaluated as a diagnostic tool in patients with all types of malignant tumors. PET assesses *in vivo* metabolism of positron-emitting radiolabeled tracers like [^{18}F] flouro-2-deoxy-D-glucose (FDG), a glucose analogue that accumulates in various malignant tumors because of their high glucose metabolic rates. FDG-PET does not provide anatomic detail to assess resectability of hilar cholangiocarcinomas or intrahepatic malignancies, but it may prove useful in detecting distant metastatic disease that would preclude a curative resection. In patients with primary sclerosing cholangitis, FDG-PET studies may be able to detect small hilar and intrahepatic cholangiocarcinomas and thus may be useful in therapeutic and transplant decision-making in these patients (72).

The final radiologic study to consider is celiac and superior mesenteric arteriography with late-phase portography. Arteriography in patients with hilar cholangiocarcinoma is important because extensive encasement of the hepatic arteries or portal vein precludes curative resection. Combining the findings on cholangiography with vascular involvement by tumor on arteriography has been found to have a greater than 80% accuracy in predicting unresectability (73). However, occasionally a patient will have compression or displacement of vascular structures rather than true malignant invasion or encasement. A high-resolution, thin-section CT scan with intravenous bolus contrast administration can demonstrate hepatic artery and portal vein involvement by a hilar tumor and obviate the need for more invasive angiographic studies. We obtain an arteriogram in less than 5% of our patients with hilar cholangiocarcinoma.

The role of laparoscopy as part of the diagnostic and staging evaluation of patients with hilar cholangiocarcinoma is being evaluated at our institution. Several patients with seemingly resectable tumors have avoided an exploratory laparotomy when peritoneal tumor implants were found with laparoscopy. Additionally, positive cytologic specimens obtained from laparoscopic washings may identify patients at high risk of developing peritoneal carcinomatosis. Lastly, laparoscopic ultrasonography can be used to exclude the presence of noncontiguous liver metastases or extensive hilar tumor infiltration in patients with extrahepatic bile duct cancers (74).

Treatment of intrahepatic cholangiocarcinoma

The majorities of patients with intrahepatic cholangiocarcinoma present with large tumors and usually have evidence of regional lymph node, pulmonary, and/or bone metastases at the time of diagnosis. In patients who present with jaundice from large intrahepatic cholangiocarcinomas, death usually ensues within a year of diagnosis.

Patients with an elevated serum bilirubin level associated with an intrahepatic cholangiocarcinoma will rarely be candidates for an attempt at curative resection because of coexistent hepatic artery and portal vein invasion, extensive lymph node metastases, bilobar liver involvement by tumor, and/or distant metastases (75). Intrahepatic cholangiocarcinomas may be detected before they metastasize or cause jaundice in 30-45% of patients (75,76). These patients should be considered for operation because long-term survival has been reported in a proportion of the patients undergoing curative liver resection for intrahepatic cholangiocarcinoma (4,75-82). A study of 19 patients who underwent resection of intrahepatic cholangiocarcinoma demonstrated that patients with no porta hepatis lymph node metastases had a 3-year survival rate of 64% compared with 0% for patients with nodal metastases (80). A larger cohort of 32 patients who underwent resection of intrahepatic cholangiocarcinomas confirmed the negative prognostic impact of regional lymph node metastases and large size (>5 cm diameter) of the primary tumor (81). The 5-year overall survival rates reported for patients who underwent a margin-negative liver resection for intrahepatic cholangiocarcinoma range from 20-48%, with regional lymph node metastases, presence of satellite tumor nodules, portal vein invasion by tumor, and large tumors identified as poor prognostic indicator (75-81). Large size of the primary tumor is a poor prognostic indicator because of the increased frequency of vascular and lymphatic invasion by the tumor as well as growth along neighboring bile duct walls (82).

Orthotopic liver transplantation has been described in patients with intrahepatic cholangiocarcinoma (81,83-85). The 1-year survival in series prior to 1990 was 29.4%, with only two of the patients undergoing liver transplantation alive 5 years following the transplant (85). Almost 90% of the patients who survived at least 90 days after the liver transplant died of recurrent cholangiocarcinoma, frequently at extrahepatic sites. Recent small series of patients describe 5-year post-transplantation survival rates up to 53% (83,84). The improved survival is based on careful selection of cholangiocarcinoma patients for liver transplantation, specifically by not transplanting patients with lymph node metastases or invasion of major intrahepatic or extrahepatic blood vessels.

Hilar bile duct cholangiocarcinoma

In 1890, Fardel first described a primary malignancy of the extrahepatic biliary tract (86). A report in 1957 described three patients with small adenocarcinomas involving the confluence of the left and right hepatic ducts (87). Such primary cholangiocarcinomas arising at the bifurcation of the extrahepatic biliary tree are known commonly as Klatskin's tumors, following his report in 1965 of a larger series of patients with these lesions (88).

Cholangiocarcinomas arising in the hilar bile ducts are relatively rare lesions. Extrahepatic biliary cancer has an incidence of 0.01-0.46% in autopsy series (89). Of 17,500 projected new cases of primary hepatobiliary cancers that occur annually in the United States, approximately 2,000 are Klatskin's tumors (90).

PROGNOSTIC FACTORS

In contrast to reports from two or three decades ago, most patients with hilar cholangiocarcinoma are now diagnosed premortem. The most important factors affecting prognosis is resectability of the tumor. Patients who undergo curative resection (margin-negative) have 3-year survival rates from 40-87% and 5-year survival rates between 10% and 73% (91-94). The wide range of survival rates is explained by variations in the incidence of factors that portend a poor prognosis in the various series. Significant determinants of improved prognosis in patients undergoing curative resection include well-differentiated tumors, absence of lymph node metastases, absence of direct tumor extension into the liver, papillary histology (vs. nodular or sclerotic), serum bilirubin at presentation of less than 9 mg/dl, and a near-normal or normal performance status (91). Palliative resection, surgical bypass procedures, and various types of intubation and drainage procedures are associated with 3-year survival rates of 0-4% (92). Hilar cholangiocarcinomas have a poorer prognosis than do carcinomas arising in the middle or distal thirds of the extrahepatic bile duct, which is related directly to presentation of hilar tumors at a more locally advanced stage with bilobar liver involvement by tumor and resultant lower rates of curative resection (95, 96). However, like hilar cholangiocarcinoma, the presence of regional lymph node metastases reduces the 5-year overall survival rate following resection of middle or distal third bile duct cancer to 21% compared to the 65% survival rate in patients with node negative disease (96).

Pathologic features of the bile duct cancer are predictors of outcome. Prognosis is affected adversely if the tumor infiltrates through the serosa of the bile duct, invades directly into the liver, demonstrates vascular invasion, or has metastasized to regional lymph nodes (97). Histologic type and grade also are important factors. Patients with the relatively unusual papillary bile duct adenocarcinoma have the most favorable prognosis, with 3-year survival rates up to 75% (92,97,98). Patients with the more common nodular or sclerotic types of hilar cholangiocarcinoma have 3-year survival rates of less than 30%. A pathologic study that correlated gross tumor type with patterns of spread provides evidence that may explain the observed differences in survival outcomes. Papillary and superficial nodular tumors spread predominantly by mucosal extension, rarely invading deeper layers of the bile duct wall or lymphatic channels, whereas nodular infiltrating or diffuse infiltrating tumors spread by direct or lymphatic extension in the submucosa (99). The distance of mucosal or submucosal spread away from the gross tumor can be as great as 30 mm, but there were no local or anastomotic recurrences if at least a 5 mm tumor-free margin was attained. Patients with well or moderately differentiated carcinomas have a 3-year survival rate of up to 51%, whereas no patient with a poorly differentiated carcinoma survived longer than 2 years (97).

TREATMENT

Resection.   Resection of a hilar cholangiocarcinoma affords the patient the best chance for significant survival; however, 5-year survival rates after resection of hilar cancers are 40% in the most hopeful reports and 10% or less in other accounts. Long-term survival rates after resection of middle or distal common bile duct cholangiocarcinomas, the latter requiring pancreaticoduodenectomy, are generally higher compared to hilar tumors (3). This is most likely related to higher rates of margin-negative resection with middle or distal extrahepatic bile duct tumors and the absence of direct tumor extension into the liver.

The patterns of failure after curative extrahepatic bile duct resection for hilar cholangiocarcinoma have been described in a few series of patients (Table 2) (100). Locoregional tumor recurrence developed in a high percentage of patients, with failure in the liver (62%), tumor bed (42%), and regional lymph nodes (20%). The caudate lobe is the most frequent site of liver recurrence. Regional lymph nodes include porta hepatis, retroduodenal, and perigastric node groups along the gastrohepatic ligament. Distant metastasis develops in the majority of patients who exhibit a locoregional recurrence but was the site of first failure in only 24%.

Table 2.   Sites of tumor recurrence after curative resection of proximal hilar cholangiocarcinomas

Site	Frequency (%)
Liver	62
Tumor bed	42
Regional lymph nodes	20
Peritoneum	16
Lungs	71
Bone	31
Skin	7

Detailed anatomic studies have offered an explanation for the high incidence of liver and local recurrence following resection of a hilar cholangiocarcinoma. In a series of 25 patients undergoing surgery for hilar cholangiocarcinoma, direct invasion of hepatic parenchyma at the hilum was noted in 12 patients (46.2%), with 11 patients (42.3%) also having carcinoma extending into the bile ducts draining the caudate lobe or directly invading the caudate lobe parenchyma (101). A study of 106 adult human cadavers showed that 97.2% had bile ducts draining the caudate lobe that entered directly into the main left hepatic duct, right hepatic duct, or both (102). These caudate lobe bile ducts frequently enter the main left or right hepatic ducts within 1 cm of the proper hepatic duct. Thus, a carcinoma arising at the confluence of the right and left hepatic ducts need not be of a large size to extend into the bile ducts draining the caudate lobe.

Because cholangiocarcinoma is known to spread along the wall of the bile ducts and because the caudate lobe and hepatic hilum are frequent sites of tumor recurrence following extrahepatic duct resection, a number of authors now recommend more aggressive resections to include the caudate lobe and hepatic hilar parenchyma (102-108). An understanding of the Bismuth-Corlette classification of hilar cholangiocarcinoma is useful in planning the extent and site of liver resection (109). The improved equipment and understanding of techniques requisite for a safe liver resection allow performance of aggressive extended resections with little or no increase in operative morbidity and mortality. The median survival associated with a more radical surgical approach has varied from 10 to 37 months, with 5-year survival rates of 20-44% and 10-year survival rates as high as 14% (102-108). These studies clearly show that liver resection is worthwhile only if completely tumor-negative resection margins can be attained, because there were no 5-year survivors with positive resection margins. While aggressive surgical resection of hilar cholangiocarcinomas, including hepatic resection, provides the best chance for long-term patient survival, these operative procedures are associated with significant risk. The operative mortality rate in modern series ranges from 5-12%, with postoperative liver failure following an extensive liver resection being the most common cause of death (102-108). Surgical complications are reported in 25-45% of the surviving patients. Infectious complications are the most common postoperative problem, and preoperative placement of biliary stents with resultant contamination of the obstructed biliary tree increases the incidence of infection (110). Very extensive operations that include major hepatectomy, resection of the extrahepatic bile ducts, and en-bloc pancreaticoduodenectomy have been used in patients with hilar cholangiocarcinoma (111). Given the operative mortality rate of at least 30% and a 100% rate of complications combined with rare survival for more than 2 years, such ultraradical procedures are of dubious value.

A multi-modality approach to reduce locoregional recurrence rates and improve survival after resection has been reported (112). Of 53 patients who underwent resection of a hilar cholangiocarcinoma, 38 received postoperative external-beam radiotherapy to the resection bed at a dose of 50-60 Gy. In addition, 27 of these 38 patients received brachytherapy with iridium-192 seeds temporarily loaded into their transhepatic biliary stents in the area of the hepaticojejunostomies. These 27 patients received 20 Gy of internal radiation after completion of external-beam radiotherapy. There was no significant difference in the 1-, 2-, and 3-year survivals for patients who underwent resection with or without radiotherapy, but there were no survivors past 3 years in the group without radiotherapy. The 5- and 10-year survival rates in the group receiving radiotherapy were 11% and 5%, respectively. Stented hepaticojejunostomies allow access to the remaining biliary tree following resection of hilar cholangiocarcinomas and can be used for diagnostic and therapeutic purposes (113).

We recently reviewed our experience in patients with extrahepatic cholangiocarcinoma treated at the University of Texas M.D. Anderson Cancer Center (114). Of 91 patients evaluated between 1983 and 1996, 51 (56%) presented with unresectable disease and 40 (44%) underwent resection. The median survival for the resected patients was 22.2 months versus 10.7 months in patients with unresectable disease (P<0.0001). Nine patients, five with hilar and four with distal common duct cholangiocarcinoma, were treated with preoperative chemoradiation therapy (continuous intravenous infusion of 5-fluorouracil at 300 mg/m^2/day combined with external beam irradiation). Three of these nine patients had a pathologic complete response to chemoradiation treatment; the remaining six patients had varying degrees of histologic response to treatment. The rate of margin-negative resection was 100% for the preoperative chemoradiation group compared to 54% for the group not receiving preoperative treatment (P<0.01). The patients treated with preoperative chemoradiation had no operative or postoperative complications related to treatment, thus it appears that neoadjuvant chemoradiation for extrahepatic bile duct cancer can be performed safely, produces significant anti-tumor response, and may improve the ability to achieve tumor-free resection margins.

Liver transplantation.   Total hepatectomy with immediate orthotopic liver transplantation (OLT) has been described in patients with hilar cholangiocarcinoma (81,83,84,115-128). The 90-day mortality from hemorrhage, sepsis, and graft rejection was 23.1%. Of the patients who survived more than 3 months following transplantation, the median survival was 11 months in series prior to 1992, but has improved to 23 months in recent series. In the older series of patients, the 5-year survival rate was 5.0%. In patients who died more than 3 months after transplantation, death was due to tumor recurrence in 85.4%. The 5-year survival rate following OLT for extrahepatic cholangiocarcinoma in current studies is 25%, and in the highly selected subset of patients with stage I-or II-disease, 5-year survival is 73% (128). Nonetheless, due to the poor results in most reports, many transplant centers no longer perform liver transplants in patients with hilar cholangiocarcinoma. Liver transplantation for hilar cholangiocarcinoma should probably only be considered as part of a prospective protocol evaluating multimodality treatment.

Palliation.   In general, curative surgical resection is possible in less than 30% of patients with hilar cholangiocarcinoma (91-94,129). Patients deemed unresectable based on the findings of diagnostic studies, can avoid laparotomy by placing percutaneous external drains or endoscopically placed endoprostheses (130,131). Conventional 10- or 12-French polyethylene endoprostheses have a high rate of occlusion and cholangitis (132). However, new expandable metal wall stents appear to have improved long-term patency rates and may be used to deliver palliative high-dose rate endoluminal brachytherapy (133, 134). When unresectability is determined at the time of laparotomy, a decision must be made on a surgical bypass versus an operative intubation to provide drainage of the obstructed biliary tree. It is clear that techniques for surgical bypass, operative intubation, and percutaneous external drainage are equivalent in partial or complete relief of jaundice in 70-100% of patients (91). Seemingly, the only potential advantage to the patient who undergoes surgical bypass instead of operative intubation is the absence of an external drainage catheter in the former group.

The advantage of not having an external biliary drainage catheter or an internal endoscopically placed biliary endoprosthesis should not be underestimated because it is known that the incidence of cholangitis and occlusion or displacement of the catheter or endoprosthesis ranges from 28% to almost 100% (130-132,135). The assessments of quality of life in patients with hilar cholangiocarcinoma who undergo surgical bypass, operative intubation, or percutaneous drainage have not demonstrated a distinct advantage for one type of palliative treatment (91,136). However, some studies suggest that the duration of well-being is longest in patients undergoing surgical bypass procedure (136-139). There is no significant difference in survival related to the type of palliative procedure employed to relive biliary obstruction; the median survival in patients undergoing palliative drainage is 8 months or less. However, effective palliation of biliary obstruction in patients with unresectable hilar cholangiocarcinomas is important because 50% will survive for at least 1 year, 20% will live for 2 years, and 10% will live 3 years or longer (140).

Chemotherapy. Given the high percentage of unresectable hilar cholangiocarcinomas, various chemotherapeutic regimens and radiotherapeutic regimens have been used in the hope of providing improved palliation and prolongation of survival. Adjuvant radiotherapy also has been employed following resection of tumors to reduce locoregional recurrence and potentially to improve survival (112). Unfortunately, reports describing chemotherapy or radiotherapy for hilar cholangiocarcinoma rarely describe the treatment results in more than 10-20 patients.

A 1988 review of systemic chemotherapy for bile duct cancer noted that 97 patients had been treated with nine different treatment programs (141). Mitomycin C, doxorubicin, and 5-fluorouracil are the agents that have shown the greatest activity against cholangiocarcinoma. The collective partial response rate in the 97 patients was 29%, with no complete responses. The median survival of these patients receiving systemic chemotherapy ranged between 6 and 11 months. No reports since 1988 have indicated a better response rate with systemic chemotherapy. With no significant increase in survival and considering the quality-of-life issues related to chemotherapeutic toxicity, systemic chemotherapy has not demonstrated a distinct advantage in patients with hilar cholangiocarcinoma.

Regional chemotherapy by hepatic artery infusion has some potential advantages over systemic chemotherapy. The proximal bile duct receives its arterial blood supply from the hepatic artery so that an increased concentration of drug can be delivered directly to the region of the tumor, including the liver. By using drugs such as 5-fluorouracil and floxuridine, systemic exposure to drug is limited because of the high rate of hepatic extraction of these agents. There are reports of 46 hilar cholangiocarcinoma patients who have been treated by hepatic artery chemotherapy infusion (141,142). The partial response rate for the entire group of patients was

43%, but there were no complete responses and no significant prolongation of survival. Hepatic artery infusion chemotherapy may have a role in palliation of patients with hilar cholangiocarcinoma, but currently available drugs do not provide improved survival.

Radiotherapy. Radiotherapy for bile duct cancer is yet more confusing due to the various types, doses, routes of administration, and association with resected and unresected tumors, all in small numbers of patients. Internal radiation with iridium-192 wires or seeds may have a palliative role in improving the patency of obstructed bile ducts; however, the number and frequency of episodes of cholangitis were not reduced, so the overall benefit is uncertain (143). Internal radiation has been associated with prolongation of survival to an average of 16 months, and occasionally patients with unresectable disease survived more than 5 years (144-146). Although the use of external-beam radiotherapy alone to treat patients with unresectable hilar cholangiocarcinoma has not provided significant differences in overall patient survival, rare long-term survivals have been reported (147). Intraoperative radiotherapy also has been evaluated in association with resectable and unresectable tumors (148,149). Again, there is a suggestion of a slight prolongation of survival in patients with unresectable tumors, but the most interesting use of intraoperative radiotherapy may be as an immediate surgical adjuvant in the resected high-risk tumor bed.

At the University of Texas M.D. Anderson Cancer Center, we have employed a treatment technique of four-field irradiation directed to the porta hepatis to a dose of 45 Gy. Patients receive 5-FU by continuous intravenous infusion during the 5-week course of external-beam irradiation. Further radiotherapy is administered by a reduced treatment field using an arc rotation to deliver an additional dose of 15-20 Gy to the primary target volume (150). We have used this treatment plan for patients who have had a surgical biliary bypass procedure and do not have transcutaneous biliary drainage catheters. This radiation technique envelops the target and a small portion of the duodenum with a high dose. However, in patients with existing external biliary drainage tubes, a combination of external beam plus endoluminal boost irradiation is an attractive treatment program. The favored treatment sequence is to start with external-beam irradiation to obtain tumor regression, which provides a better dose distribution from the endoluminal boost irradiation to treat any residual tumor. We currently use high-dose rate iridium-192 (^{192}Ir) implants in a fractionated treatment schedule of 4 Gy daily for 5 consecutive days. The fractionated high-dose rate treatment, along with the favorable dose distribution obtained with endoluminal therapy, may decrease late-occurring duodenitis. For patients in whom there are technical or medical limitations for fractionated therapy, a single 20 Gy boost with the high-dose technique can be used.

The use of endoluminal ^{192}Ir alone for palliative treatment of patients with unresectable hilar bile duct cancers has been reported (151). Endoluminal doses ranged from 15 Gy to 35 Gy when combined with external-beam irradiation (usually 45-50 Gy), or when endoluminal doses of up to 60 Gy were used alone. The dose reference point may vary from 0.5 cm to 1.0 cm from the central catheter. The total nominal doses of external-beam plus endoluminal boost irradiation are between 60 Gy and 70 Gy to the tumor, and although this range exceeds the liver and small intestine tolerance, the highest doses are confined to a small volume of tissue. The median survival for patients treated by this endoluminal method, with or without external-beam irradiation, is 15-18 months. Several patients survived for more than 4 years after treatment; however, the majority of patients failed locally.

Complications with the endoluminal boost have been related mainly to cholangitis, which occurs to some degree in nearly all patients. Septic cholangitis and death occur in less than 15% of the patients because antibiotic therapy is usually effective. Prophylactic antibiotics are not recommended because flora colonizing the catheter tract became drug resistant. A better approach to reduce sepsis is to remove the drainage catheter after therapy whenever there is cholangiographic evidence of bile duct patency following treatment.

Another specialized technique that has been used for boost treatments of biliary tract cancers is electron beam intraoperative radiotherapy (EB-IORT) (152). This technique improves the dose distribution by concentrating treatment directly on the target volume, while the uninvolved liver, adjacent duodenum, and stomach are excluded from the treatment field during surgery. Nine patients with advanced proximal biliary cancers were treated with EB-IORT in one report (153). Patients were considered for IORT if they had residual gross or microscopic disease confined to the region of the porta hepatis, or if there was adjacent hepatic parenchymal involvement by tumor. The field size was 7-10 cm in diameter, and the IOR dose was 10-22 Gy. In five patients, additional external-beam irradiation was given. An analysis of the patients treated with EB-IORT was made with concurrent groups who were treated without radiation or with external-beam irradiation with or without ^{192}Ir endoluminal boost irradiation. There was a significant improvement in median survival for the patients receiving high-dose irradiation, regardless of boost technique, compared with those who were not irradiated (13 vs. 4.6 months, respectively). Duodenitis occurred in most of the patients who received any form of irradiation, and portal vein thrombosis was observed in one patient who was treated with EB-IORT.

REFERENCES

1. Anthony PP. Tumours and tumour-like lesions of the liver and biliary tract. In MacSween RNM, Anthony PP, Scheuer PJ (eds). Pathology of the Liver, 2nd ed. Edinburgh: Churchill Livingstone, 1987, p. 574.
2. Thuluvath PJ, Rai R, Venbrux AC, Yeo CJ. Cholangiocarcinoma: A review. Gastroenterologist 5:306-315, 1997.
3. Nakeeb A, Pitt HA, Sohn TA, et al. Cholangiocarcinoma: A spectrum of intrahepatic, perihilar, and distal tumors. Ann Surg 224:463-475, 1996.
4. The Liver Cancer Study Group of Japan. Primary liver cancer in Japan. Cancer 54:1747-1755, 1984.

5. Sorensen HT, Friis S, Olsen JH, et al. Risk of liver and other types of cancer in patients with cirrhosis: A nationwide cohort study in Denmark. Hepatology 28:921-925, 1998.
6. Schwartz DA. Cholangiocarcinoma associated with liver fluke infection: A preventable source of morbidity in Asian immigrants. Am J Gastroenterol 81:76-79, 1986.
7. Kurathong S, Lerdverasirikul P, Wonkpaitoon V, et al. *Opisthorchis viverrini* infection and cholangiocarcinoma. A prospective, case-controlled study. Gastroenterology 89:151-156, 1985.
8. Nakashima T, Okuda K, Kojiro M, et al. Primary liver cancer coincident with *Schistosomiasis japonica*. A study of 23 necropsies. Cancer 36:1483-1489, 1975.
9. Kim KH, Kim CD, Lee HS, et al. Biliary papillary hyperplasia with clonorchiasis resembling cholangiocarcinoma. Am J Gastroenterol 94:514-517, 1999.
10. Nakanuma Y, Terada T, Tanka Y. Are hepatolithiasis and cholangiocarcinoma aetiologically related? A morphological study of 12 cases of hepatolithiasis associated with cholangiocarcinoma. Virchows Arch A Pathol Anat Histopathol 406:45-58, 1985.
11. Thamavit W, Phamarapravati N, Sahaphong S, et al. Effects of dimethylnitrosamine on induction of cholangiocarcinoma in *Opisthorchis viverrini*-infected Syrian golden hamsters. Cancer Res 38:4634-4639, 1978.
12. Prempracha N, Tengchaisri T, Chawengkirttikul R, et al. Identification and potential use of a soluble tumor antigen for the detection of liver-fluke-associated cholangiocarcinoma induced in a hamster model. Int J Cancer 57:691-695, 1994.
13. Landais P, Drunfeld JP, Droz D, et al. Cholangiocellular carcinoma in polycystic kidney and liver disease. Arch Intern Med 144:2274-2276, 1984.
14. Voyles CR, Smadja C, Shands W, Blumgart LH. Carcinoma in choledochal cysts. Age-related incidence. Arch Surg 118:986-988, 1983.
15. Imamura M, Miyashita T, Tani T, et al. Cholangiocellular carcinoma associated with multiple liver cysts. Am J Gastroenterol 79:790-795, 1984.
16. Dayton MT, Longmire WP, Tompkins RK. Caroli's disease: A premalignant condition? Am J Surg 145:41-48, 1983.
17. Wee A, Ludwig L, Coffey RJ, et al. Hepatobiliary carcinoma associated with primary sclerosing cholangitis and chronic ulcerative colitis. Hum Pathol 16:719-726, 1985.
18. Chen PH, Lo HW, Wang CS, et al. Cholangiocarcinoma in hepatolithiasis. J Clin Gastroenterol 6:539-547, 1984.
19. Koga A, Ichimiya H, Yamaguchi, et al. Hepatolithiasis associated with cholangiocarcinoma, possible etiologic significance. Cancer 55:2826-2829, 1985.

20. Yoshimoto H, Ikeda S, Tanaka M, Matsumoto S. Intrahepatic cholangiocarcinoma associated with hepatolithiasis. Gastrointest Endosc 31:260-263, 1985.

21. Chen MF, Jan YY, Wang CS, et al. A reappraisal of cholangiocarcinoma in patients with hepatolithiasis. Cancer 71:2461-2465, 1993.

22. Chijiiwa K, Ichimaya H, Kuroki S, et al. Late development of cholangiocarcinoma after the treatment of hepatolithiasis. Surg Gynecol Obstet 177:279-282, 1993.

23. Robertson JF, Raine PA. Choledochal cyst: A 33 year review. Br J Surg 75:799-801, 1988.

24. Lipsett PA, Pitt HA, Colombani PM, et al. Choledochal cyst disease. A changing pattern of presentation. Ann Surg 220:644-652, 1994.

25. Cherqui D, Tantawi B, Alon R, et al. Relationships between sclerosing cholangitis, inflammatory bowel disease, and cancer in patients undergoing liver transplantation. Surgery 118:615-619, 1995.

26. Rosen CB, Nagorney DM, Wiesner RH, et al. Cholangiocarcinoma complicating primary sclerosing cholangitis. Ann Surg 213:21-25, 1991.

27. Van Laethem JL, Deviere J, Bourgeois N, et al. Cholangiographic findings in deteriorating primary sclerosing cholangitis. Endoscopy 27:223-228, 1995.

28. Nichols JC, Gores GJ, LaRusso NF, et al. Diagnostic role of serum CA 19-9 for cholangiocarcinoma in patients with primary sclerosing cholangitis. Mayo Clin Proc 68:874-879, 1993.

29. Ramage JK, Donaghy A, Farrant JM, et al. Serum tumor markers for the diagnosis of cholangiocarcinoma in primary sclerosing cholangitis. Gastroenterology 108:865-869, 1995.

30. Ito Y, kojiro J, Nakashima T, Mori T. Pathomorphologic characteristics of 102 cases of thorotrast-related hepatocellular carcinoma, cholangiocarcinoma and hepatic angiosarcoma. Cancer 62:1153-1162, 1988.

31. Rubel LR, Ishak KG. Thorotrast-associated cholangiocarcinoma. An epidemiologic and clinicopathologic study. Cancer 50:1408-1415, 1982.

32. Sell S, Dunsford HA. Evidence for the stem cell origin of hepatocellular carcinoma and cholangiocarcinoma. Am J Pathol 134:1347-1363, 1989.

33. Okada Y, Jinno K, Moriwaki S, et al. Expression of ABH and Lewis blood group antigens in combined hepatocellular-cholangiocarcinoma. Possible evidence for the hepatocellular origin of combined hepatocellular-cholangiocarcinoma. Cancer 60:345-352, 1985.

34. Goodman ZD, Ishak KG, Longloss JM, et al. Combined hepatocellular-cholangiocarcinoma. A histologic and immunohistochemical study. Cancer 55:124-135, 1985.

35. Ding SF, Delhanty JD, Bowles L, et al. Loss of constitutional heterozygosity on chromosomes 5 and 17 in cholangiocarcinoma. Br J Cancer 67:1007-1010, 1993.

36. Sturm PDJ, Baas IO, Clement MJ, et al. Alterations of the *p53* tumor-suppressor gene and K-*ras* oncogene in perihilar cholangiocarcinomas from a high-incidence area. Int J Cancer 78:695-698, 1998.
37. Wattanasirichaigoon S, Tasanakhajorn U, Jesadapatarakul S. The incidence of K-*ras* codon 12 mutations in cholangiocarcinoma detected by polymerase chain reaction technique. J Med Assoc Thai 81:316-323, 1998.
38. Petmitr S, Pinlaor S, Thousungnoen A, et al. K-*ras* oncogene and *p53* gene mutations in cholangiocarcinoma from Thai patients. Southeast Asian J trop Med Public Health 29:71-75, 1998.
39. Terada T, Ashida K, Endo K, et al. c-erbB-2 protein is expressed in hepatolithiasis and cholangiocarcinoma. Histopathology 33:325-331, 1998.
40. Celli A, Que FG. Dysregulation of apoptosis in the cholangiopathies and cholangiocarcinoma. Sem Liver Dis 18:177-185, 1998.
41. Pitt H, Dooley W, Yeo C, Cameron J. Malignancies of the biliary tree. Curr Probl Surg 32:1-90, 1995.
42. Jalanko H, Kuusela P, Roberts P, et al. Comparison of a new tumor marker, CA 19-9T, with α-fetoprotein and carcinoembryonic antigen in patients with upper gastrointestinal disease. J Clin Pathol 37:218-222, 1984.
43. Oldenburg WA, Van Heerden PA, Sizemore GW, et al. Hypercalcemia and primary hepatic tumors. Arch Surg 117:1363-1366, 1992.
44. Davis JM, Sadasivan R, Dwyer T, et al. Case report: Cholangiocarcinoma and hypercalcemia. AM J Med Sci 307:350-352, 1994.
45. Weinbren K, Mutum SS. Pathological aspects of cholangiocarcinoma. J Pathol 139:217-238, 1983.
46. Aoki K, Takayasu K, Kawano T, et al. Combined hepatocellular carcinoma and cholangiocarcinoma: Clinical features and computed tomographic findings. Hepatology 18:1090-1095, 1993.
47. Yamamoto M, Takasaki K, Yoshikawa T, Ueno K, Nakano M. Does gross appearance indicate prognosis in intrahepatic cholangiocarinoma? J Surg Oncol 69:162-167, 1998.
48. Bonetti F, Chilosi M, Posa R, et al. Epithelial membrane antigen expression in cholangiocarcinoma. A useful immunohistochemical tool for differential diagnosis with hepatocarcinoma. Virchows Arch A Pathol Anat Histopathol 401:307-313, 1983.
49. Pastolero GC, Wakabayashi T, Oka T, Mori S. Tissue polypeptide antigen: A marker antigen differentiating cholangiolar tumors from other hepatic tumors. Am J Clin Pathol 87:168-173, 1987.
50. Sasaki A, Kawano K, Aramaki M, et al. Immunohistochemical expression of cyto keratins in intrahepatic cholangiocarcinoma and metastatic adenocarcinoma of the liver. J Surg Oncol 70:103-108, 1999.
51. Colli A, Cocciolo M, Mumoli N, et al. Peripheral intrahepatic cholangiocarcinoma: ultrasound findings and differential diagnosis from hepatocellular carcinoma. Eur J Ultrasound 7:93-99, 1998.
52. Kuszyk BS, Soyer P, Bluemke DA, Fishman EK. Intrahepatic cholangiocarcinoma: The role of imaging in detection and staging. Critical Rev in Diag Imaging 38:59-88, 1997.

53. Feydy A, Vilgrain V, Denys A, et al. Helical CT assessment in hilar cholangiocarcinoma: Correlation with surgical and pathologic findings. AJR 172:73-77, 1999.
54. Tillich M, Mischinger HJ, Preisegger KH, et al. Multiphasic helical CT in diagnosis and staging of hilar cholangiocarcinoma. AJR 171:651-658, 1998.
55. Han JK, Choi BI, Kim TK, Kim SW, Han MC, Yeon KM. Hilar cholangiocarcinoma: Thin-section spiral CT findings with cholangiographic correlation. Radiographics 17:1475-1485, 1997.
56. Okuda K, Ohto M, Tsuchiya Y. The role of ultrasound, percutaneous transhepatic cholangiography, computed tomographic scanning, and magnetic resonance imaging in the preoperative assessment of bile duct cancer. World J Surg 12:18-26, 1988.
57. Garber ST, Donald JJ, Lees WR. Cholangiocarcinoma: Ultrasound features and correlation of tumor position with survival. Abdom Imaging 18:66-69, 1993.
58. Neumaier CE, Bertolotto M, Perrone R, Martinoli C, et al. Staging of hilar cholangiocarcinoma with ultrasound. J Clin Ultrasound 23:173-178, 1995.
59. Kusano T, Shimabukuro M, Tamai O, et al. The use of intraoperative ultrasonography for detecting tumor extension in bile duct carcinoma. Int Surg 82:44-48, 1997.
60. Fujita N, Noda Y, Kobayashi G, et al. Staging of bile duct carcinoma by EUS and IDUS. Endoscopy 30:A132-A134, 1998.
61. Choi BI, Kim TK, Han JK. MRI of clonorchiasis and cholangiocarcinoma. J MRI 8:359-366, 1998.
62. Worawattanakul S, Semelka RC, Noone TC, et al. Cholangiocarcinoma: Spectrum of appearances on MR images using current techniques. Magnetic Resonance Imaging 16:993-1003, 1998.
63. Neri E, Boraschi P, Braccini G, et al. MR virtual endoscopy of the pancreaticobiliary tract. Magnetic Resonance Imaging 17:59-67, 1999.
64. Elias E, Hamlyn AN, Jain S, et al. A randomized trial of percutaneous transhepatic cholangiography with the Chiba needle versus ERCP for bile duct visualization in jaundice. Gastroenterology 71:439-443, 1976.
65. Tanaka M, Ogawa Y, Matsumoto S, et al. The role of endoscopic retrograde cholangiopancreatography in preoperative assessment of bile duct cancer. World J Surg 12:27-32, 1988.
66. Yamakawa T, Esguerra R, Kaneko H, et al. Percutaneous transhepatic endoprosthesis in malignant obstruction of the bile duct. World J Surg 12:78-84, 1988.
67. Pitt HA, Gomes AS, Lois JF, et al. Does preoperative percutaneous biliary drainage reduce operative risk or increase hospital cost? Ann Surg 201:545-553, 1985.
68. McPherson GAD, Benjamin IS, Hodjson HJF, et al. Preoperative percutaneous transhepatic biliary drainage: The results of a controlled trial. Br J Surg 71:371-375, 1984.

69. Cameron JL, Broe P, Zuidema GD. Proximal bile duct tumors: Surgical management with silastic transhepatic biliary stents. Ann Surg 196:412-419, 1982.

70. Crist DW, Kadir S, Cameron JL. The value of preoperatively placed percutaneous biliary catheters in reconstruction of the proximal part of the biliary tree. Surg Gynecol Obstet 165:421-424, 1987.

71. Soehendra N, Grimm H. Endoscopic retrograde drainage for bile duct cancer. World J Surg 12:85-90, 1988.

72. Keiding S, Hansen SB, Rasmussen HH, et al. Detection of cholangiocarcinoma in primary sclerosing cholangitis by positron emission tomography. Hepatology 28:700-706, 1998.

73. Voyles CR, Bowley NJ, Allison DJ, et al. Carcinoma of the proximal extrahepatic biliary tree, radiologic assessment and therapeutic alternatives. Ann Surg 197:188-194, 1983.

74. Van Delden OM, de Wit LT, van Dijkum EJ, et al. Value of laparoscopic ultrasonography in staging of proximal bile duct tumors. J Ultrasound Med 16:7-12, 1997.

75. Roayaie S, Guarrera JV, Ye MQ, et al. Aggressive surgical treatment of intrahepatic cholangiocarcinoma: Predictors of outcomes. J Am Coll Surg 187:365-372, 1998.

76. Lieser MJ, Barry K, Rowland C, et al. Surgical management of intrahepatic cholangiocarcinoma: A 31-year experience. J Hep Bil Pancr Surg 5:41-47, 1998.

77. Sixth report. Liver Cancer Study Group of Japan. Primary liver cancer in Japan. Cancer 60:1400-1411, 1987.

78. Liguory C, Canard JM. Tumours of the biliary system. Clin Gastroenterol 12:269-295, 1983.

79. Harrison LE, Fong Y, Klimstra DS, et al. Surgical treatment of 32 patients with peripheral intrahepatic cholangiocarcinoma. Br J Surg 85:1068-1070, 1998.

80. Chou FF, Sheen-Chen SM, Chen CL, et al. Prognostic factors of resectable intrahepatic cholangiocarcinoma. J Surg Oncol 59:40-44, 1995.

81. Pichlmayr R, Lamesch P, Weimann A, Tusch G, Ringe B. Surgical treatment of cholangiocellular carcinoma. World J Surg 19:83-88, 1995.

82. Sasaki A, Aramaki M, Kawano K, et al. Intrahepatic peripheral cholangiocarcinoma: Mode of spread and choice of surgical treatment. Br J Surg 85:1206-1209, 1998.

83. Sansalone CV, Colella G, Caccamo L, et al. Orthotopic liver transplantation for primary biliary tumors: Milan multicenter experience. Transplant Proc 26:3561-3563, 1994.

84. Goldstein RM, Stone M, Tillery GW, et al. Is liver transplantation indicated for cholangiocarcinoma? Am J Surg 166:768-771, 1993.

85. Curley SA, Levin B, Rich TA. Liver and bile ducts. In Abeloff MD, Armitage JO, Lichter AS, Niederhuber JE (eds). Clinical Oncology. London: Churchill Livingston, 1995, p. 1305-1372.

86. Fardel D. Malignant neoplasms of the extrahepatic biliary ducts. Ann Surg 76:205-211, 1922.

87. Altmeier WA, Gall EA, Zinninger MM, et al. Sclerosing carcinoma of the major intrahepatic bile ducts. Arch Surg 75:450-454, 1957.

88. Klatskin G. Adenocarcinoma of the hepatic duct at its bifurcation within the porta hepatis. Am J Med 38:241-248, 1965.

89. Sako K, Seitzinger GL, Garside E. Carcinoma of the extrahepatic bile ducts: Review of the literature and report of six cases. Surgery 41:416-422, 1957.

90. Landis SH, Murray T, Bolden S, Wingo PA. Cancer Statistics, 1999. CA-A Cancer Journal for Clinicians 49:8-31, 1999.

91. Bismuth H, Castaing D, Traynor O. Resection or palliation: Priority of surgery in the treatment of hilar cancer. World J Surg 12:39-47, 1988.

92. Nagorney DM, Donohue JH, Farnell MB, et al. Outcomes after curative resections of cholangiocarcinoma. Arch Surg 128:871-879, 1993.

93. Nimura Y, Kamiya J, Nagino M, et al. Aggressive surgical treatment of hilar cholangiocarcinoma. J Hep Bil Pancr Surg 5:52-61, 1998.

94. Burke EC, Jarnigan WR, Hochwald SN, et al. Hilar cholangiocarcinoma: Patterns of spread, the importance of hepatic resection for curative operation, and a presurgical clinical staging system. Ann Surg 228:385-394, 1998.

95. Chung C, Bautista N, O'Connell TX. Prognosis and treatment of bile duct carcinoma. Am Surg 64:921-925, 1998.

96. Kayahara M, Nagakawa T, Ohta T, et al. Role of nodal involvement and the periductal soft-tissue margin in middle and distal bile duct cancer. Ann Surg 229:76-83, 1999.

97. Tompkins RK, Thomas D, Wile A, et al. Prognostic factors in bile duct carcinoma. Ann Surg 194:447-457, 1981.

98. Ouchi K, Suzuki M, Hashimoto L, et al. Histologic findings and prognostic factors in carcinoma of the upper bile duct. Am J Surg 157:552-556, 1989.

99. Sakamoto E, Nimura Y, Hayakawa N, et al. The pattern of infiltration at the proximal border of hilar bile duct carcinoma: A histologic analysis of 62 resected cases. Ann Surg 227:405-411, 1998.

100. Mittal B, Deutsch M, Iwatsuki S. Primary cancers of the extrahepatic biliary passages. Int J Radiat Oncol Biol Phys 11:849-854, 1985.

101. Mizumoto R, Kawarada Y, Suzuki H. Surgical treatment of hilar carcinoma of the bile duct. Surg Gynecol Obstet 162:153-158, 1986.

102. Mizumoto R, Suzuki H. Surgical anatomy of the hepatic hilum with special reference to the caudate lobe. World J Surg 12:2-10, 1988.

103. Bengmark S, Ekberg H, Evander A, et al. Major liver resection for hilar cholangiocarcinoma. Ann Surg 207:120-125, 1988.

104. White TT. Skeletization resection and central hepatic resection in the treatment of bile duct cancer. World J Surg 12:48-51, 1988.

105. Pinson CW, Rossi RL. Extended right hepatic lobectomy, left hepatic lobectomy, and skeletonization resection for proximal bile duct cancer. World J Surg 12:52-59, 1988.

106.Washburn WK, Lewis WD, Jenkins RL. Aggressive surgical resection for cholangiocarcinoma. Arch Surg 130:270-276, 1995.

107.Baer HU, Stain SC, Dennison AR, Eggers B, Blumgart LH. Improvements in survival by aggressive resections of hilar cholangiocarcinoma. Ann Surg 217:20-27, 1993.

108.Nagino M, Nimura Y, Kamiya J, et al. Segmental liver resections for hilar cholangiocarcinoma. Hepatogastroenterology 45:7-13, 1998.

109.Bismuth H, Corlette MB. Intrahepatic cholangioenteric anastomosis in carcinoma of the hilus of the liver. Surg Gynecol Obstet 140:170-178, 1975.

110.Hochwald SN, Burke EC, Jarnagin WR, et al. Association of preoperative biliary stenting with increased postoperative infectious complications in proximal cholangiocarcinoma. Arch Surg 134:261-266, 1999.

111.Tsukada K, Yoshida K, Aono T, Koyama S, Shirai Y, Uchida K, Muto T. Major hepatectomy and pancreatoduodenectomy for advanced carcinoma of the biliary tract. Br J Surg 81:108-110, 1994.

112.Cameron JL, Pitt HA, Zinner MJ, et al. Management of proximal cholangiocarcinomas by surgical resection and radiotherapy. Am J Surg 159:91-98, 1990.

113.Alexandre JH, Dehni N, Bouillot JL. Stented hepaticojejunostomies after resection for cholangiocarcinoma allow access for subsequent diagnosis and therapy. Am J Surg 169:428-429, 1995.

114.McMasters KM, Tuttle TM, Leach SD, et al. Neoadjuvant chemoradiation enhances margin-negative resection rates for extrahepatic cholangiocarcinoma. Am J Surg 174:605-609, 1997.

115.Ringe B, Wittekind C, Bechstein WO, et al. The role of liver transplantation in hepatobiliary malignancy. Ann Surg 209:88-98, 1989.

116.O'Grady JG, Polson RJ, Rolles K, et al. Liver transplantation for malignant disease. Ann Surg 207:373-379, 1988.

117.Funovics JM, Fritsch A, Herbst F, et al. Primary hepatic cancer – the role of limited resection and total hepatectomy with orthotopic liver replacement. Hepatogastroenterology 35:316-320, 1988.

118.Iwatsuki S, Gordon RD, Shaw BW, Starzl TE. Role of liver transplantation in cancer therapy. Ann Surg 202:401-407, 1985.

119.Koneru B, Cassavilla A, Bowman J, et al. Liver transplantation for malignant tumors. Gastroenterol Clin North Am 17:177-193, 1988.

120.Yokoyama I, Todo S, Iwatsuki S, Starzl TE. Liver transplantation in the treatment of primary liver cancer. Hepatogastroenterology 37:188-193, 1990.

121.Yokoyama I, Sheahan DG, Carr B, et al. Clinicopathologic factors affecting patient survival and tumor recurrence after orthotopic liver transplantation for hepatocellular carcinoma. Transpl Proc 24:2194-2196, 1991.

122.Olthoff KM, Millis JM, Rosove MH, et al. Is liver transplantation justified for the treatment of hepatic malignancies? Arch Surg 125:1261-1268, 1990.

123. Jenkins RL, Pinson CW, Stone MD. Experience with transplantation in the treatment of liver cancer. Cancer Chemother Pharmacol 23(Suppl):S104-S109, 1989.

124. Margeiter R. Indications for liver transplantation for primary and secondary liver tumor. Transpl Proc 18(Suppl 3):74-80, 1986.

125. Angrisano L, Jurewicz WA, Clements DG, et al. Liver transplantation for liver cancer. Transpl Proc 18:1218-1225, 1986.

126. Ismail T, Angrisani L, Gunson BK, et al. Primary hepatic malignancy: The role of liver transplantation. Br J Surg 77:983-987, 1990.

127. Van Thiel DH, Carr B, Iwatsuki S, et al. Liver transplantation for alcoholic liver disease, viral hepatitis, and hepatic neoplasms. Transpl Proc 23:1917-1921, 1991.

128. Iwatsuki S, Todo S, Marsh JW, et al. Treatment of hilar cholangiocarcinoma (Klatskin tumors) with hepatic resection or transplantation. J Am Coll Surg 187:358-364, 1998.

129. Langer JC, Langer B, Taylor BR, et al. Carcinoma of the extrahepatic bile ducts: results of an aggressive surgical approach. Surgery 98:752-759, 1985.

130. Lameris JS, Stoker J, Dees J, et al. Non-surgical palliative treatment of patients with malignant biliary obstruction – the place of endoscopic and percutaneous drainage. Clin Radiol 38:603-608, 1987.

131. Huibregtse K, Tytgat GN. Palliative treatment of obstructive jaundice by transpapillary introduction of large bore bile duct endoprosthesis. Gut 23:371-375, 1982.

132. O'Brien S, Hatfield ARW, Carig PI, Williams SP. A three-year follow-up of self-expanding metal stents in the endosc, opic palliation of long term survivors with malignant biliary obstruction. Gut 36:618-621, 1995

133. Shim CS, Lee YH, Cho YD, et al. Preliminary results of a new covered biliary metal stent for malignant biliary obstruction. Endoscopy 30:345-350, 1998.

134. Kubota Y, Takaoka M, Kin H, et al. Endoscopic irradiation and parallel arrangement of wallstents for hilar cholangiocarcinoma. Hepatogastroenterology 45:415-419, 1998.

135. Mueller PR, van Sonnenberg E, Ferrucci JT, Jr. Percutaneous biliary drainage: Technical and catheter-related problems in 200 procedures. AJR 138:17-23, 1982.

136. Lai ECS, Tompkins RK, Roslyn JJ, et al. Proximal bile duct cancer: Quality of survival. Ann Surg 205:111-118, 1987.

137. Malangoni MA, McCoy DM, Richardson JD, Flint LM. Effective palliation of malignant biliary duct obstruction. Ann Surg 201:554-559, 1985.

138. Nordaback IH, Pitt HA, Coleman J, Venbrux AC, et al. Unresectable hilar cholangiocarcinoma: Percutaneous versus operative palliation. Surgery 115:597-603, 1994.

139. Guthrie CM, Banting SW, Garden OJ, Carter DC. Segment III cholangiojejunostomy for palliation of malignant hilar obstruction. Br J Surg 81:1639-1641, 1994.

140. Farley DR, Weaver AL, Nagorney DM. 'Natural history' of unresected cholangiocarcinoma: Patient outcome after noncurative intervention. Mayo Clin Proc 70:425-429, 1995.

141. Oberfield RA, Rossi RL. The role of chemotherapy in the treatment of bile duct cancer. World J Surg 12:105-108, 1988.

142. Curley SA, Cameron JL. Hilar bile duct cancer: A diagnostic and therapeutic challenge. Cancer Bull 44:309-315, 1992.

143. Meyers WC, Jones RS. Internal radiation for bile duct cancer. World J Surg 12:99-104, 1988.

144. Karani J, Fletcher M, Brinkley D, et al. Internal biliary drainage and local radiotherapy with iridium-192 wire in treatment of hilar cholangiocarcinoma. Clin Radiol 36:603-606, 1985.

145. Johnson DW, Safai C, Goffinet DR. Malignant obstructive jaundice: Treatment with external-beam and intracavity radiotherapy. Int J Radiat Biol Phys 11:411-416, 1985.

146. Mornex F, Ardiet JM, Bret P, et al. Radiotherapy of high bile duct carcinoma using intracatheter iridium 192 wire. Cancer 54:2069-2073, 1984.

147. Hishikawa Y, Shimada T, Miura T, et al. Radiation therapy of carcinoma of the extrahepatic bile ducts. Radiology 146:787-789, 1983.

148. Busse PM, Stone MD, Sheldon TA, et al. Intraoperative radiation therapy for biliary tract carcinoma: Results of a 5-year experience. Surgery 105:724-733, 1989.

149. Iwasaki Y, Todoroki T, Fukao K, et al. The role of intraoperative radiation therapy in the treatment of bile duct cancer. World J Surg 12:91-98, 1988.

150. Rich TA. Treatment planning for tumors of the gastrointestinal tract. In Paliwal BR, Griem ML (eds). Syllabus: A Categorical Course in Radiation Therapy Treatment Planning. Illinois: RSNA Division of Editorial and Publishing Services, 1986, p. 47.

151. Nunnerly HB. Interventional radiology and internal radiotherapy for bile duct tumors. In Preece PE, Cushieri A, Rosin RD (eds). Cancer of the Bile Ducts and Pancreas. Philadelphia: W.B. Saunders, 1989, p 93.

152. Rich TA. Intraoperative radiotherapy: A review. Radiother Oncol 6:207-221, 1986.

153. Deziel DJ, Kiel KD, Kramer TS, et al. Intraoperative radiation therapy in biliary tract cancer. Am Surg 54:402-407, 1988.

8
GALLBLADDER CANCER

Lillian G. Dawes, M.D.
University of Michigan, Ann Arbor, MI

INTRODUCTION

The gallbladder lies between the right and left lobe of the liver and attaches to the liver at the under surface of segment IV and V. In this protected position, it acidifies, concentrates and stores bile. When stimulated to contract the gallbladder delivers bile salts and other biliary components into the intestine where these substances aid in the absorption of nutrients.

Benign and malignant lesions in the gallbladder can remain silent for a considerable amount of time. In the case of gallstones this is not a problem for therapy is not indicated until symptoms are manifest. Unfortunately this is not true for gallbladder cancer. Too often the symptoms of gallbladder cancer, jaundice, pain or a mass are associated with advanced disease. This may at least in part explain the dismal prognosis of this disease. Surgical therapy is the best treatment with no effective chemotherapy regimen to date. Although rare, comprising only 2% of gastrointestinal malignancies, gallbladder cancer remains a challenge for the future.

PRESENTATION

Gallbladder cancer has an incidence of about 2.5 per 100,000 population. It is more frequent in females and the female/male ratio is 3:1. Cancer of the gallbladder primarily occurs in the elderly and the mean age at presentation is 65. Ten percent of gallbladder cancers are serendipitously found at the time of cholecystectomy for presumed symptomatic cholelithiasis. This scenario can lead to finding of an early gallbladder cancer and often has the best prognosis

Most gallbladder cancers are locally aggressive and symptoms from this local extension of tumor are what bring individuals to medical attention. Common symptoms are jaundice, pain or a mass. Weight loss and fatigue are frequent with larger tumors.

Gallbladder cancer often obstructs the cystic duct and can erode into the common bile duct. Jaundice occurs when the gallbladder cancer grows to obstruct the bile duct. When the tumor obstructs the cystic duct, acute cholecystitis can result. Ten percent of all gallbladder cancers present with acute cholecystitis. Since the majority of patients with gallbladder cancer are over the age of sixty, elderly patients with acute cholecystitis and jaundice should have additional evaluation (1). If the possibility of a gallbladder cancer is high, an open procedure should be considered. There is also an association of Mirizzi's syndrome with gallbladder cancer (2). Mirizzi's syndrome occurs when an impacted large stone in the cystic duct obstructs the hepatic bile duct. Consideration for the possibility of gallbladder cancer should be given prior to operation on patients with this finding.

Intermittent right upper quadrant pain can be the presenting symptom with gallbladder cancer. This pain can be similar to biliary colic. Whether the pain is from the cancer or from coexistent gallstones is not always possible to discern since 90% of the patients with gallbladder cancer also have gallstones. The incidence of gallbladder cancer increases as the size of the gallstone increases and gallstone disease increases the risk of gallbladder cancer (3,4). This finding has lead to the postulate that chronic inflammation from irritation by the gallstones may have a causative role in gallbladder cancer. With the low incidence of gallbladder cancer, however, cholecystectomy is not indicated in asymptomatic patients with gallstones based on risk of development of gallbladder cancer. The exception to this would be if the stone disease were associated with a calcified gallbladder wall, or "porcelain gallbladder". A porcelain gallbladder has a high risk of harbouring a cancer. The incidence of finding this association varies from 25 to 60% in the literature.

A mass can be palpated in the right upper quadrant when the tumor grows away from the liver. Fatigue, loss of appetite and weight loss is common with direct tumor extension into the liver or with liver metastasis.

PATHOLOGY

The majority of gallbladder cancers are adenocarcinomas. This histology is seen in 80-90% of cancers in the gallbladder. Adenocarcinomas can be subdivided into papillary, serous, colloid or glandular carcinomas. Papillary adenocarcinomas tend to a more favorable prognosis. A small percentage of gallbladder cancers are adenosquamous or sqaumous carcinomas. Up to ten percent are anaplastic carcinomas. Lymphomas and carcinoids of the gallbladder have been reported. Cystic malignancies, such as mucinous cystadenomas or mucinous cystadenocarcinomas of the gallbladder, are extremely rare. Metastatic tumor to the gallbladder is uncommon but can occur.

Gallbladder cancers are often sessile tumors (5). The cancers tend to spread along the mucosa or muscularis. The gallbladder wall is usually thickened and irregular. Occasionally gallbladder cancer is seen in a polyp. Gallbladder polyps are most often benign and are usually cholesterol or inflammatory polyps (6). Polyps that are malignant are often solitary while cholesterol or inflammatory polyps are usually multiple. Seventy-four gallbladders that contained polyps were reviewed after cholecystectomy by Shinkai et.al (6). When there were fewer than three polyps in the gallbladder, there was a 37% incidence of gallbladder cancer in polyps whose size ranged from 5mm to 10mm (7). Only 6% had a neoplasm if the lesion was less than 5mm. When a gallbladder polyp is over 10mm in size, the incidence of malignancy increases (8). When gallbladder polyps are large, consideration should be given to the possibility of a malignancy. Removal of the gallbladder is indicated for polyps that are 1cm or greater in size (9). Cholecystectomy should be considered with solitary polyps 5mm to 10mm in size. If not surgically removed, these polyps should be closely monitored for growth. Polyps less than 5mm most likely are benign and can be followed.

Lymph node spread is common in gallbladder cancer and cancer in the lymph nodes is a prognostic factor. Pericholedochal nodes are commonly involved, as is the cystic lymph node (10). Other lymph nodes that can be involved with tumor spread of gallbladder cancer are the retroportal, posterior-superior pancreaticoduodenal and celiac or periaortic lymph nodes (listed in order of frequency). The incidence of lymph node metastasis correlates with tumor size (10). Small tumors or T1 tumors will infrequently have lymph node metastasis. T2-T4 tumors often have lymph node metastasis. These findings are considered when planning operative treatment.

The venous drainage of the gallbladder is through small venules into the liver. This most likely explains the frequent finding of direct extension with tumor growth into the liver bed.

DIAGNOSIS

Ultrasound is often the first test performed in the evaluation of jaundice or right upper quadrant pain, common symptoms with gallbladder cancer. On ultrasound gallbladder cancers appear as thickening of the gallbladder wall or as a mass lesion compressing or growing into the bile duct. Often associated gallstones are seen and at times, inflammatory changes can be difficult to distinguish from gallbladder cancer. Endoscopic ultrasound may be helpful to distinguish benign polyps and adenomyosis from adenomas and adenocarcinomas (8).

Computed Axial Tomography (CAT scan) is a useful test in the evaluation of gallbladder cancer. Direct extension of tumor into the liver is common, and the liver is the most frequent site of metastasis of gallbladder cancer. A CAT scan is a good method for detection of this metastasis or local spread (11). Magnetic Resonance Imaging (MRI) can also be used (12) but has no clear advantage over CAT scans at present.

Figure 1

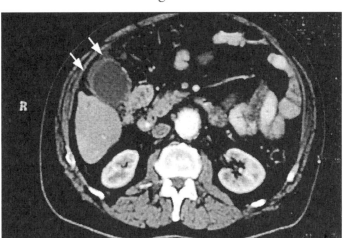

Gallbladder cancer on CAT scans can appear as a irregular thickened gallbladder wall as
illustrated here. This thickening can be difficult at times to distinguish from chronic inflammation.

To evaluate the extent of invasion into the biliary tree; endoscopic retrograde
cholangiopancreatography (ERCP) is useful. Should unresectable or nonsurgical
disease be found, this avenue also is useful for the placement of stents for palliation.
An alternative test to look at the biliary tree is now being investigated, MR
cholangiography (13). The advantage of this modality is that it is non-invasive and
does not require the use of iodinated contrast. Additional information on the extent
of the tumor is also available with magnetic resonance imaging. With improvement
of techniques and increased availability, this may in the future play a larger role in
the evaluation of the obstructed biliary tree (14).

Once the gallbladder cancer has been imaged by one of the above modalities, a
histologic diagnosis is needed. Should the patient be deemed an operative candidate
with localized disease, obtaining tissue for microscopic examination could be done
at the time of surgical exploration. For situations where it is unclear whether an
operation is going to be performed or the patient has unresectable disease, fine
needle aspiration is often helpful. Fine needle aspiration of the gallbladder has been
shown to give a diagnosis in over 80% of the time. Biopsies or bile cytology can
also be done at the time of ERCP.

STAGING

There are two classifications used to stage gallbladder cancer, the Nevin staging
system and TNM staging. The TNM staging system is the preferred method so that
the staging is more consistent with the staging of other malignancies. The Nevin

staging system was developed prior to the development of the TNM staging system. This classification has five stages. Stage 1 is disease localized to the mucosa. Stage II includes tumors that invade into the submucosa and muscularis. Stage III is when the tumor invades through the serosa or invades into the liver for a distance less than 2 cm. Stage IV shows tumors invasion into surrounding organs or more than 2 cm into the liver. Stage V corresponds to metastatic disease.

The TNM staging system, which is used more often today, classifies a gallbladder cancer on the basis of the tumor size (T), the nodal status (N) and the presence of metastasis (M). The American Joint Committee on Cancer (AJCC) periodically reviews this classification and the listed designations for T, N and M are those listed in the 1997 published guidelines. The categories for the tumor size are listed in Table 1 below.

Table 1: TNM Staging Classification: Primary Tumor (T) designations

T	DEFINITION OF PRIMARY TUMOR
TX	Primary tumor cannot be assessed
T0	No evidence of primary tumor
Tis	Carcinoma in situ
T1	Tumor invades lamina propria or muscle layer T1a Tumor invades lamina propria T1b Tumor invades muscle layer
T2	Tumor invades perimuscular connective tissue, no extension beyond serosa or into liver.
T3	Tumor perforates the serosa (visceral peritoneum) or directly invades one adjacent organ, or both (extension 2 cm or less into liver)
T4	Tumor extends more than 2 cm into liver, and/or into two or more adjacent organs (stomach, duodenum, colon, pancreas, etc.)

Nodal disease is N1 if localized to cystic and choledochal or hilar lymph nodes. N2 refers to nodal disease along the celiac axis, superior mesenteric or peripancreatic region. M is a measure for metastasis, i.e. when disease has spread to other organs distant from the site of the original tumor.

Stage 1 includes T1 tumors without lymph node metastasis (T1, N0, M0). Stage II is T2 tumors without lymph node metastasis (T2, N0, M0). Stage III has T1, T2 tumors with N1 lymph node metastasis or T3 tumors, either with or without N1 lymph node metastasis. Stage IV is divided into two categories, IVA or IVB. Stage IVA is T4 tumors with or without lymph node metastasis. Stage IVB includes gallbladder cancers that have N2 lymph node involvement or with distant metastasis. Since gallbladder cancer is a rare disease, an accurate staging system is important to compare treatment results. Unfortunately most patients with gallbladder cancer have Stage IV disease.

SURGERY

Complete surgical excision of gallbladder cancer remains the best treatment and the only treatment that will result in long term survival. With the paucity of effective alternative therapy there is debate as to how aggressive surgical therapy should be in situations where there is only a small chance of cure. Since gallbladder cancer is relatively rare, there are no large prospective, randomized trials to guide therapy. For earlier stage tumors aggressive therapy has been shown to improve survival. Earlier detection of gallbladder cancer remains the best chance for to improve the outcome of this disease.

Tumors that involve only the mucosa or the lamina propria (T1a) or confined to the muscle layer of the gallbladder, T1b tumors, are effectively treated with cholecystectomy alone. Most of these patients will be cured of their cancer. Once the tumor erodes beyond the muscularis into the perimuscular connective tissue (T2) the survival drops off. Cholecystectomy alone is inadequate therapy for T2 tumors. As mentioned previously, T2 tumors often have lymph node metastasis. A lymph node dissection including the lymph nodes commonly involved with gallbladder cancer, along with a wedge resection of the liver has been shown to improve survival (15,16). This procedure has been termed "extended" or "radical" cholecystectomy. In an extended cholecystectomy a 2 to 3 centimeter margin of liver extending from the gallbladder bed is resected along with the gallbladder. The cystic, pericholedochal, retroportal, posterior superior pancreatic, hepatic artery and celiac nodes are dissected. If a cholecystectomy had been already performed and the gallbladder cancer was an incidental finding, re-operation to do a wedge resection of the gallbladder fossa and a lymph node dissection should be done with T2 tumors.

Yamaguchi et al looked at the anatomic distances from the neck of the gallbladdder to the right hepatic duct and to the bifurcation of the anterior and posterior branch of the right hepatic duct. These were 1.6 and 5.9mm respectively (17). This study demonstrates that the neck of the gallbladder is close to the hepatic hilum. For gallbladder cancers in this area, a more extensive surgical excision may need to be considered. If the cystic duct margin is positive, resection of a portion of the common bile duct with choledochojejunostomy may be needed to obtain negative margins.

With T2 gallbladder cancers (16), 5-year survival improved from 28% with cholecystectomy alone to 91% with extended cholecystectomy and this compared to 67% with hepatectomy. The incidence of lymph node metastasis strongly influences the survival and the lymph node dissection done with extended cholecystectomy has an important impact on the improvement in survival. Unlike T1 tumors that do not usually have lymph node metastasis, T2 tumors have lymph node involvement with tumor in approximately sixty percent of the cases. If limited to the N1 lymph nodes i.e. the portal, common hepatic artery and hilar nodes the prognosis is good. Tumor in the celiac or superior mesenteric nodes (N2) carries a grave prognosis, as does disease in the periaortic lymph nodes (18).

For T3 and T4 tumors, surgical margins are often positive and the 1 year survival is seen in only a small percentage of patients. For T3 tumors without lymph node involvement an extended cholecystectomy may be warranted (19). In considering a formal hepatic lobectomy to potentially cure gallbladder cancer, an extended right hepatic lobectomy often is required since the gallbladder lies between the right and left hepatic lobes. Although this has been done for locally advanced gallbladder cancer, there are only a handful of survivors reported. Ogura et al have described a central bisegmentectomy of the liver along with resection of the caudate lobe of the liver for gallbladder cancer (20). Part of this procedure involves removal of the extrahepatic bile duct to get a complete lymph node dissection. Combined pancreaticoduodenectomy and hepatectomy for locally advanced gallbladder cancer is an option if the cancer can be completely excised. Shirai et al (21) report 5 (29%) of 17 patients with a 5-year survival after this procedure. Although the only chance of long-term survival rests in complete excision of gallbladder cancer, most patients with this large of a tumor will only present after a short time with metastatic disease. The choice of major hepatic resection for gallbladder cancer should be carefully considered and the potential risk versus potential benefit should be evaluated. If N2 lymph node involvement is present the prognosis even with resection is poor. At the time of exploration for more radical resection, inspection for the presence of celiac, superior mesenteric or periaortic lymph nodes should be done. If cancer were present in these nodes, radical surgery would not be indicated.

LAPAROSCOPY AND GALLBLADDER CANCER

Laparoscopic cholecystectomy is the treatment of choice for symptomatic gallstone disease. The safety of removing cancer with the laparoscopic approach has been questioned. Metastasis of gallbladder cancer at port sites has been seen after laparoscopic removal of an incidental gallbladder cancer (7,22,23). This raises the question whether laparoscopy has a negative impact on survival and whether an open operation should be done if a gallbladder cancer is suspected. In a retrospective study from Sweden during a time period when 11,976 laparoscopic cholecystectomies were done, 447 gallbladder cancers were detected. Fifty-five (20%) were done laparoscopically and 9 (16%) had port site metastasis (7). Others have not observed a high incidence of port site metastasis with gallbladder cancer discovered at time of laparoscopic cholecystectomy (24). The depth of invasion of the gallbladder cancer most likely has an influence on the occurrence of port site metastasis. The incidence of port site metastasis with pT1 tumors following laparoscopic removal is rare. The incidence of abdominal wall recurrences may be more a reflection of aggressive disease rather than a result of laparoscopy (25).

When the gallbladder cancer is diagnosed preoperatively, an open operation is indicated. If a gallbladder cancer is found in a gallbladder removed for symptomatic gallstone disease, no adverse effect of the laparoscopic approach has been seen with pTis or pT1 or early gallbladder cancer (26). With reoperation for a wedge liver resection and lymph node dissection, resection of the port sites can be done at the same time (26). Resection of the port sites may reduce the incidence of abdominal wall recurrence. Laparoscopic removal of a gallbladder cancer found incidentally at the time of cholecystectomy has not been shown to adversely affect survival (27).

CHEMOTHERAPY/ RADIATION THERAPY

Since gallbladder cancer is frequently unresectable, chemotherapy is often given. Unfortunately the response to most chemotherapeutic regimens is poor. Chemotherapy treatment trials for biliary neoplasms often have small numbers of patients and in general have shown response rates of less than 25% (28). 5-Fluorouracil is the most common agent used. The combination of 5-fluorouracil, doxirubicin, and mitomycin (FAM) showed a response rate of 31% but the series only included 13 patients (29). Recent reports of the use of gemcitibine (30) or 5-fluorouracil with interferon alfa-2b (28) show some response with a small number of patients. More effective chemotherapy is needed for gallbladder cancer.

Radiation likewise can be beneficial with gallbladder cancer. Some benefit from radiation therapy has been noted in small series of patients. To deliver intensive treatment to the area of the gallbladder cancer, iridium wires have been used along stents traversing the area of bile duct obstruction caused by the gallbladder cancer. Radiation therapy may also help to reduced recurrence in individuals with positive histologic margins following resection.

Adjuvant therapy with preoperative therapy has been tried to improve the results of gallbladder cancer. De Aretxabala et al treated eighteen patients with preoperative radiation therapy and continuous infusion of 5-fluorouracil for gallbladder cancer. At 24 months of follow-up seven of 13 patients were still alive (31). A prospective, randomized trial has not yet been performed.

PALLIATION

Gallbladder cancer is often found at an advanced stage. Biliary obstruction causing pruritus, jaundice and cholangitis often occurs. Relief of the biliary obstruction can be beneficial for improved quality of life and to treat sepsis. Surgical biliary drainage can be performed with success. Segment III cholangiojejunostomy can give good relief of symptoms and give prolonged benefit (32,33). Segment III cholangiojejunostomy identifies the left hepatic duct as it traverses the left lobe just underneath the falciform ligament (34). This biliary drainage procedure most often has been described for bile duct tumors especially Klatskin tumors. It is very effective for palliation of bile duct obstruction due to gallbladder cancer as well.

Improved percutaneous techniques and more durable expandable metallic stents have made it possible to effectively palliate gallbladder cancer without a surgical procedure (35). If surgical treatment is warranted for other reasons, or the patients has been explored for potential resectability, surgical drainage can be considered. Most often stents are placed endoscopically to relieve biliary obstruction caused by gallbladder cancer. This is the preferred method if possible. If the endoscopic route is not possible, then a transhepatic route can usually be successful. Combined approaches have also been used. Rarely is surgical decompression needed in patients with advanced gallbladder cancer.

SUMMARY

Gallbladder cancer often presents with advanced disease. When found early, surgery can be curative for this particular malignancy. Prognostic factors that influence the success of aggressive surgical therapy include depth of invasion, extent of hepatic infiltration, histologic grade, presence of venous, lymphatic or perineural invasion, and lymph node metastasis. Tumors with tumor limited to the subserosal layer, hepatic infiltration that is only 5mm or less, papillary or well differentiated adenocarcinomas, tumors with no venous, lymphatic or perineural invasion and lymph node metastasis limited to the hepatoduodenal ligament have the best prognosis with surgery (15,16,36). Extended cholecystectomy with lymph node dissection has improved the results of treating T2 gallbladder cancers. More extensive resections should keep the above prognostic factors in mind. When surgical resection is not possible, endoscopic stenting of the biliary tree for palliation of obstructive jaundice is effective. Earlier detection or more effective chemotherapy will be needed to significantly improve the prognosis of this disease.

REFERENCES

1. Liu, K.J., Richter, H.M., Cho, M.J., Jarad, J., Nadimpalli, V., and Donahue, P.E. Carcinoma involving the gallbladder in elderly patients presenting with acute cholecystitis. *Surgery* 122:748, 1997.
2. Redaelli, C.A., Buchler, M.W., Schilling, M.K., Krahenbuhl, L., Ruchti, C., Blumgart, L.H., and Baer, H.U. High coincidence of Mirizzi syndrome and gallbladder carcinoma. *Surgery* 121:58, 1997.
3. Chow, W., Johansen, C., Gridley, G., Mellemkjaer, L., Olsen, J., and Fraumeni, J.J. Gallstones, cholecystectomy and risk of cancers of the liver, biliary tract and pancreas. *Br J Cancer* 79:640, 1999.
4. Okamoto, M., Okamoto, H., Kitahara, R., Kobayashi, K., Karikome, K., Miura, K., Matsumoto, Y., and Fujino, M. Ultrasonographic evidence of association of polyps and stones with gallbladder cancer. *Am J Gastroenterol* 94:446, 1999.
5. Collett, J., Allan, R., Chisholm, R., Wilson, I., Burt, M., and Chapman, B. Gallbladder polyps: prospective study. *J Ultrasound Med* 17:207, 1998.
6. Shinkai, H., Kimura, W., and Muto, T. Surgical indications for small polypoid lesions of the gallbladder. *Am J Surg* 175:114, 1998.
7. Lundberg, O. and Kristoffersson, A. Port site metastases from gallbladder cancer after laparoscopic cholecystectomy. Results of a Swedish survey and review of published reports. *Eur J Surg* 165:215, 1999.

8. Sugiyama, M., Xie, X., Atomi, Y., and Saito, M. Differential diagnosis of small polypoid lesions of the gallbladder: the value of endoscopic ultrasonography. *Ann Surg* 229:498, 1999.

9. Mangel, A.W. Management of gallbladder polyps. *South Med J* 90:481, 1997.

10. Tsukada, K., Kurosaki, I., Uchida, K., Shirai, Y., Oohashi, Y., Yokoyama, N., Watanabe, H., and Hatakeyama, K. Lymph node spread from carcinoma of the gallbladder. *Cancer* 80:661, 1997.

11. Ohtani, T., Shirai, Y., Tsukada, K., Muto, T., and Hatakeyama, K. Spread of gallbladder carcinoma: CT evaluation with pathologic correlation. *Abdom Imaging* 21:195, 1996.

12. Kelekis, N.L. and Semelka, R.C. MR imaging of the gallbladder.[Review]. *Top Magn Reson Imaging* 8:312, 1996.

13. Schwartz, L.H., Coakley, F.V., Sun, Y., Blumgart, L.H., Fong, Y., and Panicek, D.M. Neoplastic pancreaticobiliary duct obstruction: evaluation with breath-hold MR cholangiopancreatography. *Am J Roentgenol* 170:1491, 1998.

14. Georgopoulos, S.K., Schwartz, L.H., Jarnagin, W.R., Gerdes, H., Breite, I., Fong, Y., Blumgart, L.H., and Kurtz, R.C. Comparison of magnetic resonance and endoscopic retrograde cholangiopancreatography in malignant pancreaticobiliary obstruction. *Arch Surg* 134:1002, 1999.

15. de Aretxabala, X., Roa, I.S., Burgos, L.A., Araya, J.C., Villaseca, M.A., and Silva, J.A. Curative resection in potentially resectable tumors of the gallbladder. *Eur J Surg* 163:419, 1997.

16. Yamaguchi, K., Chijiiwa, K., Saiki, S., Nishihara, K., Takashima, M., Kawakami, K., and Tanaka, M. Retrospective analysis of 70 operations for gallbladder carcinoma. *Br J Surg* 84:200, 1997.

17. Yamaguchi, K., Chijiiwa, K., Shimizu, S., Yokohata, K., Tsuneyoshi, M., and Tanaka, M. Anatomical limit of extended cholecystectomy for gallbladder carcinoma involving the neck of the gallbladder. *Int Surg* 83:21, 1998.

18. Shimada, H., Eno, I., Togo, S., Nakano, A., Izumi, T., and Nadagawara, G. The role of lymph node dissection in the treatment of gallbladder carcinoma. *Cancer* 79:892, 1997.

19. Chijiiwa, K. and Tanaka, M. Indications for and limitations of extended cholecystectomy in the treatment of carcinoma of the gallbladder. *Eur J Surg* 162:211, 1996.

20. Ogura, Y., Matsuda, S., Sakurai, H., Kawarada, Y., and Mizumoto, R. Central bisegmentectomy of the liver plus caudate lobectomy for carcinoma of the gallbladder. *Dig Surg* 15:218, 1998.

21. Shirai, Y., Ohtani, T., Tsukada, K., and Hatakeyama, K. Combined pancreaticoduodenectomy and hepatectomy for patients with locally advanced gallbladder carcinoma: long term results. *Cancer* 80:1904, 1997.

22. Schaeff, B., Paolucci, V., and Thomopoulos, J. Port site recurrences after laparoscopic surgery. A review. *Dig Surg* 15:124, 1998.

23. Z'graggen, K., Birrer, S., Maurer, C.A., Wehrli, H., Klaiber, C., and Baer, H.U. Incidence of port site recurrence after laparoscopic cholecystectomy for preoperatively unsuspected gallbladder carcinoma. *Surgery* 124:831, 1998.

24. Contini, S., Dalle Valle, R., and Zinicola, R. Unexpected gallbladder cancer after laparoscopic cholecystectomy: an emerging problem? Reflections on four cases. *Surg Endosc* 13:264, 1999.

25. Ricardo, A.E., Feig, B.W., Ellis, L.M., Hunt, K.K., Curley, S.A., MacFadyen, B.V., and Mansfield, P.F. Gallbladder cancer and trocar site recurrences. *Am J Surg* 174:619, 1997.

26. Yamaguchi, K., Chijiiwa, K., Ichimiya, H., Sada, M., Kawakami, K., Nishikata, F., Konomi, K., and Tanaka, M. Gallbladder carcinoma in the era of laparoscopic cholecystectomy. *Arch Surg* 131:981, 1996.

27. Suzuki, K., Kimura, T., and Ogawa, H. Is laparoscopic cholecystectomy hazardous for gallbladder cancer? *Surgery* 123:311, 1998.

28. Patt, Y.Z., Jones, D.V., Hoque, A., Lozano, R., Markowitz, A., Raijman, I., Lynch, P., and Charnsangavej, C. Phase II trial of intravenous flourouracil and subcutaneous interferon alfa-2b for biliary tract cancer. *J Clin Oncol* 14:2311, 1996.

29. Harvey, J.H., Smith, F.P., and Schein, P.S. 5-Fluorouracil, mitomycin, and doxorubicin (FAM) in carcinoma of the biliary tract. *J Clin Oncol* 2:1245, 1984.

30. Castro, M. Efficacy of gemcitabine in the treatment of patients with gallbladder carcinoma: a case report. *Cancer* 82:639, 1998.

31. de Aretxabala, X., Roa, I., Burgos, L., Cartes, R., Silva, J., Yanez, E., Araya, J.C., Villaseca M., Quijada, I., and Vittini, C. Preoperative chemoradiotherapy in the treatment of gallbladder cancer. *Am Surg* 65:241, 1999.

32. Chaudhary, A., Dhar, P., Tomey, S., Sachdev, A., and Agarwal, A. Segment III cholangiojejunostomy for carcinoma of the gallbladder. *World J Surg* 21:866, 1997.

33. Kapoor, V.K., Pradeep, R., Haribhakti, S.P., Singh, V., Sikora, S.S., Saxena, R., and Kaushik, S.P. Intrahepatic segment III cholangiojejunostomy in advanced carcinoma of the gallbladder. *Br J Surg* 83:1709, 1996.

34. Blumgart, L.H. and Kelley, C.J. Hepaticojejunostomy in benign and malignant high bile duct stricture: approaches to the left hepatic ducts. *Br.J.Surg.* 71:257, 1984.

35. Lee, B.H., Choe, D.H., Lee, J.H., Kim, K.H., and Chin, S.Y. Metallic stents in malignant biliary obstruction: prospective long-term clinical results. *Am J Roentgenol* 168:741, 1997.

36. Chijiiwa, K., Yamaguchi, K., and Tanaka, M. Clinicopathologic differences between long-term and short-term postoperative survivors with advanced gallbladder carcinoma. *World J Surg* 21:98, 1997.

9

MALIGNANT BILIARY OBSTRUCTION: ENDOSCOPIC APPROACHES

Willis G. Parsons, M.D.
Rameez Alasadi, M.D.
Northwestern University Medical School, Chicago, IL

INTRODUCTION

Malignant obstruction of the biliary tree can occur at different sites; intrahepatic, perihilar, and extrahepatic. Symptoms of biliary obstruction vary significantly from patient to patient but may include right upper quadrant abdominal pain, back or shoulder pain, pruritis, jaundice, acholic stool, dark urine, and fatigue. Less than ten percent of malignancies involving the biliary tree will present with evidence of cholangitis; typical symptoms of biliary obstruction along with fever, chills, or bacteremia. A multidisciplinary team approach involving gastroenterologists, surgeons, interventional radiologists, and oncologists is often required for managing patients with malignant biliary obstruction. This chapter will focus on endoscopic approaches for alleviating biliary obstruction, either as a palliative technique for unresectable tumors or as a bridge to surgery for potentially curable tumors.

HISTORICAL PERSPECTIVE

As greater than 85% of patients presenting with biliary obstruction from tumors will be found to have incurable malignancies, the introduction of minimally invasive, outpatient-type palliative procedures was an important milestone. Palliative endoscopic stenting for malignant biliary obstruction, first described by Soehendra et al in 1980, is now widely applied (1). The early experience with endoscopic biliary stent placement was, however, variably successful. It is important to note that the techniques of ERCP (endoscopic retrograde cholangiopancreatography) were first being introduced in the United States only five years prior to Soehendra's publication. Despite twenty-five years of evolving technology including the development of video duodenoscopes, hydrophilic guide wires, and metal self-expanding biliary stents, the most important factor determining the outcome of endoscopic biliary stenting is the training and ability of the endoscopist. Early reports came from the pioneers in the field and were not reproduced by community hospital gastroenterologists. The advent of advanced endoscopy fellowship training programs, live endoscopy courses, and ERCP workshops have increased the percentage of successful outcomes to the point that, in most hospitals, endoscopic biliary decompression is the first modality attempted in patients with incurable peri-ampullary maliganancies with obstructive jaundice. PTC (percutaneous transhepatic cholangiography) with the associated techniques of external-internal biliary drain insertion or metal biliary stent placement is typically reserved for failures of endoscopic stenting in peri-ampullary tumors or as part of a multi-modality approach in patients with hilar strictures.

The traditional surgical approach toward the palliation of jaundiced patients with unresectable malignancies with via biliary-enteric bypass (hepatojejunostomy or cholecystojejunostomy) is no longer widely performed as endoscopic biliary stent placement has been demonstrated to be as effective in resolving jaundice but with less morbidity, mortality, and cost as well as with a shorter hospital stay. In a large randomized, controlled trial, Smith et al reported 14% procedure-related mortality for patients who underwent biliary-enteric bypass surgery compared to 3% (p = 0.01) for the patients who underwent placement of a 10 French plastic biliary stent (2). In that study, the complication rate was 2.5-fold higher for surgically treated patients (29% vs 11%, p = 0.02) with a significantly longer median hospitalization (26 days vs 20 days, p = 0.001) (2). Although the re-intervention rate was higher in the stented group due to stent occlusion, the introduction of self-expanding metal biliary stents in 1989 with prolonged patency rates compared to plastic stents has made the difference in re-intervention rates between stent and surgical bypass groups less important.

As 15% of patients with pancreatic carcinoma will develop duodenal obstruction at some point in their course, some surgeons have advocated that all patients undergoing laparotomy have a therapeutic or prophylactic gastrojejunostomy at the time of the index operation. The morbidity of gastrojejunostomy is significant, however, prompting development of self-expanding, endoscopically placed duodenal metal stents. These stents are similar in design to the biliary metal stents but expand up to 2.2 cm diameter. So-called "endoscopic double biliary bypass" is now possible in the majority of patients with unresectable peri-ampullary malignancy who develop gastric outlet obstruction in addition to biliary obstruction.

The choice of performing ERCP versus PTC depends on local expertise, the clinical situation, and the location of biliary obstruction. ERCP is less invasive than PTC, with less procedure related complications and is better tolerated by patients. The overall technical success rate for endoscopic insertion of a biliary endoprosthesis is 80%-90% (3) (4) (5) but varies significantly with the experience of the endoscopist. The success rate of ERCP decreases for obstruction at or above the hepatic duct bifurcation. Patients with distal obstruction who undergo endoscopic biliary decompression have longer median survival, better relief of jaundice, and required less antibiotic treatment when compared to patients with proximal obstruction (6).

ENDOSCOPIC TECHNIQUE

Patient preparation for ERCP includes fasting the patient for 6 hours, correction of coagulopathy or significant thrombocytopenia if possible, and administration of a prophylactic broad-spectrum antibiotic. Obstructive jaundice due to malignancy is often associated with coagulopathy. We typically correct coagulopathy with vitamin K or fresh frozen plasma if the INR is greater than 1.3. Platelet transfusions should be given if the platelet count is less than 50,000. While there are many options available, we favor a semi-synthetic penicillin derivative or a fluoroquinolone intravenously as the antibiotic administered prior to ERCP.

A careful upper endoscopy is possible and should be performed routinely using the duodenoscope at the beginning of each ERCP. Only the cervical and mid-esophagus is difficult to thoroughly view with a duodenoscope. A large diameter or "therapeutic" size duodenoscope should be used for these patients as this allows for placement of the larger 10 and 11.5 French diameter plastic stents as well as all available self-expanding metal biliary stents. Specific attention should be paid to the appearance of the duodenum and the ampulla prior to cannulation. The presence of duodenal puckering or stricturing in a patient with a peri-ampullary malignancy has been demonstrated to portend a worse prognosis than that of a patient without duodenal abnormalities (7). Endoscopic biopsies of the diseased duodenum may give a positive tissue diagnosis even when brushings of the biliary stricture are negative.

The decision whether to obtain a pancreatogram in the setting of malignant biliary obstruction is based upon the clinical scenario, the results of the CT scan, and the difficulty level of cannulating the bile duct. For example, in a patient with a mass in the head of the pancreas and obstructive jaundice, if a cholangiogram is obtained first and demonstrates a distal biliary stricture, there is little to be gained by de-cannulating the bile duct and trying to obtain a pancreatogram. The same can be said for a patient undergoing ERCP with a suspected hilar cholangiocarcinoma. If, however, the CT scan is equivocal, the patient might have chronic pancreatitis mimicking a malignancy, or the etiology of jaundice is not obvious by non-invasive imaging studies, then obtaining a complete pancreatogram is often helpful. It is important to recognize that the sensitivity of ERP for detecting pancreatic carcinoma is 95%, not 100%. Small tumors in the uncinate process or those arising in the duct of Santorini may be associated with normal pancreatography.

The biliary tree should be studied with great attention to the location of obstruction, the length of the stricture, and whether extension into the intrahepatic ducts is present. Overfilling of an obstructed bile duct should be avoided, since that may increase the risk of developing cholangitis, especially if placement of a stent is unsuccessful. The decision regarding unilateral versus bilateral cholangiography and stenting in patients with hilar cholangiocarcinoma will be discussed separately in the

Special Considerations. If a mid- or proximal bile duct stricture is present, a gallbladder carcinoma should be included in the differential diagnosis and the cystic duct and gallbladder should be examined. The cystic duct is typically obstructed in patients with gallbladder carcinoma with an associated biliary stricture. Although ERCP is not typically regarded as a staging procedure in patients with malignancy, it is just that in some patients with cholangiocarcinoma and gallbladder carcinoma.

Specifically, patients with cholangiocarcinoma and gallbladder carcinoma are not considered resectable for curative intent if bilateral stricturing is seen within the intrahepatic ducts or unilateral stricturing is present with contralateral vessel involvement on mesenteric angiography or MRA. As imaging resolution improves with MRCP (magnetic resonance cholangiopancreatography), this non-invasive modality may be able to provide the same information as ERCP. MRCP can also image completely obstructed duct systems that may not be seen at all via ERCP. In this way, MRCP may identify the most dilated system and allow for the most effective palliative drainage technique to be performed.

Once the diagnostic cholangiogram has been obtained, deep cannulation of the bile duct should be achieved, either with "free hand" technique, with the help of a guide wire, or via a pre-cut sphincterotomy. Pre-cut sphincterotomy has three-fold increased risks of complications and should only be done by experienced endoscopists (8). After inserting the catheter deep in the bile duct, the biliary stricture is traversed using a hydrophilic-coated guide wire. Many experts perform bilateral biliary stent placement for hilar strictures, which requires placement of two wires, one in each duct system.

Performing a sphincterotomy is not necessary for placement of a single biliary stent of 10 French diameter or smaller. However, performing a sphincterotomy will facilitate placement of tissue sampling devices into the bile duct and will facilitate subsequent stent exchanges if necessary. We routinely perform a biliary sphincterotomy in these patients. Usually a partial sphincterotomy is sufficient for this purpose, which usually has a lower complication rate when compared to a complete sphincterotomy done in the setting of stone extraction or sphincter dysfunction, for example.

Tissue sampling should also be undertaken at the time of ERCP unless a positive tissue diagnosis is already known (9). This may be attempted using different types of sampling devices, including wire guided brush or a brush with spring wire tip, aspirating needle, or small biopsy forceps. The sensitivity of brush cytology can approach 50% to 60% for primary bile duct malignancies but is significantly lower for metastatic malignancy causing obstructive jaundice (10). The sensitivity can be increased to as high as 86% if a combination of different tissue sampling modalities are used (11) (9) A "three-in-one device" to allow for biliary stricture brushing, needle aspiration, and biopsies was developed by Wilson-Cook, Inc. (Winston-Salem, NC) and allows for "complete" tissue sampling in ten minutes with a combined yield for detecting malignancy of 69% (12).

Dilating tight strictures facilitates the insertion of biliary stents and also increases the yield of endoscopic tissue sampling. Most endoscopists use either graduated dilation catheters or high pressure balloons to dilate biliary strictures. The dilation catheters lose their dilating vector force the further away the stricture is from the ampulla of Vater. As a result, hilar strictures are usually more effectively dilated with a balloon catheter. However, routine stricture dilation is not necessary. We reserve formal dilation maneuvers for patients with hilar strictures undergoing bilateral stent placement and for patients with tight strictures that preclude easy negotiation with an 8 French diameter wire-guided brush cytology device.

Polyethylene biliary stents with an outside diameter of 10 or 11.5 French are commonly used to relieve biliary obstruction (Figure 1A-1C). Smaller diameter stents such as 7 or 8.5 French should be avoided if possible as they occlude much more quickly than the larger stents. Teflon stents are available but have not been shown to remain patent longer that polyethylene stents (13). Plastic stents are available in different lengths and configurations (straight, curved, single pigtail, double pigtail). The approximate stent length needed is measured with the aid of graduated markings on the tip of the guide wire, by centimeter spaced numbers etched onto the guide wire (Tracer Metro guide wire, Wilson-Cook, Inc.), or by measuring the distance between the stricture and the papilla on a developed x-ray film after adjusting for 30% magnification.

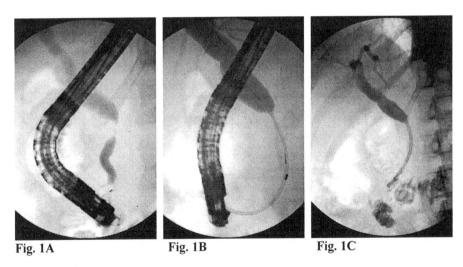

Fig. 1A   **Fig. 1B**   **Fig. 1C**

Figure 1. Endoscopic retrograde cholangiogram of a patient with head of pancreas carcinoma and obstructive jaundice. Figure 1A demonstrates a mid-common bile duct stricture with proximal biliary dilatation. Figure 1B: tissue sampling of the biliary stricture using a wire-guided brush. Figure 1C: placement of a 10 French diameter polyethylene stent through the biliary stricture.

After selecting the appropriate stent size, a stent is placed across the stricture using the conventional three-layer "pusher device" or by using the One Action Stent Introduction System (OASIS Wilson-Cook, Inc.) which is easier and quicker to use (14).

In some instances where retrograde biliary decompression is difficult, a "rendezvous" procedure can be performed (15). This requires a team effort, with an interventional radiologist performing PTC usually with transabdominal ultrasonographic guidance. The guidewire is then negotiated through the biliary stricture, across the biliary sphincter, and into the duodenum. Next, the radiologist passes a standard catheter over the guide wire, to protect the liver, in an anterograde fashion across the biliary stricture. Once the wire is in the duodenum, a snare is passed through the working channel of the duodenoscope, to grasp the wire and pull it out to be used for stent placement through the endoscope in the standard way. If palliation is the goal, then a one-step procedure can be performed with the placement of a metal stent percutaneously rather than via the combined rendezvous method.

RESULTS OF PLASTIC BILIARY STENT PLACEMENT

It is important to distinguish between technical and clinical success of invasive procedures. In regards to biliary stenting in patients with malignant biliary obstruction, technical success can be defined as proper placement of a stent across a biliary stricture whereas clinical success can be defined as relief of jaundice and pruritis. Several large series from expert centers have reported a technical success rate for palliative endoscopic biliary stenting of 80-90% (3) (4) (5). The primary reason for technical failure by experts is lack of access to the ampulla of Vater, due to duodenal stricture or obstruction, peri-ampullary distortion due to tumor, or ampullary tumor invasion. While ampullary access problems can also thwart attempts by non-experts, the inability to cannulate the bile duct or to negotiate a guide wire through the malignant biliary stricture are two common reasons for technical failure by non-experts. The vast majority of patients who undergo technically successful biliary stenting will enjoy relief of jaundice and pruritis as well as some improvement in their overall sense of well being. Luman et al reported a prospective study of 47 patients with malignant biliary obstruction who underwent placement of plastic biliary endoprostheses (16). Using symptom and quality of life questionnaires administered before and after stenting, they demonstrated that stenting significantly decreases jaundice, pruritis, anorexia, and diarrhea and improves sleep patterns. In addition, they demonstrated that stenting improved emotional, cognitive, and global health scores. In some series, however, approximately 10% of patients did not enjoy clinical success after proper stent placement. Reasons for clinical failure include death prior to resolution of jaundice, liver failure due to prolonged biliary obstruction prior to proper stenting, the presence of delta-bilirubin (serum bilirubin conjugated to albumin) which greatly slows the resolution of jaundice after stenting, and hyper-acute obstruction of the stent by viscous bile, biliary sludge, or mucin.

If a plastic biliary stent is placed to relieve jaundice in a patient with malignant biliary obstruction, the endoscopist should place a 10 or 11.5 French diameter stent. Multiple studies have demonstrated an average patency rate of three months for these large diameter endoprotheses. In addition, there is clear data demonstrating that the smaller diameter plastic biliary stents (7 and 8.5 French) occlude faster and, as a result, require more frequent stent exchanges compared with 10 and 11.5 French diameter stents. Placement of the larger diameter plastic biliary stents does require a so-called "therapeutic" size duodenoscope with a larger diameter channel.

COMPLICATIONS OF BILIARY STENT PLACEMENT

The complications of biliary stent placement can be categorized as those specific to ERCP and those related to stenting.

Complications specific to ERCP:

Acute pancreatitis

Post-ERCP pancreatitis is defined as new or increased abdominal pain consistent with pancreatitis, lasting at least 24 hours after ERCP, with an associated elevation in serum amylase of at least 2.5 to 3 fold above normal (17). Although there may well be multiple factors that contribute to the development of post-ERCP pancreatitis, there is no doubt that multiple pancreatic duct injections as well as trauma and edema at the pancreatic orifice predispose to this complication. Therefore, the endoscopist should be very cautious not to overfill the pancreatic duct and to limit pancreatic duct manipulations as much as possible. Placement of a 5 French pancreatic duct stent may decrease the risk of developing post ERCP pancreatitis, (18). Although there is data suggesting that the administration of the protease inhibitor Gabexate prior to ERCP decreases the rate of post-ERCP pancreatitis, this has not yet become part of clinical practice in the United States (19) (20). Possibly due to the obstruction or near obstruction of the main pancreatic duct in patients with pancreatic cancer, post-ERCP pancreatitis is infrequently seen in this group.

Surprisingly, there is only a little difference in the occurrence of post-ERCP pancreatitis between diagnostic and therapeutic ERCP. The risk of post-ERCP pancreatitis after diagnostic ERCP has been reported to vary between 1-3% (21). The risk of pancreatitis following endoscopic biliary sphincterotomy is 1% to 5% (18) (22). The best study on post-ERCP complications comes from Freeman et al. as this represents a prospective, multicenter (community and university hospitals) study (8). They found a 4.9% rate of post-ERCP pancreatitis after biliary sphincterotomy, an overall 9% rate of any complication after ERCP, and a 24% rate of a complication after needle-knife papillotomy. The rate of post-ERCP pancreatitis is 1.8 to 8% after pancreatic sphincterotomy (23) (24) (18) (25). It is fortunate that most cases of post-ERCP pancreatitis are mild, self-limited, and require only supportive care. Approximately 75% of cases of post-ERCP pancreatitis are classified as mild, requiring a hospitalization of three days or less (17).

Bleeding and perforation

Bleeding after sphincterotomy occurs in 1% to 3% in most series, with an associated mortality rate less than 1% (17) (26). Bleeding after endoscopic sphincterotomy is usually mild (hemoglobin drop <3 gm) and self-limited. For significant bleeding requiring blood transfusion, a duodenoscopy should be performed. Post-sphincterotomy bleeding usually occurs at the apex of the sphincterotomy site and can be treated with injection of dilute epinephrine using a bowed sphincterotome or a Howell needle (HBAN-22, Wilson-Cook, Inc.). Cautery of the bleeding site should be reserved for bleeding that continues despite epinephrine injection, as this technique is more likely to result in either pancreatitis or perforation compared to injection techniques. Rarely, angiographic embolization or surgical intervention is needed to control post-sphincterotomy bleeding.

The risk of retroperitoneal perforation is less than 1% in the majority of series (17). This complication occurs almost exclusively in patients who undergo sphincterotomy. Although this complication can be recognized during the procedure, more often than not it is recognized after the ERCP as upper abdominal or back pain accompanied by fever and leukocytosis. Although pancreatitis can be present in addition to a retroperitoneal perforation, most patients will have normal or only mildly elevated serum amylase. As plain abdominal radiographs will often be unremarkable, a CT scan of the abdomen and pelvis should be ordered if there is a clinical suspicion of a retroperitoneal perforation. Management includes NPO, nasogastric tube to low intermittent suction, broad-spectrum intravenous antibiotics, and surgical consultation (27) (28). It is estimated that 20-30% of patients with a post-sphincterotomy retroperitoneal perforation will require surgery. The indications for surgery for this complication are retroperitoneal abscess formation, intractable pain, and sepsis.

Peritoneal perforation is a rare complication of ERCP. This can occur either by the duodenoscope perforating the duodenum at the superior duodenal angle, at the site of an invading tumor, or at the site of a coincident pyloric channel or duodenal ulcer. In addition, duodenal perforations have been reported during biliary stent exchanges, either as a complication of the distal aspect of the stent eroding into the opposing duodenal wall or due to an endoscope perforation. The vast majority of peritoneal perforations require prompt exploratory laparotomy with repair or oversewing of the defect in the duodenal wall.

Biliary obstruction and cholangitis

Transient biliary obstruction can occur after biliary sphincterotomy or after cannulation attempts due to edema at the distal aspect of the bile duct. This typically manifests as a rise in liver tests the day after the procedure, with or without associated biliary colic. If the patient is asymptomatic and afebrile, then conservative management is appropriate, as the edema will resolve over 24-72 hours. If, however, there is associated biliary colic, we keep the patient NPO and begin or continue broad-spectrum antibiotics. If there is clinical evidence of cholangitis in addition to the elevations in liver chemistries, then biliary decompression should be considered via endoscopic stent, nasobiliary drain, or percutaneous biliary drain placement in addition to administering broad-spectrum antibiotics. The incidence of cholangitis after ERCP is typically 1% but can be as high as 30% in the group of patients with Bismuth type III hilar cholangiocarcinoma. In patients with malignant biliary obstruction who undergo ERCP with opacification of the proximal biliary tree but with unsuccessful stent placement, antibiotics should be started (or continued) and an alternative drainage procedure should be pursued promptly.

Should cholangitis develop after failed endoscopic biliary stent placement in a patient with malignant biliary obstruction, then biliary decompression should be performed within 24 hours. Should expert Interventional Radiology not be available, the patient should be transferred to a referral center that possesses expertise in ERCP and Interventional Radiology. This principle should also hold true for hilar strictures when the endoscopist can place only one stent. In that case, PTC with biliary drain placement on the unstented side should be done.

Stent related complications:

Migration

Plastic biliary stent migration, either proximally or distally, may occur at a rate of 10.8% (29). Large diameter stents, short stents, the presence of a malignant stricture as well as sphincterotomy, are all reported to be predisposing factors for biliary stent migration (29). Proximally migrated stents can be successfully retrieved by various endoscopic techniques (30). It is very uncommon that surgical or percutaneous approaches are needed for stent recovery (31). On rare occasions, distal stent migration can lead to duodenal wall ulceration and bleeding. In addition, small and large intestine perforation have been reported from plastic biliary stents that have migrated out of the biliary tree and moved distally in the gut (32). While inadvertent proximal deployment of a metal biliary stent may occur in upwards of 5% of cases, migration of a metal stent after it has expanded is quite rare.

Stent Occlusion

Recurrent jaundice and various degrees of cholangitis due to stent occlusion are the major complications of endoscopic stenting for malignant biliary obstruction. Stent blockage may develop within a weeks to 6 months, depending upon the diameter of the stent placed as well as several unknown or at least unpredictable parameters such as mucus production by the tumor or the lithogenicity of bile. On rare occasions plastic biliary stents can remain patent for two years. Some experts recommend prophylactic exchange of biliary stents every 3-to 4-months to prevent cholangitis and sepsis. Frakes et al studied 50 patients with obstructive jaundice, who underwent 70 biliary stent placements, and reported low occlusion rates using 10-and 11.5-Fr stents of 4.2% and 10.8%, respectively, at 3 and 6 months intervals. Thus, he recommended that biliary stent replacement interval could be safely extended from 3 to 6 months, with subsequent decrease in procedure-related cost, and patient discomfort (33). Patients should be educated about the signs and symptoms of early stent obstruction, (i.e. low-grade fever, malaise, pruritis) and stent exchange must be performed at that time. However, this approach can be used only with very compliant and highly motivated patients.

The most common early complication of stent placement for proximal biliary stenosis is cholangitis, which can occur in 5% of types I-and II-stenoses, and as high as 32% of type III stenosis despite pre-procedure antibiotic administration. The risk of cholangitis increases when both hepatic segments are opacified during cholangiography, but only single lobar drainage is achieved (34). The duration of antibiotic prophylaxis must be tailored according to the quality of biliary drainage accomplished (35).

Microscopic studies demonstrated that bacterial biofilm formation plays a major role in plastic biliary prostheses blockage (36) (37). Multiple attempts to improve stent patency and prevent clogging by altering the bile composition, reducing bile duct bacterial colonization (38, 39), as well as changes in the stent design, and constructing material (40) has not yet been shown to preclude stent blockage (41). It was proven in multiple studies that large caliber stents can provide a longer patency rate, but they do not prevent blockage indefinitely (42) (43) (44). It is uncertain whether an 11.5 French stent offer any significant advantage over 10 French plastic stent (45).

Acute cholecystitis after stenting the bile duct occurs rarely, especially if the stent compromises an already diseased cystic duct origin (46).

SELF-EXPANDING METAL BILIARY STENTS

To overcome the problem of short patency rate of plastic biliary stents, larger caliber self-expanding metal biliary stents were developed. The initial endoscopic placement experience was reported in 1989 (47) (48) and since then these metal stents and their delivery systems have undergone significant modifications.

 There are now six different FDA-approved metal biliary stents available for endoscopic insertion, each with their own specific properties. The two most popular metal biliary stents in the United States at the time of this writing are the Wallstent (Boston-Scientific Microvasive, Inc., Natick, MA) and the spiral Z stent (Wilson-Cook, Inc.). The Diamond (Boston-Scientific Microvasive, Inc.), Endocoil (Bard Interventional, Billerica, MA), and Za (Wilson-Cook, Inc.) stents are the metal stents constructed from Nitinol, a flexible metal alloy first developed by the United States Navy for military use. Nitinol is less radiopaque than the other available metal stents and therefore is harder to visualize fluoroscopically during deployment. The Diamond and Za stents are similar in appearance with an open mesh design. The Endocoil is a single coil of flattened Nitinol in a 10 French diameter delivery catheter. The Diamond stent has a 9.25 French delivery catheter whereas the Za stent has an 8.5 French delivery system. The Wallstent and the coated Wallstent (Boston-Scientific, Inc.) are made of Elgiloy, a superalloy composed of Nickel and Cobalt. The mesh is relatively closed in design. The coated Wallstent contains a silicone covering on all but the most proximal and distal 0.5 cm of the stent. This mesh is constrained between a hydrophilic inner and outer sheath. Withdrawing the outer sheath deploys the stent, while the inner one remains in place. Advancing the outer sheath over the inner catheter can reverse the deployment, only when less than 50% of the stent has been exposed. The delivery catheter of the Wallstent is 7.5 French in diameter. This "Unistep" delivery device has an outer diameter of 7.5 French, which allows its passage through either a diagnostic or therapeutic size duodenoscope. The Wallstent is available in 42, 68, and 80 mm lengths. Although these stents are available in both 8 and 10 mm diameters (after final deployment and expansion have occurred), most endoscopists use the larger diameter stents. Prior to stent deployment proper positioning should be undertaken keeping in mind that these stents will foreshorten by 20% to 40% while the stent is expanding in diameter. A completely expanded Wallstent is considered permanent, since it integrates into the bile duct wall by triggering an inflammatory response with subsequent fibrosis that covers the luminal aspect of the stent completely (49). This epithelization process decreases the rate of stent migration significantly.

It was concluded from multiple European open studies of endoscopically or percutaneously placed Wallstents for different types of malignant biliary obstruction that the stent is easy to insert with a technical success rate of greater than 95% (50) (51) (52) (47) (53) (Figure 2A-2C). The early complications were related to the endoscopic procedures as well as to the mechanical failure of the delivery device, which underwent subsequent modification with significant improvement. Tumor ingrowth or overgrowth was the main cause for late Wallstent occlusion, occurring in 10% of the patients. This problem was not seen previously with plastic stents. On the other hand, metal stent occlusion from biliary sludge and biofilm deposition was seen only in 2% of the cases whereas this is the primary mechanism of most plastic biliary stent occlusions.

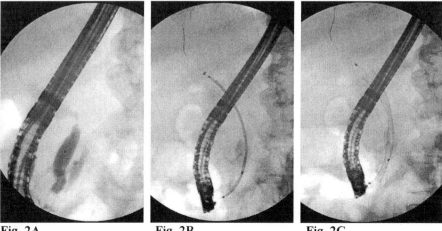

Fig. 2A   Fig. 2B   Fig. 2C

Figure 2. Endoscopic retrograde cholangiopancreatogram of a patient with unresectable head of pancreas carcinoma. Figure 2A shows a "double duct sign" with a distal bile duct stricture and a high-grade main pancreatic duct stricture. Figure 2B: a 10 x 68 mm-biliary Wallstent (Boston-Scientific Microvasive, Inc.) is placed over a 0.035 in diameter guide wire through the biliary stricture. Figure 2C: the Wallstent has been deployed across the stricture by removing the outer constraining sheath. The stent will expand to 1 cm diameter over a few days as it shrinks in length in a process process termed "foreshortening."

The spiral Z stent (Wilson-Cook, Inc.) is a stainless steel stent with an open mesh design (Figure 3A-3C). Howell et al recently reported their experience with placement of the newly modified Gianturco-Rosch Z-stent. They were able to place the Z-stent across hilar as well as common bile duct malignant obstructing lesions, using either a diagnostic or therapeutic Olympus (Olympus, Inc., Lake Placid, NY) duodenoscope, with good stent expansion confirmed by follow up abdominal x-ray films (54). In this modified type of Z stent, the stainless steel cages are arranged in a spiral fashion, distributing the eyelets in a random style producing a more flexible stent. It is available in 5.7 cm and 7.5 cm lengths and expands to 10 mm diameter. Unlike the Wallstent, the Z-stent does not foreshorten upon expansion, potentially enabling more accurate positioning of the stent across a stricture. The other advantage of the Z-stent is the absence of sharp edges at the ends of the stent, which theoretically minimizes duodenal irritation, erosion, and subsequent hemorrhage as have been reported previously with the use of the Wallstent (55). Some of the disadvantages of the earlier generation Z-stent were the lack of flexibility, the large interspace between wires that was thought to increase the rate of tumor ingrowth, and the large (10 Fr) stiff introducer catheter. The modified biliary Z stent has an 8.5 French delivery catheter.

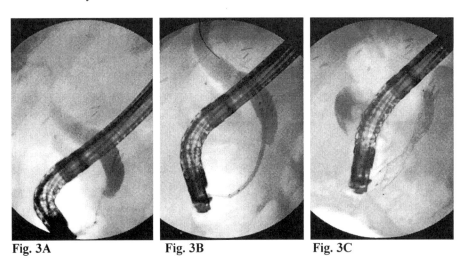

Fig. 3A   **Fig. 3B**   **Fig. 3C**

Figure 3.   Endoscopic retrograde cholangiogram of a patient with unresectable cholangiocarcinoma.   Figure 3A depicts a high grade, distal common bile duct stricture. Figure 3B: placement of a 10 x 57 mm biliary spiral Z stent (Wilson-Cook, Inc.) across the stricture. Figure 3C: after deployment of the Z stent.

A multicenter randomized controlled trial comparing the modified spiral Z-stent versus the uncoated biliary Wallstent has now been completed (56). One hundred forty-two patients with unresectable malignant biliary obstruction at least 2 cm below the bifurcation were randomized to receive an uncoated Wallstent (n = 73) or a biliary Z stent (n = 69). All patients had successful metal stent placement, although there were 5 technical problems in the Wallstent group and 7 in the Z stent group. Two-thirds of the patients are alive at the time of this writing. There was no statistically significant difference in the overall calculated patency rates between these two stents; Z-stent 151 days and Wallstent 169 days.

Metal versus plastic?

Since metal stent removal is, for all intents and purposes, not possible, only poor surgical candidates or patients with unresectable disease should be considered for metal stent placement. The prolonged patency rate and overall cost benefit are reasonable arguments for metal stent insertion in these patients.

It was found from previous studies that the patency rates for metal and plastic stents are comparable during the first 3 months (57). It is only after 3 months that the real benefit of a metal stent will be realized. In a recent study comparing metal stents with plastic stents in the palliation of patients with inoperable malignant biliary obstruction, cost analyses showed that metallic stents were advantageous in patients surviving more than 6 months, whereas a plastic stent was advantageous in patients surviving 6 months or less (58). However, it is often difficult to predict survival in patients with malignancy, making the initial selection of stent type challenging. It was determined from a retrospective analysis of 210 patients who underwent 250 Wallstent placements that the absence of liver metastases, a distal stricture less than 2 cm in length, a serum bilirubin level of less than 3.2 mg/dl, and the lack of an elevated white blood count portends a better prognosis and therefore favors the placement of a metal stent (59). In another study it was found that the tumor size plays a major role in determining prognosis of patients with malignant biliary obstruction. Patients with a tumor diameter greater than 3 cm had a poor prognosis with a median survival of 3.2 months (58). Another group of patients who clearly benefit from placement of a metal biliary stent are those who develop early plastic stent occlusion.

Multiple advantages of metal Wallstents have been noted when compared to the conventional plastic endoprostheses in three randomized trials (57) (60) (61). The biliary Wallstent was found to be easier to insert, because of its smaller and more flexible delivery catheter. It offered excellent initial drainage (90%-95%) secondary to its larger diameter augmented by increased side branch drainage through the open mesh, which is an important feature especially if the obstruction is due to a hilar stricture (62). Because of the prolonged patency rate of the metal stents, there is less need for stent exchanges, thus enhancing the overall cost benefit. The major disadvantages of metal biliary stents are their higher initial cost and the inability of removing them after complete deployment.

In a randomized trial by Davids et al (57), 105 patients with inoperable distal common bile duct malignant obstruction were assigned to undergo placement of either a self expanding metal Wallstent (n= 49) or a polyethylene stent (n= 56). The median patency rate for the metal stent was significantly longer when compared to that of the plastic stent (273 versus 126 days, respectively, p = 0.006), with a lower occlusion rate (33% versus 54%). They shared similar placement success rates, initial drainage efficacy rates, and early complication rates. The overall median patient survival was 149 days and did not differ significantly between treatment groups. There was a 28% decrease in the number of endoscopic procedures in the metal stent group, as shown by incremental cost-effectiveness analyses.

In another prospective trial by Knyrim (63), 62 patients with malignant common bile duct strictures were randomized to receive a metal biliary stent (n= 31) or an 11.5 Fr polyethylene stent (n= 31). Wallstents were placed in 70% of the metal stent group and Strecker stents (another type of metal stent, no longer available in the United States for endoscopic deployment) in the remainder. Metal stent placement was performed either endoscopically or by the combined percutaneous-endoscopic "rendezvous" technique. Early results at one month were similar in both groups. Median follow up was 5 months for both groups. There was a higher stent failure rate (43% versus 22%), a significantly higher incidence of cholangitis (36% versus 15%), a longer hospital stay (11.8 +/- 3 days versus 4 +/- 1.9 days; p = 0.02), and a higher overall cost in the polyethylene stent group compared to the metal stent group.

In the United States Wallstent study group 183 patients with unresectable malignant biliary obstruction were randomized; 94 patients received Wallstents and 89 received polyethylene stents. The stent insertion success rates were 97% and 96%, respectively, for metal and plastic stents. Within each stent group, patients were also randomized according to the site of malignant stricture with 30% hilar and 70% distal bile duct locations. Early complications (within 30 days) were comprised of 3% stent occlusion rate in the plastic group versus none in the Wallstent group and a 7% mortality rate due to advanced underlying disease. Late stent occlusion (more than 30 days) was due to sludge formation in 28% of the plastic stents and 6% in the metal stents as well as tumor ingrowth or overgrowth in the Wallstent group in 14%. There was no difference in patient survival between the two groups as shown by life table analysis. However, stent patency was longer in the Wallstent group (132 days vs 62 days). The likelihood of developing stent occlusion was 2.8 times greater for those patients who received plastic stents. The authors concluded that Wallstent placement for the treatment of malignant biliary obstruction carries significant clinical advantages over plastic stent placement including a cost advantage due to reduced need for multiple endoscopic interventions (61, 64).

Despite their prolonged patency rate compared to plastic stents, metallic stents can occlude. Multiple techniques have been described to treat this problem, which is caused, by either tumor ingrowth or overgrowth (65) (66). In a multicenter retrospective study the management of 44 occluded Wallstents in 38 patients was reported. In 19 patients a second Wallstent was placed, in 20 patients a plastic stent was inserted through the occluded Wallstent, and in 5 patients mechanical cleaning of the metal stent alone was performed. Endoscopic management was successful in 98% of the cases. Incremental cost effective analysis showed that plastic stent insertion is the most cost-effective option when a metal stent occludes.

To overcome the problem of metal stent occlusion by tumor ingrowth, polyurethane-covered metal stents have been developed (67-71). In a pilot study, 30 patients with malignant biliary obstruction received polyurethane-covered Wallstents. Patients with hilar obstructions were excluded, and all stents were inserted percutaneously. Effective biliary decompression was accomplished in all the patients without acute complications. The patency rates after 1, 3, 6, and 12 months were 96%, 69%, 47%, and 31%, respectively. The authors concluded that this new type of stent did not offer better results than those seen with uncovered metal stents. The coating did not prevent tumor ingrowth trough the covering sheath or the distal aspect of the stent, which is not covered (69). A recent study randomly assigned 50 patients with malignant biliary obstruction to receive either a polyurethane covered Diamond stent or an original uncovered Diamond stent (70). Stent patency rates at three; six, and twelve months were 100%, 83%, and 83% in the covered group, and 77%, 69%, and 52% in the uncovered group, respectively ($p = 0.055$). Potential blockage of the cystic duct or the pancreatic duct orifice were concerns regarding the use of covered metal biliary stents that have not been borne out by early clinical experience. In an effort to prevent pancreatic orifice obstruction by the coating of the Wallstent, the distal (and proximal) 5 mm of the stent are uncoated. A recent multicenter, non-randomized study reported that of 31 patients who underwent technically successful placement of a covered Wallstent for the palliation of malignant biliary obstruction, 28 stents remained patent until death or at least six months follow up (71). More data is needed with coated biliary stents prior to making conclusions about whether this modification offers a significant clinical advantage over standard, uncoated metal biliary stents.

SPECIAL CONSIDERATIONS: HILAR AND METASTATIC LESIONS

Stenting the proximal biliary tree is more challenging and is associated with lower success rates when compared to stenting of distal and mid-duct strictures. The overall endoscopic drainage success rate in proximal biliary obstruction is close to 80% in some series, but as low as 50% in others (72) (6).

An important question for physicians treating patients with advanced primary or metastatic tumors involving the liver is who will benefit from the interventions? As hepatocellular dysfunction, sepsis, and metabolic disturbances may contribute to the development of jaundice, it is not surprising that biliary stent placement does not resolve the jaundice in all patients. Furthermore, heroic efforts to place one or more stents in a jaundiced, pre-terminal patient are neither reasonable nor compassionate. Generally speaking, patients are more likely to benefit from biliary decompression if their Karnofsky score is 60 or higher (patient requires occasional assistance but is able to care for most personal needs).

In an effort to further define which patients with hepatocellular carcinoma and jaundice might benefit from stenting, Martin et al. retrospectively analyzed 26 patients at the University of Pittsburgh Medical Center who underwent ERCP after CT or ultrasound (73). Eleven of 26 patients had a dominant biliary stricture on ERCP; all 11 underwent placement of either plastic or metal stents. Six of 11 (55%) stented patients had a significant decline in serum bilirubin and three became eligible for further chemotherapy. All six responders to stenting had biliary dilation on prior CT or ultrasound. The authors concluded that ERCP and stenting provided no benefit in the absence of biliary dilation on CT or ultrasound.

The success rate of endoscopic palliation of proximal biliary obstruction depends upon the endoscopist's skill, type of tumor, and location. Polydorou et al. evaluated 190 patients who underwent endoscopic stent insertion for unresectable proximal malignant biliary obstruction, either from primary or metastatic cancer. A successful single stent insertion was achieved in 89% of the cases, resulting in clinical success in 82%. Endoscopic-percutaneous technique was used in 7% of patients, and further stents were placed in 4% of the cases when cholestasis failed to improve or cholangitis developed secondary to an undrained liver segment. He reported an overall technical success rate of 93% for Bismuth type I hilar stenosis (nonobstructed primary confluence), 94% type II (obstruction limited to primary confluence), and 84% type III (primary confluence obstructed with extension to right or left secondary confluence), with an overall drainage success rate of 91%, 83%, and 73% of patients, respectively. Early complication rates were 7% Type I, 14% Type II, and 31% Type III (72).

In another study, placement of a large bore plastic endoprosthesis for palliation of proximal malignant biliary obstruction was successful in 66 of 92 patients (74%) and was clinically effective in 49 (53%) (6). Cholangitis was the main procedure related complication, occurring in 25 patients. No combined endoscopic-percutaneous modality was used in this study. Results varied greatly according to location of stenosis: successful drainage was achieved in 86% of Bismuth type I patients but in only 15% of Bismuth type III patients. Multivariate analysis demonstrated that the independent prognostic factors of 30-day mortality were the development of post-ERCP cholangitis and the absence of successful drainage. They concluded that endoscopic drainage should be avoided in Bismuth type III patients.

Perhaps the most careful study to date regarding the issue of whether drainage of both lobes of the liver is necessary in bifurcation tumors comes from the Wellesley Hospital in Toronto, Canada (34). In this retrospective review of 141 patients (43 Bismuth type I, 58 type II, 40 type III), plastic stents were placed in all but three patients. The Bismuth types II and III patients were further divided into three groups: group A, one lobe opacified with same lobe drained; group B, both lobes opacified with both lobes drained; and group C, both lobes opacified with one lobe drained. Stents were replaced when there was clinical evidence of occlusion or at 3- to 4-month intervals. Percutaneous drainage was performed for failure to place one stent endoscopically, in patients with persistent jaundice or cholangitis despite unilateral stent placement, or at the discretion of the physician. Overall median survival for types I, II, and III patients was 160, 131, and 62 days, respectively. Among type II and III patients the median survivals of groups A, B, and C were 145, 225, and 46 days, respectively. Survival was significantly longer in-group A vs. group C, group B vs. group C, and group A + B vs. group C. There was no difference in groups A + B versus type I. In addition, when comparing single drain only (group A + C, 80 days) versus double drains (group B, 225 days), there was a significant survival advantage. The authors concluded that in bifucation tumors the best survival was noted in those with bilateral drainage, and the worst survival in those with cholangiographic opacification of both lobes but drainage of only one. This paper underlines the importance of bilateral stenting for hilar obstruction, the need for percutaneous drainage in some patients, and the notion that non-experts should not be performing these complex, technically difficult procedures.

As no randomized trials are currently available to guide us, the available data favors bilateral stenting in patients with unresectable malignancy with hilar obstruction. We have adopted a policy of attempting bilateral endoscopic stent placement in all such patients. For Bismuth types II and III patients, this may well involve maneuvers to place a guidewire into a completely obstructed system. A recently developed multi-port catheter (Haber Ramp catheter, Wilson-Cook Medical, Inc.) is helpful in placing guidewires bilaterally in hilar strictures. In cases of malignant biliary obstruction secondary to hilar tumors placing bilateral metal biliary stents can be technically difficult. However this problem can be overcome by either placing a guide wire in each system prior to the insertion of the delivery device, or by advancing a guide wire through the mesh of previously placed stent into the opposite intrahepatic duct, followed by dilating the mesh with a balloon catheter before inserting the second delivery system. The Howell biliary introducer with needle (HBIN-35, Wilson-Cook Medical, Inc.) is another device that has been used to gain access into the contralateral intrahepatic biliary tree in patients with hilar obstruction (74). It is important to avoid placement of the delivery system tip within a small intrahepatic duct, since this may prevents full expansion of the deployed stent, and subsequent removal of the delivery device since its tip is a little larger than a collapsed stent. On rare occasions when firm traction fails to remove the catheter, using the catheter as nasobiliary drain for several hours while allowing the stent to expands a little more, usually succeed in removing the entrapped tip (75) (52). The optimal situation for placement of bilateral metal biliary stents is in a side-by-side configuration, after first having placed guide wires bilaterally (Figure 4A-4D). The side-by-side configuration makes re-intervention much easier, should recurrent jaundice or cholangitis prompt repeat ERCP. If possible, side-by-side metal stent deployment should be done so as to leave the distal aspects of the metal stents flush with each other. Then, at the time of re-intervention, it is relatively easy to preferentially select one or the other stent using a triple-lumen stone extraction balloon, pre-loaded with an angled-tip guide wire. We routine perform balloon dilation of the hilar stricture(s) over each guide wire, and then proceed with stenting. If both systems are dilated equally, the left system should be stented first, as this usually is the more technically difficult system to stent. After deployment of the first metal stent, should placement of the second stent's delivery catheter fail, then we will attempt the so-called "Y" stenting configuration, with the second stent penetrating through the mesh of the first stent. Because of its more open cage design compared to the Wallstent, the spiral Z stent is ideal for this application (Figure 5A-5B). However, re-intervention, whether it is attempted endoscopically or percutaneously, is technically cumbersome as the cages and barbs of the two stents are now interlocked. As a result, restoration of bilateral biliary patency via internal stenting often fails and the patient may require at least one external biliary drain. Should only unilateral endoscopic stenting be successful, we proceed with percutaneous drainage (and usually percutaneous metal stenting) of the other side.

Although no comparative study exists regarding plastic versus metal stenting of hilar strictures, there is a growing trend among referral centers to place bilateral metal stents as soon as the patient has been deemed unresectable for curative intent. One major potential advantage of metal biliary stents in patients with hilar strictures is that many more biliary radicals can be drained due to the open lattice design of these stents compared to standard plastic stents.

Fig. 4A   **Fig. 4B**

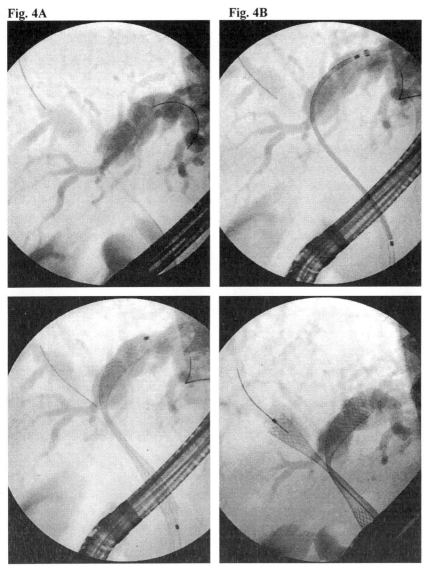

Fig. 4C   **Fig. 4D**

Figure 4. Endoscopic retrograde cholangiogram of a patient with pancreatic tail carcinoma with metastases to the porta hepatis causing a hilar stricture. Figure 4A shows placement of two 0.035 in guide wires into the left and right hepatic ducts. Figure 4B: placement of a 10 x 68 mm biliary Wallstent across the hilar stricture going into the left system while maintaining guide wire access into the right. Figure 4C: deployment of the left sided biliary Wallstent. Figure 4D: after deployment of the second Wallstent in the right system. Note the criss-crossing pattern after deployment of bilateral, side-by-side metal biliary stents.

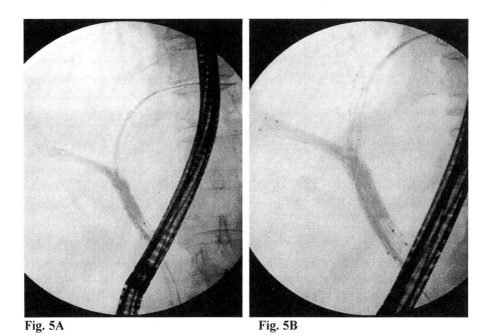

Fig. 5A   **Fig. 5B**

Figure 5. Endoscopic retrograde cholangiogram of a patient with unresectable hilar cholangiocarcinoma. Figure 5A shows a deployed spiral Z stent across the hilar stricture and into the right hepatic duct as well as an undeployed Z stent placed through the open mesh of the first stent moving into the left hepatic duct. Figure 5B: after deployment of the second Z stent. Note the "Y" configuration after deployment of bilateral, "stent through a stent" metal biliary stents.

CONCLUSIONS

As the vast majority of patients with malignant biliary obstruction have incurable disease, palliative endoscopic biliary stent placement has become an integral part of management. Endoscopic biliary stent placement may be performed on an outpatient basis, is successful in 90% of cases of peri-ampullary malignancy, and is associated with less than 10% morbidity. Endoscopic biliary stenting relieves jaundice and pruritis as well as improves overall quality of life. Randomized controlled trials have demonstrated that endoscopic stenting is as effective as surgical biliary bypass, but with lower morbidity, mortality, and cost. Self-expanding metal biliary stents provide more durable relief of biliary obstruction compared with plastic stents and have been demonstrated to be more cost-effective by decreasing the need for stent exchanges. Jaundice related to hilar cholangiocarcinoma and metastatic tumors to the porta hepatis and liver is more difficult to manage, with lower success rates of endoscopic stenting compared to peri-ampullary tumors as well as with a significant risk of procedure related cholangitis. A multidisciplinary approach involving

Interventional Radiology and Gastroenterology is essential in the management of patients with proximal biliary obstruction. Bilateral metal biliary stent placement is becoming the gold standard of drainage in patients with incurable hilar malignancy. As inadequate biliary drainage of proximal biliary obstruction is associated with shorter patient survival, these patients are best managed in referral centers with expertise in complex endoscopic and percutaneous procedures.

REFERENCES

1. Soehendra N, Reynders-Frederix V. Palliative bile duct drainage - a new endoscopic method of introducing a transpapillary drain. *Endoscopy*. 1980;12:8.
2. Smith AC, Dowsett JF, Russell RC, Hatfield AR, Cotton PB. Randomised trial of endoscopic stenting versus surgical bypass in malignant low bileduct obstruction. *Lancet*. 1994;344:1655.
3. Huibregtse K, Katon RM, Coene PP, Tytgat GN. Endoscopic palliative treatment in pancreatic cancer. *Gastrointest Endosc*. 1986;32:334.
4. Siegel JH, Snady H. The significance of endoscopically placed prostheses in the management of biliary obstruction due to carcinoma of the pancreas: results of nonoperative decompression in 277 patients. *Am J Gastroenterol*. 1986;81:634.
5. Brandabur JJ, Kozarek RA, Ball TJ, Hofer BO, Ryan JA, Jr., Traverso LW, Freeny PC, Lewis GP. Nonoperative versus operative treatment of obstructive jaundice in pancreatic cancer: cost and survival analysis. *Am J Gastroenterol*. 1988;83:1132.
6. Ducreux M, Liguory C, Lefebvre JF, Ink O, Choury A, Fritsch J, Bonnel D, Derhy S, Etienne JP. Management of malignant hilar biliary obstruction by endoscopy. Results and prognostic factors. *Dig Dis Sci*. 1992;37:778.
7. Parsons WG, Hanson BL, Howell DA. Duodenal involvement by pancreatic adenocarcinoma at initial ERCP: Outcome of endoscopic therapy. *Gastrointest Endosc*. 1995;41:A524.
8. Freeman ML, Nelson DB, Sherman S, Haber GB, Herman ME, Dorsher PJ, Moore JP, Fennerty MB, Ryan ME, Shaw MJ, Lande JD, Pheley AM. Complications of endoscopic biliary sphincterotomy [see comments]. *N Engl J Med*. 1996;335:909.
9. Parsons WG, Howell D. Progress in tissue sampling at ERCP. In: Cotton PB, Tygat GN, Williams CB, eds. *Annual of Gastrointestinal Endoscopy*. 8 ed. London: Current Science; 1995.
10. Scudera PL, Koizumi J, Jacobson IM. Brush cytology evaluation of lesions encountered during ERCP. *Gastrointest Endosc*. 1990;36:281.
11. Ponchon T, Gagnon P, Berger F, Labadie M, Liaras A, Chavaillon A, Bory R. Value of endobiliary brush cytology and biopsies for the diagnosis of malignant bile duct stenosis: results of a prospective study. *Gastrointest Endosc*. 1995;42:565.

12. Howell DA, Parsons WG, Jones MA, Bosco JJ, Hanson BL. Complete tissue sampling of biliary strictures at ERCP using a new device. *Gastrointest Endosc*. 1996;43:498.
13. Meyerson SM, Geenen JE, Catalano MF, Schmalz MJ, Genen DJ, al. e. "Tannenbaum" Teflon stents vs traditional polyethylene stents for treatment of malignant biliary strictures: A multicenter prospective randomized trial. *Gastrointest Endosc*. 1998;47:A394.
14. Lawrie BW, Pugh S, Watura R. Bile duct stenting: a comparison of the One-Action Stent introduction system with the conventional delivery system. *Endoscopy*. 1996;28:299.
15. Tsang TK, Crampton AR, Bernstein JR, Buto S, Cahan JA. Percutaneous-endoscopic biliary stenting in patients with occluded surgical bypass. *Am J Med*. 1990;88:344.
16. Luman W, Cull A, Palmer KR. Quality of life in patients stented for malignant biliary obstructions. *Eur J Gastroenterol Hepatol*. 1997;9:481.
17. Cotton PB, Lehman G, Vennes J, Geenen JE, Russell RC, Meyers WC, Liguory C, Nickl N. Endoscopic sphincterotomy complications and their management: an attempt at consensus. *Gastrointest Endosc*. 1991;37:383.
18. Sherman S, Lehman GA. ERCP- and endoscopic sphincterotomy-induced pancreatitis [published erratum appears in Pancreas 1992;7(3):402]. *Pancreas*. 1991;6:350.
19. Andriulli A, Leandro G, Niro G, Mangia A, Festa V, Gambassi G, Villani MR, Facciorusso D, Conoscitore P, Spirito F, De Maio G. Pharmacologic treatment can prevent pancreatic injury after ERCP: a meta-analysis [see comments]. *Gastrointest Endosc*. 2000;51:1.
20. Cavallini G, Tittobello A, Frulloni L, Masci E, Mariana A, Di Francesco V. Gabexate for the prevention of pancreatic damage related to endoscopic retrograde cholangiopancreatography. Gabexate in digestive endoscopy-- Italian Group [see comments]. *N Engl J Med*. 1996;335:919.
21. Parsons WG, Carr-Locke DL. *Endoscopic retrograde cholangiopancreatography*. In: Beger, ed. The Pancreas: A Clinical Textbook, first edition. Oxford: Blackwell Science; 1998.
22. Leese T, Neoptolemos JP, Baker AR, Carr-Locke DL. Management of acute cholangitis and the impact of endoscopic sphincterotomy. *Br J Surg*. 1986;73:988.
23. Kozarek RA, Ball TJ, Patterson DJ. Endoscopic approach to pancreatic duct calculi and obstructive pancreatitis. *Am J Gastroenterol*. 1992;87:600.
24. Sauerbruch T. Endoscopic management of bile duct stones. *J Gastroenterol Hepatol*. 1992;7:328.
25. Elton E, Howell DA, Parsons WG, Qaseem T, Hanson BL. Endoscopic pancreatic sphincterotomy: indications, outcome, and a safe stentless technique. *Gastrointest Endosc*. 1998;47:240.
26. Foutch PG. A prospective assessment of results for needle-knife papillotomy and standard endoscopic sphincterotomy. *Gastrointest Endosc*. 1995;41:25.

27. Aliperti G. Complications related to diagnostic and therapeutic endoscopic retrograde cholangiopancreatography. *Gastrointest Endosc Clin N Am.* 1996;6:379.

28. Gould J, Train JS, Dan SJ, Mitty HA. Duodenal perforation as a delayed complication of placement of a biliary endoprosthesis. *Radiology.* 1988;167:467.

29. Johanson JF, Schmalz MJ, Geenen JE. Incidence and risk factors for biliary and pancreatic stent migration. *Gastrointest Endosc.* 1992;38:341.

30. Tarnasky PR, Cotton PB, Baillie J, Branch MS, Affronti J, Jowell P, Guarisco S, England RE, Leung JW. Proximal migration of biliary stents: attempted endoscopic retrieval in forty-one patients. *Gastrointest Endosc.* 1995;42:513.

31. Brown KA, Carpenter S, Barnett JL, Williams DM. Proximal migration of a biliary stent: treatment by combined percutaneous/endoscopic approach. *Gastrointest Endosc.* 1995;41:611.

32. Storkson RH, Edwin B, Reiertsen O, Faerden AE, Sortland O, Rosseland AR. Gut perforation caused by biliary endoprosthesis. *Endoscopy.* 2000;32:87.

33. Frakes JT, Johanson JF, Stake JJ. Optimal timing for stent replacement in malignant biliary tract obstruction. *Gastrointest Endosc.* 1993;39:164.

34. Chang WH, Kortan P, Haber GB. Outcome in patients with bifurcation tumors who undergo unilateral versus bilateral hepatic duct drainage. *Gastrointest Endosc.* 1998;47:354.

35. Motte S, Deviere J, Dumonceau JM, Serruys E, Thys JP, Cremer M. Risk factors for septicemia following endoscopic biliary stenting. *Gastroenterology.* 1991;101:1374.

36. Speer AG, Cotton PB, MacRae KD. Endoscopic management of malignant biliary obstruction: stents of 10 French gauge are preferable to stents of 8 French gauge. *Gastrointest Endosc.* 1988;34:412.

37. Leung JW, Ling TK, Kung JL, Vallance-Owen J. The role of bacteria in the blockage of biliary stents. *Gastrointest Endosc.* 1988;34:19.

38. Ghosh S, Palmer KR. Prevention of biliary stent occlusion using cyclical antibiotics and ursodeoxycholic acid. *Gut.* 1994;35:1757.

39. Barrioz T, Ingrand P, Besson I, de Ledinghen V, Silvain C, Beauchant M. Randomised trial of prevention of biliary stent occlusion by ursodeoxycholic acid plus norfloxacin [see comments]. *Lancet.* 1994;344:581.

40. Coene PP, Groen AK, Cheng J, Out MM, Tytgat GN, Huibregtse K. Clogging of biliary endoprostheses: a new perspective. *Gut.* 1990;31:913.

41. Matsuda Y, Shimakura K, Akamatsu T. Factors affecting the patency of stents in malignant biliary obstructive disease: univariate and multivariate analysis. *Am J Gastroenterol.* 1991;86:843.

42. Siegel JH, Lichtenstein JL, Pullano WE, Ramsey WH, Rosenbaum A, Halpern G, Nonkin R, Jacob H. Treatment of malignant biliary obstruction by endoscopic implantation of iridium 192 using a new double lumen endoprosthesis. *Gastrointest Endosc.* 1988;34:301.

43.   Siegel JH. Improved biliary decompression with large caliber endoscopic prostheses. *Gastrointest Endosc.* 1984;30:21.

44.   Pedersen FM. Endoscopic management of malignant biliary obstruction. Is stent size of 10 French gauge better than 7 French gauge? *Scand J Gastroenterol.* 1993;28:185.

45.   Kadakia SC, Starnes E. Comparison of 10 French gauge stent with 11.5 French gauge stent in patients with biliary tract diseases. *Gastrointest Endosc.* 1992;38:454.

46.   Leung JW, Chung SC, Sung JY, Li MK. Acute cholecystitis after stenting of the common bile duct for obstruction secondary to pancreatic cancer. *Gastrointest Endosc.* 1989;35:109.

47.   Huibregtse K, Cheng J, Coene PP, Fockens P, Tytgat GN. Endoscopic placement of expandable metal stents for biliary strictures-- a preliminary report on experience with 33 patients. *Endoscopy.* 1989;21:280.

48.   Neuhaus H, Hagenmuller F, Classen M. Self-expanding biliary stents: preliminary clinical experience. *Endoscopy.* 1989;21:225.

49.   Bethge N, Sommer A, von Kleist D, Vakil N. A prospective trial of self-expanding metal stents in the palliation of malignant esophageal obstruction after failure of primary curative therapy. *Gastrointest Endosc.* 1996;44:283.

50.   Lammer J, Klein GE, Kleinert R, Hausegger K, Einspieler R. Obstructive jaundice: use of expandable metal endoprosthesis for biliary drainage. Work in progress. *Radiology.* 1990;177:789.

51.   Neuhaus H, Hagenmuller F, Griebel M, Classen M. Percutaneous cholangioscopic or transpapillary insertion of self- expanding biliary metal stents [see comments]. *Gastrointest Endosc.* 1991;37:31.

52.   Bethge N, Wagner HJ, Knyrim K, Zimmermann HB, Starck E, Pausch J, Vakil N. Technical failure of biliary metal stent deployment in a series of 116 applications. *Endoscopy.* 1992;24:395.

53.   Huibregtse K, Carr-Locke DL, Cremer M, Domschke W, Fockens P, Foerster E, Hagenmuller F, Hatfield AR, Lefebvre JF, Liquory CL, et al. Biliary stent occlusion--a problem solved with self-expanding metal stents? European Wallstent Study Group. *Endoscopy.* 1992;24:391.

54.   Howell DA, Nezhad SF, Dy RM. Endoscopically placed Gianturco endoprosthesis in the treatment of malignant and benign biliary obstruction. *Gastrointest Endosc Clin N Am.* 1999;9:479.

55.   Ee H, Laurence BH. Haemorrhage due to erosion of a metal biliary stent through the duodenal wall. *Endoscopy.* 1992;24:431.

56.   Howell D, Shah RJ, Desilets DJ, Parsons WG, Lehman GA, Sherman S, Baillie J, Branch MS, Chuttani R, Pleskow D, Bosco JJ. Multicenter randomized comparative trial of the new spiral Z-stent compared to Wallstent: final results of the ZOOM trial. *Gastrointest Endosc.* 2001;In press.

57.   Davids PH, Groen AK, Rauws EA, Tytgat GN, Huibregtse K. Randomised trial of self-expanding metal stents versus polyethylene stents for distal malignant biliary obstruction [see comments]. *Lancet.* 1992;340:1488.

58.   Prat F, Chapat O, Ducot B, Ponchon T, Pelletier G, Fritsch J, Choury AD, Buffet C. A randomized trial of endoscopic drainage methods for inoperable malignant strictures of the common bile duct [see comments]. *Gastrointest Endosc.* 1998;47:1.

59.   Hoepffner N, Foerster E, C., EiBing D, Domschke W. Prognostic factors for the palliative treatment of malignant biliary obstruction with Wallstents. *Gastrointest Endosc.* 1995;41:A416.

60.   Knyrim K, Wagner HJ, Starck E, Herberg A, Pausch J, Vakil N. [Metal or plastic endoprostheses in malignant obstructive jaundice. A randomized and prospective comparison]. *Dtsch Med Wochenschr.* 1992;117:847.

61.   Carr-Locke DL, Ball T, Connors PJ, Cotton PB, Geenen DJ, Hawes RH, Jowell P, Kozarek R, Lehman G, Meier R, Ostroff JW, Shapiro MJ, Silvis SE, Vennes J. Multicenter, Randomized Trial of Wallstent Biliary Endoprosthesis versus Plastic Stents. *Gastrointestinal Endoscopy.* 1993;39:A310.

62.   Nicholson AA, Royston CM. Palliation of inoperable biliary obstruction with self-expanding metal endoprostheses: a review of 77 patients. *Clin Radiol.* 1993;47:245.

63.   Knyrim K, Wagner HJ, Pausch J, Vakil N. A prospective, randomized, controlled trial of metal stents for malignant obstruction of the common bile duct. *Endoscopy.* 1993;25:207.

64.   Carr-Locke DL, Roston AD. Endoscopic Therapy for Malignant Biliary Obstruction. In: Jacobson IM, ed. *ERCP and Its Applications.* Philadelphia: Lippincott-Raven; 1998:225.

65.   Tham TC, Carr-Locke DL, Vandervoort J, Wong RC, Lichtenstein DR, Van Dam J, Ruymann F, Chow S, Bosco JJ, Qaseem T, Howell D, Pleskow D, Vannerman W, Libby ED. Management of occluded biliary Wallstents. *Gut.* 1998;42:703.

66.   Jackson JE, Roddie ME, Chetty N, Benjamin IS, Adam A. The management of occluded metallic self-expandable biliary endoprostheses. *AJR Am J Roentgenol.* 1991;157:291.

67.   Born P, Rosch T, Bruhl K, Ulm K, Sandschin W, Frimberger E, Allescher H, Classen M. Long-term results of endoscopic treatment of biliary duct obstruction due to pancreatic disease. *Hepatogastroenterology.* 1998;45:833.

68.   Rossi P, Bezzi M, Salvatori FM, Panzetti C, Rossi M, Pavia G. Clinical experience with covered wallstents for biliary malignancies: 23-month follow-Up. *Cardiovasc Intervent Radiol.* 1997;20:441.

69.   Hausegger KA, Thurnher S, Bodendorfer G, Zollikofer CL, Uggowitzer M, Kugler C, Lammer J. Treatment of malignant biliary obstruction with polyurethane-covered Wallstents. *AJR Am J Roentgenol.* 1998;170:403.

70.   Isayama H, Komatsu Y, Tsujino T, al. e. A prospective randomized study of "covered" vs "uncovered" metallic stent for diatal malignant biliary obstruction. *Gastrointest Endosc.* 2000;51:191.

71. Ponnudurai R, Haber GB, Kortan P, al. e. A new covered biliary Wallstent: effectiveness in the palliation of malignant obstructive jaundice; results from a multicenter trial. *Gastrointest Endosc.* 2000;51:5641.
72. Polydorou AA, Cairns SR, Dowsett JF, Hatfield AR, Salmon PR, Cotton PB, Russell RC. Palliation of proximal malignant biliary obstruction by endoscopic endoprosthesis insertion. *Gut.* 1991;32:685.
73. Martin JA, Slivka A, Rabinovitz M, Carr BI, Wilson J, Silverman WB. ERCP and stent therapy for progressive jaundice in hepatocellular carcinoma: which patients benefit, which patients don't? *Dig Dis Sci.* 1999;44:1298.
74. Silverman W, Slivka A. New technique for bilateral metal mesh stent insertion to treat hilar cholangiocarcinoma. *Gastrointest Endosc.* 1996;43:61.
75. Jowell PS, Cotton PB, Huibregtse K, France HG, Jr., Erickson RV, Aas J, Ostroff JW, Gordon RL. Delivery catheter entrapment during deployment of expandable metal stents. *Gastrointest Endosc.* 1993;39:199.

10
BIOLOGY OF LIVER METASTASES

**Russell S. Berman, M.D., Charles A. Portera, Jr.,M.D.
and Lee M. Ellis, M.D.**

The University of Texas M.D. Anderson Cancer Center, Houston, TX

INTRODUCTION

Metastasis is the major cause of death from cancer. By the time many cancers are diagnosed, metastasis has already occurred and the presence of multiple metastases makes complete eradication by surgery, radiation, chemotherapy, or biotherapy nearly impossible. As with other cancers, current therapies for distant metastatic disease have had minimal impact on outcome. Modifications of current treatment regimens are unlikely to significantly impact the natural history of liver metastases. Therefore, a better understanding of the biology of metastasis and the molecular events leading to the metastatic phenotype is essential if new and innovative anti-neoplastic therapeutic approaches are to be developed. This review will highlight the molecular and biologic alterations that occur in tumors that lead to the development of liver metastasis. Although numerous tumors have the potential to metastasize to the liver, metastases from colon cancer will be used as a paradigm for liver metastasis in this review.

THE METASTATIC CASCADE

Metastasis of cancer is a highly selective, nonrandom process consisting of a series of linked, sequential steps and favoring the survival of a subpopulation of metastatic cells preexisting within the primary tumor mass (1) (Figure 1). For a tumor cell to be able to form a metastasis, it must express a complex phenotype that begins with the invasion of the surrounding normal stroma either by a single tumor cell with increased motility or by groups of cells from the primary tumor. Once the invading cells penetrate the vascular or lymphatic channels, cells may detach and be transported within the circulatory system. Tumor emboli must survive the host's immune defenses and the turbulence of the circulation, arrest in the capillary bed of compatible organs, extravasate into the organ parenchyma, proliferate, and establish a micrometastasis. Growth of these small tumor lesions requires the development of a vascular supply (angiogenesis) and continuous evasion of host defense cells. Failure to complete one or more steps of the process (e.g., inability to grow in a distant organ's parenchyma) eliminates the cells. To produce clinically relevant metastases, the successful metastatic cell must therefore exhibit a complex phenotype that is regulated by transient or permanent changes in different genes at the DNA and/or mRNA level(s) (1, 2).

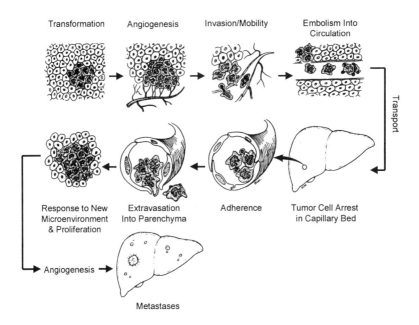

Figure 1.   The pathogenesis of cancer metastasis. To produce metastases, tumor cells must detach from the primary tumor, invade the extracellular matrix (ECM) and enter the circulation, survive in the circulation to arrest in the capillary bed, adhere to subendothelial basement membrane, gain entry into the organ parenchyma, respond to paracrine growth factors, proliferate and induce angiogenesis, and evade host defenses.   The pathogenesis of metastasis is therefore complex and consists of multiple sequential, selective, and interdependent steps whose outcome depends on the interaction of tumor cells with homeostatic factors.   (Modified from Fidler IJ, Molecular Biology of cancer: invasion and metastasis. In De Vita JR. Hellman, S, Rosenberg SA, eds. Cancer Principles and Practice of Oncology, 1997, 135-152.)

It is now widely accepted that many malignant tumors contain heterogeneous subpopulations of cells.   This heterogeneity is exhibited in a wide range of genetic, biochemical, immunologic, and biologic characteristics, such as growth rate, antigenic and immunogenic status, cell surface receptors and products, enzymes, karyotypes, cell morphology, invasiveness, drug resistance, and metastatic potential. It is likely that specific tumor cells or colonies within the larger heterogeneous tumor specimen are the forerunners of distant metastases (3).

Successful metastasis depends in part on the interaction of favored tumor cells with a compatible milieu provided by a particular organ environment (4).   In humans and in experimental rodent systems, numerous examples exist in which malignant tumors metastasize to specific organs (1).   Two arguments have been advanced previously to explain organ-specific metastasis.   In 1889, Paget proposed that the growth of metastases is influenced by the interaction of particular tumor cells (the "seed") with unique organ environments (the "soil") and thus that metastases result only when the seed and soil are compatible (5). Ewing, 40 years later, challenged Paget's "seed and soil" theory and hypothesized that metastatic dissemination occurs by purely mechanical factors that are a result of the anatomic structure of the vascular system (6). These explanations have been evoked separately or together to explain the secondary site preference of certain types of neoplasms. In a review of clinical studies on secondary site preferences of malignant neoplasms, Sugarbaker concluded that common regional metastasis could be attributed to anatomic or mechanical considerations, such as efferent venous circulation or lymphatic drainage to regional lymph nodes, but that distant organ colonization by metastatic cells from various cancers was attributable to their own patterns of site specificity (7). Other investigators have confirmed these observations, both experimentally (8) and clinically (9). Thus, the microenvironment of each organ can influence the implantation, invasion, survival, and growth of particular tumor cells, with the importance of each individual interaction varying among different tumor systems.

The liver is the most common site of distant metastasis from colorectal cancer because of both anatomic and biologic determinants. The liver filters the venous drainage from the intraabdominal viscera, including the distal esophagus, stomach, spleen, small bowel, colon, rectum, adrenals, pancreas, gallbladder, and biliary tree. In addition, the liver receives 30% of the cardiac output. Thus, the volume of blood filtered by the liver is second only to that filtered by the lungs. Physiologically, numerous cell types capable of providing a rich milieu for tumor cell growth occupy the liver. Tumor cells that survive the systemic circulation may eventually reach the liver. If the tumor cells express the appropriate phenotype, allowing progression through all stages of the metastatic cascade, then the result is a metastasis.

LIVER METASTASIS AND ANGIOGENESIS

The realization that the growth and spread of tumors are dependent on angiogenesis has created new avenues of research designed to help us to better understand cancer biology and to facilitate the development of new therapeutic strategies. Since Folkman's initial discovery that tumors are angiogenesis dependent (10), a myriad of positive and negative regulators of angiogenesis have been discovered. The survival of tumors and thus their metastasis are dependent upon the balance of endogenous angiogenic and anti-angiogenic factors such that the outcome favors increased angiogenesis (Table 1) (11). Of the angiogenic factors identified, vascular endothelial growth factor (VEGF) has been the one most frequently associated with tumor progression and metastasis (12, 13). Angiogenesis consists of sequential processes emanating from microvascular endothelial cells (10). To generate capillary sprouts, endothelial cells must proliferate, migrate, and penetrate host stroma, the direction of migration generally pointing toward the source of angiogenic molecules. The capillary sprout subsequently expands and undergoes morphogenesis to yield a capillary. Although most solid tumors are highly vascular, their vessels are not identical to normal vessels of normal tissue. There are differences in cellular composition, permeability, blood vessel stability, and regulation of growth (10).

Table 1. *Endogenous angiogenic and anti-angiogenic factors*

Stimulatory	Inhibitory
Acidic and basic fibroblast growth factor	Angiostatin
Angiogenin	Endostatin
Angiopoietin	Interferon -α, -β
Hepatocyte growth factor	Interferon inducible protein –10
Interleukin -8	Platelet factor 4
Placenta growth factor	Prolactin fragment
Platelet-derived endothelial cell growth factor	Thrombospondin
Transforming growth factor -α, -β	Tissue inhibitor of metalloproteinase
Tumor necrosis factor -α	Vasculostatin
Vascular endothelial growth factor/ vascular permeability factor	Others
Others	

In our initial studies, our laboratory set out to determine if vessel counts correlated with the presence of metastases in patients with colon cancer (12). A secondary aim was to determine if expression of specific angiogenic factors correlated with vessel counts and metastases. Paraffin-embedded specimens of human colon cancers (and adenomas) from patients operated on at The University of Texas M. D. Anderson Cancer Center were studied. Sections were stained with antibodies to factor VIII (highlighting endothelial cells), and vessels were counted. Ten adenomas, 28 non-metastatic colon tumors, and 24 primary colon tumors that had metastasized were studied. We found that vessel counts in

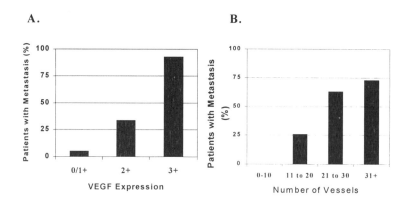

Figure 2. Relationship between VEGF expression and metastasis (A), and

vessel count and metastasis (B) in primary human colon carcinomas.   The prevalence of metastatic disease increases as the intensity of VEGF staining in primary tumors increases (A).   Similarly, incrases in vessel counts in primary colon cancers correspond to increases in the prevalence of metastsis (B). (Modified from Takahashi et al., Cancer Res 55:3964-3968, 1995).

primary colon tumors that had metastasized were significantly higher than vessel counts in non-metastatic colon tumors and adenomas (12). There was a statistically significant correlation between VEGF expression and vessel count but no correlation between vessel count and basic fibroblast growth factor expression. These data demonstrate that vessel counts and VEGF expression in human colon cancers correlate with metastasis formation (Figure 2).

Since VEGF expression in the primary tumor correlates with both metastatic disease and vessel count, it was necessary to confirm the biology of the ligand/receptor system. Therefore, we stained tumor endothelium with antibodies to the VEGF receptor *KDR*. The presence of *KDR* on tumor endothelium correlated with vessel count and VEGF expression (12). In addition, a greater percentage of primary colon tumors that had metastasized exhibited positive staining of tumor endothelium compared with non-metastatic colon tumors or adenomas.

Our laboratory then sought to determine if vessel counts and VEGF expression could serve as prognostic markers in node-negative colon cancer.   Paraffin-embedded tumor specimens from 27 patients who presented with node-negative colon cancer and who had been followed for at least 5 years were studied (14). Eight patients developed distant metastases. The prognostic significance of VEGF expression and vessel count was compared with that of other clinicopathologic prognostic factors. Three factors (VEGF expression, vessel count, and perineural invasion) correlated with time to recurrence. As in the previous study, VEGF expression significantly correlated with vessel count. Patients with high vessel count and high VEGF expression had a significantly worse prognosis than patients with lower vessel counts or lower VEGF expression.

Anti-angiogenic therapy is perhaps the most active field of anticancer research. However, the mechanism of action of many agents being investigated in preclinical and clinical trials is not known.   A more effective approach to anti-angiogenic therapy might be to target a specific angiogenic factor and develop therapies to inhibit the activity of this factor. VEGF is one potential target for anti-angiogenic therapy.   Currently, potential therapies to inhibit VEGF expression include VEGF antibodies or antibodies to the VEGF receptor, specific tyrosine kinase inhibitors of the VEGF receptor, VEGF anti-sense DNA, ribozymes, or soluble receptors of VEGF. In our laboratory, we have studied two strategies for inhibiting the growth of liver metastasis in an *in vivo* colon cancer model. One strategy was to utilize a specific antibody that binds to the VEGF receptor and blocks ligand interaction. Tumor cells were injected in the spleens of mice to produce liver metastases, and therapy was begun with control, 5-fluorouracil, or VEGF receptor antibody 7 days later.   Liver weights, as a gross measure of hepatic tumor burden, were significantly decreased in the mice receiving anti-VEGF therapy compared to liver weights in the other two groups.

Immunohistochemical analysis demonstrated that vessel counts in the group treated with VEGF receptor antibody were significantly less than in the other groups, and a great deal of necrosis was noted in the anti-VEGF therapy group compared with the other groups. Cell proliferation in all groups was relatively similar. However, specific staining for apoptosis (TUNEL) demonstrated increased levels of tumor cell apoptosis in the group treated with VEGF receptor antibody.

A second strategy to inhibit angiogenesis was to utilize a specific tyrosine kinase inhibitor to the VEGF receptor. Similarly to the previous study, liver weight was decreased in the group treated with the tyrosine kinase receptor antagonist compared to the control group. In this study, blocking VEGF activity decreased the number of hepatic metastasis. Anti-VEGF therapy led to a great deal of tumor cell apoptosis in hepatic metastasis. It appears that blocking VEGF activity not only decreases further tumor growth, but also may actually lead to endothelial cell apoptosis that leads to a second wave of tumor cell apoptosis. Others have also demonstrated that blocking VEGF activity (with VEGF antibodies) decreases the growth of hepatic metastasis in mice (13).

Numerous anti-angiogenic agents are currently under clinical investigation, including agents that inhibit matrix breakdown, agents that block activators of angiogenesis, inhibitors of endothelial cell survival signals, inhibitors of endothelial cell growth, and agents that are anti-angiogenic in vitro and in vivo, but whose mechanism of action is unknown. For a detailed list of current anti-angiogenic compounds in clinical trials, access the Website http://cancertrials.nci.nih.gov/NCI_CANCER_TRIALS/zones/PressInfo/Angio/table.html.

GROWTH FACTORS AND GROWTH FACTOR RECEPTORS

The presence of a tumor cell in a distant organ does not automatically lead to the development of a clinically relevant distant metastasis. Less than 1% of all circulating cancer cells are capable of forming a metastatic focus. For a tumor cell that has implanted at a distant site to form a viable metastatic lesion, it must be capable of responding appropriately to environmental stimuli. Proliferation, which is a necessary step in the development of clinically relevant metastases, may occur secondary to constitutively activated oncogenes (e.g., k-ras and src) or microenvironmental stimuli such as growth factors. Growth factors act by binding to specific tyrosine kinase receptors. It is the activation of these receptors that leads to the transcription of genes that regulate cellular proliferation and metastatic tumor growth. Growth factor ligands implicated in the growth of colorectal liver metastases include epidermal growth factor (EGF) (15), hepatocyte growth factor (HGF) (15), and insulin-like growth factor-I (IGF-I) (16).

The receptors for EGF (EGF-R), HGF (c-*met*), and IGF-I (IGF-I-R) are members of the tyrosine kinase receptor family. Tyrosine kinase receptors are cell membrane proteins composed of three domains: an extracellular domain is responsible for binding the receptor's ligand; a transmembrane domain anchors the protein to the membrane; and a cytosolic domain has catalytic activity and leads to tyrosine phosphorylation and activation (Figure 3). Binding of a receptor's ligand to the extracellular domain causes the tyrosine kinase receptor to dimerize. This dimerization stimulates the protein kinases, located on each receptor monomer, to phosphorylate a distinct set of tyrosine residues in the cytoplasmic portion of its dimerized partner. The phosphorylation of tyrosine residues leads to downstream effects capable of altering cell function (17).

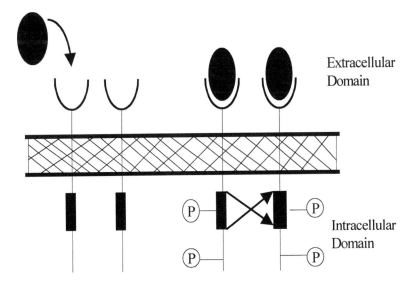

Figure 3 Receptor tyrosine kinases. Receptor tyrosine kinases exist as monomers until activated by their specific ligands. Once activated by their ligands, the receptors dimerize and then induce specific catalytic activity. Each catalytic domain in turn phosphorylates tyrosine residues in the cytoplasmic domain of its dimerized partner, which then in turn initiates specific downstream effects.

Epidermal Growth Factor

The EGF axis is composed of the EFG-R and its ligands, EGF and transforming growth factor alpha (TGF-α). Both EGF and TGF-α play important roles in the growth and proliferation of normal colonic epithelial cells (18). The role of the EGF axis in tumor progression and metastasis depends on the aberrant activation of EGF-R. Levels of expression of EGF-R in primary cultures of established human colorectal carcinoma cell lines are significantly higher in cell lines established from patients with Duke's stage D lesions than in cell lines established from patients with Duke's stage B lesions. *In vivo* studies, increased levels of EGF-R correlated directly with the ability to produce hepatic metastases (19). Others have demonstrated that EGF-R density in the cell lines derived from more "aggressive" colorectal carcinomas is significantly higher than in those derived from less aggressive tumors (15). These studies suggest that EGF-R, and its ligand, are important for the growth and metastasis of colorectal carcinoma. This hypothesis has been evaluated in an *in vivo* model by the treatment of established colorectal carcinoma in nude mice with a monoclonal antibody against the EGF-R (C225) alone or in combination with chemotherapy. C225 significantly inhibited tumor growth and prolonged the lifespan of treated mice compared to control mice. The combination of C225 with chemotherapy resulted in a near total regression of the tumor burden (20). These studies indicate the potential usefulness of EGF-R blockade either alone or as an adjunct to conventional chemotherapy in the treatment of human colorectal carcinoma. In addition, there are several tyrosine kinase inhibitors specific to the EGF-R being evaluated in pre-clinical and clinical trials.

Insulin-like Growth Factor

Another receptor-ligand system implicated in the progression and metastasis of colorectal carcinoma is the insulin-like growth factor (IGF) system. The IGF system is composed of three ligands (IGF-I, IGF-II and insulin), three receptors (IGF-IR, IGF-IIR, and insulin receptor), and at least six structurally and functionally distinct IGF binding proteins (21). IGF-I, IGF-II, and insulin have significant structural homology. Because of the similarities between these ligands, a small but significant amount of "cross talk" occurs between the ligands and their receptors. For example, IGF-IR binds IGF-II with a 2-10-fold lower affinity than it binds IGF-I, while IGF-IIR binds IGF-I with a 100-1000 times lower affinity than it binds IGF-II and does not recognize insulin (22). All three ligands stimulate mitogenesis based solely on their ability to activate the IGF-IR (23). In addition, IGF-IR has been shown to protect tumor cells from apoptosis both *in vitro* and *in vivo*. IGF-IIR is structurally distinct from IGF-IR and is also known as the mannose-6-phosphate receptor. The receptor is known to have no tyrosine kinase activity, and its biologic function remains unknown (21).

IGF's circulate in the plasma complexed to a family of binding proteins (BP). The functions of IGF-BP's appear to be diverse but remains to be clarified. IGF-BP3, the most common circulating IGF-BP, modulates the activity of IGF-I by binding to it and transporting it from the circulatory system to the cell surface receptor. As long as IGF-I is bound to IGF-BP3 it is inactive, but after dissociation from IGF-BP3, IGF-I can bind to and activate IGF-IR.

Controversy exists about the precise role of activation of the IGF system in colorectal cancer cell proliferation. In some studies, IGF-I has been shown to be a potent stimulator of colorectal carcinoma cellular proliferation. Paradoxically, IGF-BP3 has also been shown to inhibit cellular proliferation (24). While the exact role of IGF-BP3 in the induction of cellular proliferation has yet to be defined, it is clear that IGF-I is a potent stimulator of cellular proliferation and that proliferation rates can be affected by the presence or absence of IGF-BP3.

Our laboratory has demonstrated that IGF-I functions as a survival factor for human colon carcinoma cells. IGF-I treatment of colon cancer cells led to an up-regulation of the anti-apoptotic factor Bcl-X_L, which decreased cell kill by 5-

fluouracil *in vitro*. Therefore, blocking IGF-IR signaling may sensitize colon cancer cells to DNA-damaging agents.

IGF-I and its receptor may also be involved in the induction of colon cancer angiogenesis. We have found that treatment of human colorectal carcinoma cell lines with IGF-I induced VEGF mRNA and protein expression (25). Cumulative studies thus suggest that IGF-I is capable of stimulating colorectal carcinoma progression *in vivo* through multiple pathways, including cell proliferation, angiogenesis, and survival. These pathways are all inherently involved in metastasis formation. At present no pharmacologic strategies are available to inhibit IGF-IR function. However, dominant negative transfection of the IGF-IR leads to inhibition of tumor cell growth *in vivo*, suggesting that interference with IGF-IR signaling is a promising strategy for anti-neoplastic therapy for colorectal liver metastases.

INVASION AND METASTASIS

The ability of tumor cells to invade is a prerequisite for successful metastasis. For a tumor cell to form a metastasis, it must be able to traverse the basement membrane (BM) and ECM. The process of invasion is so critical to tumor progression that depth of tumor penetration on routine histopathologic evaluation is a major determinant in staging and treatment algorithms. This is especially true for colon cancer, in which tumor cells must invade through the muscularis mucosa and into the submucosa to gain access to the lymphatic channels or blood vessels.

The complex interaction between tumor cells and the host microenvironment can significantly influence tumor progression and metastatic potential (26). Numerous mechanisms of tumor cell invasion of host tissue have been described (27). Mechanical pressure induced by a rapidly growing neoplasm may force tumor cells along tissue planes that offer minimal resistance (28). Increased cell motility may also increase tumor cell invasiveness (27). A third mechanism for invasion involves degradation of the BM and ECM, which function as barriers between epithelial cells and the stroma. This degradation of the ECM and BM is the focus of intense research on invasive mechanisms involved in tumor progression and metastasis.

Role of Basement Membrane and Extracellular Matrix

The ECM and BM are a mixture of connective tissue components including collagen, laminin, proteoglycan and other molecules (29) and are produced not only by host epithelial and stromal cells but also by tumor cells. Collagen acts as the structural support for the BM, whereas laminin plays a role in cellular adhesion (29). The BM and ECM are generally believed to act as a barrier between tumor cells and normal host cells, with invasion required for tumor cells to spread locally (i.e.-through the bowel wall to contiguous structures) or to metastasize by gaining access to blood or lymphatic vessels. Studies examining the role of the BM in colon cancer have confirmed this. In the normal colon, collagen type IV-producing fibroblasts are in close association with colonocytes, forming an intact BM (30). Fibroblasts in colon cancer, however, lose their close association with epithelial cancer cells. This loss of epithelial-mesenchymal association leads to defective type IV collagen production and a defective BM (30). Fibroblasts in colon cancer have also been shown to have features of myofibroblasts and can produce lytic enzymes capable of degrading the BM and ECM. Thus, not only is there a defective BM in colon cancer, but also the cells responsible for defective matrix may help promote degradation of the BM and ECM (30).

Matrix Metalloproteinases

Among the most extensively studied of the degradative enzymes are the matrix-degrading metalloproteinases (MMPs) (Table 2). The MMPs comprise a family of enzymes that degrade the ECM and BM at a physiologic pH and are produced by host connective tissue or tumor cells (31). The MMPs play a role in normal physiologic tissue turnover as well as in pathologic conditions such as arthritis and malignancy. There are at least 17 MMPs grouped into four subfamilies: the collagenases, the gelatinases, the stromelysins, and the metalloelastases (32). There are also three MMP-specific inhibitors known as tissue inhibitors of metalloproteinases (TIMPs). The balance of activity of MMPs and TIMPs is likely to influence the invasive phenotype. Studies in colon cancer have demonstrated that the expression of four MMPs (stromelysins-1,-2 and -3 and matrilysin) is increased in tumors (32). Furthermore, the expression of matrilysin correlates with tumor progression. Interestingly, expression of stromelysin-1 and -3 in the stromal cells surrounding the malignancy also correlates with tumor progression (32).

Table 2. Major matrix-degrading metalloproteinases

Collagenases	Gelatinases	Stromelysins	Metalloelastase
MMP-1	MMP-2	MMP-3	MMP-12
MMP-5	MMP-9	MMP-10	
		MMP-11	
		MMP-7	

Other MMPs have been implicated in colon cancer progression as well. Increased expression of M_r 72,000 type IV collagenase has been shown in colon carcinoma cells when compared to normal colon cells (33). Studies using orthotopic injections of human colon cancer into nude mice have also shown that increased type IV collagenase expression correlates with metastatic ability (34). However, despite the fact that metastatic human colon cancer cells were able to grow after heterotopic subcutaneous implantation, they were not invasive and did not express type IV collagenase (34). Thus, the site of tumor growth modulates the invasive phenotype of colon cancer cells.

Urokinase type plasminogen activator (uPA) is a serine protease that promotes cancer invasion and metastasis by converting plasminogen into plasmin, which helps to degrade the ECM and activate proteases (35). uPA content and cell surface expression of the uPA receptor have been implicated in invasion and metastasis in colon cancer (36). The enzymes hyaluronidase (37) and thrombospondin (38) have also been implicated in tumor cell invasion.

The tissue inhibitors of metalloproteinases (TIMPs) serve to balance MMP activity in physiologic processes. Synthetic inhibitors of MMPs have been developed in an attempt to inhibit pathologic invasion. The synthetic matrix metalloproteinase inhibitor batimastat, or BB-94, has been used to study the effects of MMP inhibitors in colon cancer. Human colorectal cancer cell lines were injected systemically or into the peritoneal cavity of nude mice followed by treatment with batimastat. Batimastat significantly reduced the number of liver tumors compared to treatment with vehicle only. When lung-invasive colorectal tumor cells (AP5LV) were injected, batimastat decreased tumor burden in the lung but did not decrease the number of metastatic nodules (39). In another study, fragments of human colon cancer were orthotopically implanted in the colon of nude mice. Treatment with batimastat resulted in decreased median weight of primary tumors and a decreased incidence of local and regional invasion. There was also a survival advantage in the batimastat-treated group (40). However, early clinical trials have been associated with joint pains that have necessitated many patients withdrawing from studies (41). Other anti-invasive agents are currently being investigated with the goal to limit toxicity while maintaining efficacy. Reports from these trials are not yet available.

Cyclooxygenase

Recently, there has been interest in cyclooxygenase expression and inhibition in colorectal cancer. This interest was sparked by studies demonstrating a decreased mortality rate from colon cancer in users of aspirin and other non-steroidal anti-inflammatory drugs (NSAIDS) which inhibit COX-1 and COX-2 (42)). Furthermore, NSAID administration has been associated with polyp regression in patients with familial adenomatous polyposis syndrome (43). Whereas COX-1 is expressed in normal intestinal tissue, COX-2 levels are not normally detectable. However, COX-2 levels are elevated in up to 85% of colorectal cancers (44). Transfected Caco-2 human colorectal cancer cells with COX-2 were more invasive when compared to control or to parental Caco-2 cells. There was also activation of MMP-2 and an increase in MMP-2 RNA levels. Treatment of the cells with sulindac, an NSAID and therefore a COX-2 inhibitor, resulted in a decrease in invasiveness (45). The ability of COX inhibitors to decrease tumor invasion makes this class of compounds attractive as a potential novel therapy in the prevention of both primary and metastatic tumors.

ADHESION MOLECULES

Adhesion molecules play a vital role at numerous stages of tumor progression and metastasis formation. Based on their biochemical structure, adhesion molecules can be classified into four groups: integrins, cadherins, selectins, and immunoglobulin-like proteins. Invasion of the BM and ECM cannot take place without adhesion. Although invasion is considered one step of the metastatic cascade, it can be divided into numerous substeps in which adhesion molecules play distinct and differing roles. First, tumor cells must attach to the BM and ECM to initiate degradation through the previously discussed mechanisms (46). The integrin family of adhesion molecules acts as cell surface receptors to bind to the laminin, fibronectin, and collagen component of the ECM, and many integrins are expressed on the surface of human colon carcinoma cells (47-49). Tumor cell adhesion to BM laminins has been recognized as a critical step in the invasion process, and recent studies show that the invading front of numerous carcinomas is rich in the expression of certain laminins (50). Laminin-5, also, has been shown to increase cell migration (51).

Poorly differentiated colon carcinomas have been shown to express the α6β4 integrin, an adhesion molecule implicated in tumor progression (52). The integrins play an extremely active role in invasion and have been shown to bind to MMP-2. Also, the uPAR has been demonstrated to bind directly to the integrins (52). Once tumor cells have adhered to the ECM and BM and have produced degradative substances, the tumor cells must then detach to migrate into the stroma. In this setting, a decrease in integrin expression to promote detachment from the primary tumor correlates with tumor progression (49). Similarly, decreased expression of the E-cadherin/α-catenin cell-cell adhesion complex facilitates detachment of tumor cells from primary lesions and is associated with higher metastatic potential, poor differentiation, and worse prognosis in colon cancer (53). The impact of E-cadherin and the catenins on metastatic potential has been confirmed in several studies (54, 55).

Adhesion is also critical for tumor cells to arrest in the microvasculature of the distant metastatic site. Embolized tumor cells often circulate as clumps of cells adherent to other tumor cells (cohesion) or platelets. This ability to clump during tumor cell embolization may increase trapping of tumor cells in the microcirculation of distant organs such as the liver, thereby increasing metastatic potential. Studies have shown that carcinoembryonic antigen, a member of the immunoglobulin supergene adhesion molecule family and a useful clinical tumor marker in colorectal cancer may facilitate adhesion of tumor cells to other tumor or host cells (56). Furthermore carcinoembryonic antigen administration facilitates liver colonization in nude mice secondary to increased arrest of tumor cells in the liver (57). However, arrest of tumor cells alone does not guarantee survival and formation of metastasis (58). Cell surface adhesion molecules must also attach the arrested tumor cells to hepatic or other distant organ endothelial cells or ECM. Tumor cells with up-regulated specific adhesion molecules may have an advantage in the metastatic process. For colon cancer, these specific adhesion molecules include CD44 (59), the ganglioside GM2 (60), and the carbohydrate antigens (61). Members of the integrin family have also been shown to facilitate dynamic attachment and detachment of tumor cells to endothelial cells under the laminar flow conditions present in the microcirculation, a process known as "rolling" (62). A recent investigation using *in vivo* video microscopy determined that integrin-mediated adhesion is important in the extravasation of cancer cells from the hepatic microcirculation and into the mouse hepatic parenchyma (62).

The selectins are a group of adhesion receptors that play an important role in inflammation, during which endothelial cells express E-selectin, resulting in the slowing down or "rolling" of leukocytes by interaction with cell surface carbohydrates. In colon cancer, E-selectin has been determined to mediate similar adhesive interactions between tumor and endothelial cells (63). E-selectin-mediated binding correlates with metastatic potential (63).

Migration and Motility

Tumor cell migration is a critical process that allows cells to gain access to the circulation. It is regulated by factors that affect motility. The migration and motility of cells is stimulated by cytokines known as scatter factors. The prototype protein of this group of factors is HGF (64), a protein produced in large quantities by the liver.

Hepatocyte Growth Factor

HGF is a naturally occurring peptide produced mainly by cells of mesodermal origin and not by normal colonic epithelium. The receptor for HGF (c-*met*) is located in the cellular membrane and has intrinsic tyrosine kinase activity. The over-expression of c-*met*, plays an important role in the progression of human colorectal carcinoma. The addition of exogenous HGF to primary colon carcinoma cell lines increases *c-met* activation and induces human colorectal carcinoma cell motility (65).

Recently, there has been increasing evidence that HGF also contributes to the formation of hepatic metastases in patients with colorectal carcinoma. Levels of c-*met* mRNA have been shown to be higher in hepatic metastases than in primary colorectal tumors (66).   Only about 50% of primary colorectal carcinomas overexpress *c-met* (67).   However, in approximately 70% of liver metastases, the level of *c-met* gene is higher when compared to the primary colorectal lesions from the same patient. Collectively, these studies suggest that overexpression of the c-*met* gene is important in the selection of cells which have the capability to migrate and form distant metastases.

Transforming Growth Factor

Transforming growth factor beta (TGF-β) is a potent inhibitor of the growth of normal colonic epithelial cells, but it has also been implicated in the enhancement of colon cancer cell migration and motility. Decreasing TGF-β activity utilizing neutralizing antibodies and anti-sense constructs for TGF-β can reverse cell growth and invasion (68, 69). Studies suggest that elevated levels of TGF-β provide a selective advantage for more aggressive colon cancer cells by stimulating their growth and motility.   Immunohistochemical evaluation of paired primary and metastatic cells has shown that higher levels of TGF-β protein are present in metastatic cancers than in primary tumors or normal mucosa (70). Because TGF-β correlates with more aggressive tumors and the metastatic phenotype, TGF-β may be a useful prognostic indicator in patients with colorectal carcinoma.

APOPTOSIS AND METASTASIS

On a simple level, cancer can be viewed as the result of an inappropriate net gain of transformed cells. The appreciation of the role of apoptosis in both normal and abnormal physiology has resulted in the revision of the traditional cancer model that centered exclusively on cellular proliferation. Uncontrolled cellular proliferation, decreased cell death, or both are responsible for the net gain of abnormal cells known as cancer. Apoptosis was first described to introduce a distinct physiologic process of cellular suicide or "programmed cell death." Apoptosis is critical for normal homeostasis and the apoptotic machinery is present in almost all eukaryotic cells. The activation of death-inducing factors or the withdrawal of survival factors can trigger the apoptotic process (Figure 4).

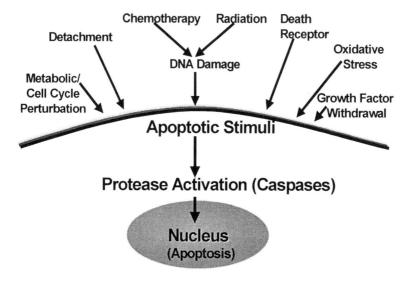

Figure 4. Common triggers of apoptosis. Apoptosis is essential to both physiologic and pathologic processes including cancer. Numerous extrinsic and intrinsic triggers of apoptosis result in activation of common intracellular pathways that lead to a caspase cascade, which ultimately leads to DNA fragmentation and cellular disassembly.

Although different triggers of apoptosis may result in activation of distinct intracellular apoptotic signaling pathways, the family of cysteine aspartate proteases, known as caspases, is responsible for both the initiation and execution of apoptosis. To accomplish this, there exist both initiator and effector caspases that cleave substrates at aspartate residues and are themselves activated by cleavage on aspartate residues, resulting in a proteolytic cascade. This caspase cascade leads to cellular disassembly (71). Finally, apoptotic bodies are formed with intact plasma membranes.   Phagocytosis by neighboring cells and macrophages eliminates these apoptotic bodies without any inflammation (72).

A complex balance of pro- and anti-apoptotic factors tightly controls the process of apoptosis (Table 3). Cancer cells can exploit these factors to bypass the normal physiologic checkpoints that would trigger defective cells to undergo apoptosis. The mechanisms used by tumors to evade apoptosis are elaborate and are summarized in a recent review article (71).   The up-regulation of anti-apoptotic genes and the down-regulation of pro-apoptotic genes are mechanisms to avoid apoptosis.   Alterations in the Bcl-2 family of proteins, a major apoptosis-regulatory protein family, often occur in cancers. There are currently approximately 16 known Bcl-2 family members in humans, both pro- and anti-apoptotic.   In addition, some factors may mediate both pro- and anti-apoptotic pathways depending on activation by phosphorylation.   An additional mechanism to down-regulate pro-apoptotic genes includes phosphorylation of the pro-apoptotic BAD by Akt, thereby preventing BAD from dimerizing with Bcl-2/Bcl-X_L (71).   Other tumor mechanisms to suppress apoptosis include expression of the inhibitors of apoptosis family of proteins. One such protein, survivan, is overexpressed in human cancers (73). Tumor cells can also avoid apoptosis by overexpressing anti-apoptotic death effector domains (74), by down-regulating Fas receptors, by mutating Fas, or by increasing expression of decoy receptors (71).

Table 3. Apoptotic factors

Apoptosis Suppressors	Apoptosis Promoters
Bcl-2	Bax
Bcl-X_L	Bak
Bcl-ω	BAD
Mcl-1	Bik
Bfl-1	Bid
Brag-1	Bcl-X_S
A-1	Hrk

Colon Cancer and Apoptosis

Colon cancer provides an excellent model to study the complex alterations in apoptosis in cancer. The availability of tissues from the continuum of normal colonic epithelium to adenomas to invasive carcinomas to metastatic lesions allows for examination of mediators of apoptosis along the entire spectrum of neoplastic progression.   Early neoplastic transformation may be associated with increased rates of both apoptosis and proliferation. However, at the adenoma-to-carcinoma transition, decreased levels of apoptosis have been associated with expression of mutant p53, demonstrating lack of function of this protein classically thought to be involved in the regulation of apoptosis and cell cycle arrest.   In addition, colon carcinomas exhibit decreased levels of apoptosis relative to earlier stages of disease progression (75).   Numerous groups have studied the expression of Bcl-2 family members during colon tumorigenesis. Bcl-X_L over-expression has been observed in colon adenocarcinoma and in some adenomas, suggesting that up-regulation of Bcl-X_L is a relatively early event in colon cancer progression. Bcl-2 expression, however, declines during progression. This decrease in the anti-apoptotic Bcl-2 is contrary to previous findings of elevated Bcl-2 expression in both adenomas and adenocarcinoma (75). This discrepancy in study findings may be due to the fact that Bcl-2 expression may be influenced by tumor differentiation, a parameter not always examined in the study of human specimens. Decreased Bcl-2 expression may be a late event associated with less differentiated tumors (76). Decreased expression of the pro-apoptotic gene Bak also may be associated with tumor progression. Although levels of Bax expression are not associated with tumor progression (76), mutation of Bax may mediate apoptosis (77).

Metastatic Colon Cancer and Apoptosis

Tumor progression to the metastatic phenotype has also been associated with alterations in apoptosis. Highly metastatic breast (human) and melanoma (human and mouse) cell lines have shown resistance to apoptosis compared to their poorly metastatic counterparts (78). Additionally, overexpression of the anti-apoptotic protein Bcl-2 in murine melanoma cells increases pulmonary metastases compared to the parental cells, which have low Bcl-2 expression and low metastatic potential (79). Alterations in apoptotic pathways in metastatic colon cancer have not been as clear-cut. Apoptotic rates in lymph node and liver metastases from colon cancer have been demonstrated to be higher than those in primary lesions (80). Our laboratory analyzed proliferation and cell death in paired primary tumors and liver metastases in 16 patients with colon cancer. Proliferative indices were higher in the primary tumors. Furthermore, when the ratio of the mean apoptotic index to the mean proliferative index was compared, net cell death was paradoxically higher in the hepatic metastatic lesions (81). We also found that Bcl-2 expression was decreased in the liver metastases. In accompanying *in vitro* studies, apoptosis was induced by staurosporine, a protein kinase inhibitor, in the paired colorectal cancer cell lines SW480 (primary) and SW620 (metastatic). Counterintuitive to the original working hypothesis, the metastatic cell line was significantly more sensitive to staurosporine-induced apoptosis than the primary cell line was (81). We therefore compared intrinsic expression of the Bcl-2 family members in the matched primary and metastatic colorectal cancer cell lines. Levels of the anti-apoptotic Bcl-X_L protein were lower and levels of the pro-apoptotic Bax and Bak proteins were higher in the metastatic cell lines (81).

Anoikis and Colon Cancer Metastasis

The data on apoptosis in metastatic colorectal cancer present a confusing, if not paradoxical, picture. In an effort to clarify the role of apoptosis in the metastatic process, our laboratory has begun to investigate matrix-independent survival in metastatic colorectal cancer cells. During the metastatic cascade, cancer cells must establish extracellular matrix (ECM) -independent survival during passage through the circulation in order to form a metastatic focus at a distant site. Therefore, investigating colon cancer cells in suspension may be more informative than studying already established metastatic foci *in vivo* or adherent metastatic cells *in vitro*. Anoikis, or detachment-induced apoptosis, is a normal physiologic mechanism discovered in epithelial cells that were experimentally dissociated from their ECM (82). In normal physiology, anoikis prevents cells from colonizing elsewhere after they have been detached (82). Resistance to anoikis may result in the ability of cells to survive independent of their normal matrix, a condition required for metastasis formation. *In vitro* studies support the hypothesis that resistance to anoikis plays a significant role in colon carcinoma metastasis. Survival of human colon carcinoma cells (LIM 1863) *in vitro* is dependent on cell-cell cohesion (83). These cells grow as organoids *in vitro*. After the organoids are dissipated into a single-cell suspension, anti-integrin antibodies block reformation of organoids. This results in spontaneous apoptosis. Thus, cell-cell contact and cohesion may act as a survival mechanism for colon cancer cells (83). Preliminary work from our laboratory examined rates of anoikis in the paired colorectal cancer cell lines SW480 and SW620. We have demonstrated that the metastatic SW620 cells are significantly resistant to anoikis when compared to the primary SW480 cells after 24, 48, and 72 hours of detachment conditions (84). Resistance to anoikis would be a critical survival advantage for potentially metastatic cells.

Although a significant amount of evidence points toward increasing apoptosis resistance with increasing tumor progression, this is by no means a uniform finding. It is possible that increased apoptosis, under certain physiologic, physical, or chemotherapeutic conditions, acts as a selection factor providing clones that will ultimately progress to metastasis. If this is the case, then at specific points during tumor progression, increased apoptosis may be the price paid for cell proliferation and selection of metastatic clones. As more is understood about the mechanisms of apoptosis and anoikis resistance, anti-neoplastic and anti-metastatic therapies should emerge.

Therapeutic Implication

Chemotherapy and radiation therapy exert their antineoplastic effects largely though the induction of tumor cell apoptosis. In this capacity, apoptosis is a critical determinant of the success of most conventional antineoplastic therapies. Research is currently focusing on new chemotherapeutic agents, such as the proteosome inhibitors, that are potent triggers of apoptosis. The proteosome is a protease that is responsible for the turnover of many regulatory proteins in eukaryotic cells. *In vitro* and *in vivo* studies have demonstrated significant antineoplastic action for this class of compounds. Phase-I human trials have recently been initiated.

Understanding mechanisms of apoptosis evasion by cancer cells allows the development of new therapeutic strategies. The restoration of wild-type pro-apoptotic genes and the down-regulation or blocking of anti-apoptotic genes can be exploited for therapy, as can restoring wild-type p53 (a tumor suppressor gene critical for apoptosis and cell cycle control) in tumors with mutated p53. Blocking expression of the inhibitors of apoptosis family members and manipulating the Fas or Fas-ligand pathway are also being explored for therapeutic potential.

METASTASIS SUPPRESSOR GENES

A metastasis suppressor gene is one that, when lost, leads to the formation of metastatic disease. When a metastasis suppressor gene is re-introduced to the cell, tumor metastasis is inhibited, but primary tumor growth is unaffected.

Nm23

Nm23 was the first metastasis suppressor gene described and serves as a prototype for this class of genes. In several different tumor systems, lower levels of nm23 mRNA and protein levels have been associated with a more aggressive/metastatic phenotype *in vitro*, although a great deal of controversy exists as to *nm23's* role *in vivo*. Recent studies have suggested that *nm23* also plays a significant role in the development of the metastatic phenotype in human colorectal carcinoma. This gene has been investigated in regards to regulating both lymph node and hepatic metastases. An evaluation of 100 resected colorectal carcinoma specimens demonstrated no correlation between *nm23* protein level and tumor size. However, an inverse correlation between the level of *nm32* protein expression in the primary tumor and the presence of lymph node metastases suggested that the loss of *nm23* facilitates the formation of nodal metastases (85). Others have shown that nm23 mRNA levels in primary lesions of patients presenting with liver metastases were significantly lower than *nm23* levels in the primary lesions of patients who presented without hepatic metastases (86).

KAI1

KAI1 has been shown to be a metastasis suppressor gene in other carcinomas. For evaluation of the effect of KAI1 protein expression in colorectal carcinomas, levels of KAI1 expression were modulated utilizing stable transfectants of colorectal carcinoma cell lines. Varying levels of KAI1 were shown to have no effect on *in vitro* growth, but increased KAI1 expression decreased cellular motility and invasiveness *in vitro*. These studies imply that KAI1 is a potential regulator of both the invasive and metastatic capability of colon carcinoma and a potential target for colorectal carcinoma therapy (87).

MRP1/CD9

Another recently evaluated metastasis-related gene is the motility related protein MRP1/CD9. *In vitro* analyses utilizing human colorectal carcinoma cell lines derived from primary and metastatic colorectal cancer lesions have shown that lesions not expressing MRP1/CD9 have a significantly higher frequency of vascular invasion and liver metastases than do lesions that expressing MRP1/CD9 (88). In a follow-up study, the levels of MRP1/CD9 expression in paired groups of primary colorectal carcinoma and hepatic metastases were evaluated by immunohistochemical staining. The authors found significantly lower levels of MRP1/CD9 expression in the hepatic metastases than in the primary lesions (89). These data support the role of MRP1/CD9 as a metastasis suppressor gene in colorectal cancer.

SUMMARY

A primary goal of cancer research is an increased understanding of the molecular mechanisms mediating the process of cancer metastasis. Analyses of colon cancer cells (the seeds) and the microenvironment (the soil) have increased our understanding of the biologic mechanisms mediating metastasis formation. Insight into the molecular mechanisms regulating the pathobiology of colon cancer metastasis, as well as a better understanding of the interaction between the metastatic cell and the host environment (including the vasculature), should provide a foundation for new therapeutic approaches. To the clinician, it is readily apparent that by the time metastases form, most steps in the metastatic cascade have completed. Therefore, therapy to down-regulate or interrupt the last stages of metastasis, proliferation and angiogenesis as well as mechanisms to disrupt cell survival signals seems the most promising areas of investigation.

Acknowledgments
The authors thank Melissa Burkett for editorial assistance. This work supported in part by NIH T-32 grant (09599-08)(CAP, RB) and the Gillson-Longenbaugh Foundation and the Jon and Suzie Hall Fund For Colon Cancer Research (LME).

REFERENCES

1. Fidler IJ. Critical factors in the biology of human cancer metastasis: Twenty-eighth G.H.A. Clowes Memorial Award Lecture. Cancer Res 1990; 50:6130-6138.
2. Fidler I, Radinsky R. Genetic control of cancer metastasis (editorial). J Natl Cancer Inst 1990; 82:166-168.
3. Kerbel R. Growth dominance of the metastatic cancer cell: Cellular and molecular aspects. Adv Cancer Res 1990; 55:87-132.
4. Fidler IJ. Modulation of the organ microenvironment for treatment of cancer metastasis. J Natl Cancer Inst 1995; 87:1588-1592.
5. Paget S. The distribution of secondary growths in cancer of the breast. Lancet 1889; 1:571-573.
6. Ewing J. Neoplastic Diseases. Philadelphia: WB Saunders, 1928.
7. Sugarbaker E. Patterns of metastasis in human malignancies. Cancer Bioloy Review 1981; 2:235-278.
8. Hart I. "Seed and soil" revisited: Mechanisms of site specific metastasis to specific secondary sites. Cancer Metastasis Rev 1982; 1:5-17.
9. Tarin D, Price J, al e. Mechanisms of human tumor metastasis studied in patients with peritoneovenous shunts. Cancer Res 1984; 44.
10. Folkman J. How is blood vessel growth regulated in normal and neoplastic tissue? - G.H.A. Clowes Memorial Award Lecture. Cancer Res 1986; 46:467-473.
11. Fidler IJ, Ellis LM. The implications of angiogenesis to the biology and therapy of cancer metastasis. Cell 1994; 79:185-188.
12. Takahashi Y, Kitadai Y, Bucana CD, Cleary KR, Ellis LM. Expression of vascular endothelial growth factor and its receptor, KDR, correlates with vascularity, metastasis, and proliferation of human colon cancer. Cancer Res 1995; 55:3964-3968.
13. Warren RS, Yuan H, Matli MR, Gillett NA, Ferrara N. Regulation by vascular endothelial growth factor of human colon cancer tumorigenesis in a mouse model of experimental liver metastasis. J Clin Invest 1995; 95:1789-1797.
14. Takahashi Y, Tucker SL, Kitadai Y, et al. Vessel counts and VEGF expression as prognostic factors in node-negative colon cancer. Arch Surg 1997; 132:541-546.

15. Tong W-M, Ellinger A, Sheinin Y, Cross HS. Epidermal growth factor receptor expression in primary cultured human colorectal carcinoma cells. British Journal of Cancer 1998; 77:1792-1798.

16. Guo Y-S, Narayan S, Chandrasekhar Y, Singh P. Characterization of insulin-like growth factor I receptors in human colon cancers. Gastroenterology 1992; 102:1101-1108.

17. Yarden Y, Ullrich A. Growth factor receptor tyrosine kinases. Ann Rev Biochem 1988; 57:443.

18. Markowitz SD, Molkentin K, Gerbic C, al e. Growth stimulation by coexpression of transforming growth factor-a and epidermal growth factor receptor in normal and adenomatous human colon epithelium. J Clin Invest 1990; 86:356.

19. Radinsky R, Risin S, Fan D, et al. Level and function of epidermal growth factor receptor predict the metastatic potential of human colon carcinoma cells. Clinical Cancer Research 1995; 1:19-31.

20. Ciardiello F, Bianco R, Damiano V, et al. Antitumor activity of sequental treatment with topotecan and anti-epidermal growth factor receptor monoclonal antibody C225. Clinical Cancer Research 1999; 5:909-916.

21. Singh P, Rubin N. Insulinlike growth factors and binding proteins in colon cancer. Gastroenterology 1993; 105:1218-1237.

22. Rosenfeld RG. Biological functions of IGF receptors. In: Frisch H, Thorner MO, eds. Hormonal regulation of growth. New York: Raven, 1989:113-126.

23. Rechler MM, Nissley SP. The nature and regulation of the receptors for insulin-like growth factors. Ann Rev Physiol 1985; 47:425.

24. Michell NP, Dent S, Langman MJS, Eggo MC. Insulin-like growth factor binding proteins as mediators of IGF-I effects on colon cancer cell proliferation. Growth Factors 1996; 14:269-277.

25. Akagi Y, Liu W, Zebrowski B, Xie K, Ellis LM. Regulation of vascular endothelial growth factor expression in human colon cancer by insulin-like growth factor-I. Cancer Research 1998; 58:4008-4014.

26. Radinsky R. Paracrine growth regulation of human colon carcinoma organ-specific metastasis. Cancer Metastasis Rev 1993; 12:345-361.

27. Gutman M, Fidler IJ. Biology of human colon cancer metastasis. World J Surg 1995; 19:226-234.

28. Gabbert H. Mechanisms of tumor invasion: evidence from in vivo observations. Cancer Metastasis Rev 1985; 4:293-309.

29. Liotta LA. Tumor invasion and metastases--role of the extracellular matrix: Rhoads Memorial Award lecture. Cancer Res 1986; 46:1-7.

30. Martin M, Pujuguet P, Martin F. Role of stromal myofibroblasts infiltrating colon cancer in tumor invasion. Path Res Pract 1996; 192:712-717.

31. Matrisian LM. The matrix-degrading metalloproteinases. Bioessays 1992; 14:455-63.

32. Matrisian LM, Wright J, Newell K, Witty JP. Matrix-degrading metalloproteinases in tumor progression. Princess Takamatsu Symp 1994; 24:152-61.

33. Levy AT, Cioce V, Sobel ME, et al. Increased expression of the Mr 72,000 type IV collagenase in human colonic adenocarcinoma. Cancer Res 1991; 51:439-44.

34. Nakajima M, Morikawa K, Fabra A, Bucana CD, Fidler IJ. Influence of organ environment on extracellular matrix degradative activity and metastasis of human colon carcinoma cells. J Natl Cancer Inst 1990; 82:1890-8.
35. Dano K, Andreasen PA, Grondahl-Hansen J, Kristensen P, Nielsen LS, Skriver L. Plasminogen activators, tissue degradation, and cancer. Adv Cancer Res 1985; 44:139-266.
36. deBruin PA, Griffioen G, Verspaget HW, et al. Plasminogen activator profiles in neoplastic tissues of the human colon. Cancer Res 1988; 48:4520-4.
37. Csoka TB, Frost GI, Stern R. Hyaluronidases in tissue invasion. Invasion Metastasis 1997; 17:297-311.
38. Yamashita Y, Kurohiji T, Tuszynski GP, Sakai T, Shirakusa T. Plasma thrombospondin levels in patients with colorectal carcinoma. Cancer 1997; 82:632-638.
39. Watson SA, Morris TM, Robinson G, Crimmin MJ, Brown PD, Hardcastle JD. Inhibition of organ invasion by the matrix metalloproteinase inhibitor batimastat (BB-94) in two human colon carcinoma metastasis models. Cancer Research 1995; 55:3629-3633.
40. Wang X, Fu X, Brown PD, Crimmin MJ, Hoffman RM. Matrix metalloproteinase inhibitor BB-94 (batimastat) inhibits human colon tumor growth and spread in a patient-like orthotopic model in nude mice. Cancer Research` 1994; 55:4726-4728.
41. Wojtowicz-Praga S, Torri J, Johnson M, et al. Phase I trial of Marimastat, a novel matrix metalloproteinase inhibitor, administered orally to patients with advanced lunch cancer. J Clin Oncol 1998; 16:2150-6.
42. Thun MJ, Namboodiri MM, Heath CWJ. Aspirin use and reduced risk of fatal colon cancer. N Engl J Med 1991; 325:1593-6.
43. Giardiello FM, Hamilton SR, Krush AJ, et al. Treatment of colonic and rectal adenomas with sulindac in familial adenomatous polyposis. N Engl J Med 1993; 328:1313-6.
44. Eberhart CE, Coffey RJ, Radhika A, Giardiello FM, Ferrenbach S, DuBois RN. Up-regulation of cyclooxygenase 2 gene expression in human colorectal adenomas and adenocarcinomas. Gastroenterology 1994; 107:1183-8.
45. Tsujii M, Kawano S, DuBois RN. Cyclooxygenase-2 expression in human colon cancer cells increases metastatic potential. Proc Natl Acad Sci 1997; 94:3336-3340.
46. .Stetler-Stevenson WG, Aznavoorian S, Liotta LA. Tumor cell interactions with the extracellular matrix during invasion and metastasis. Annu Rev Cell Biol 1993; 9:541-73.
47. Koretz K, Schlag P, Boumsell L, Moller P. Expression of VLA-alpha 2, VLA-alpha 6, and VLA-beta 1 chains in normal mucosa and adenomas of the colon, and in colon carcinomas and their liver metastases. Am J Pathol 1991; 138:741-50.
48. Hemler ME, Crouse C, Sonnenberg A. Association of the VLA alpha 6 subunit with a novel protein. A possible alternative to the common VLA beta 1 subunit on certain cell lines. J Biol Chem 1989; 264:6529-35.

49. Pignatelli M, Smith ME, Bodmer WF. Low expression of collagen receptors in moderate and poorly differentiated colorectal adenocarcinomas. Br J Cancer 1990; 61:636-8.
50. Pyke C, Salo S, Ralfkiaer E, Romer J, Dano K, Tryggvason K. Laminin-5 is a marker of invading cancer cells in some human carcinomas and is coexpressed with the receptor for urokinase plasminogen activator in budding cancer cells in colon adenocarcinomas. Cancer Res 1995; 55:4132-9.
51. Kikkawa Y, Umeda M, Miyazaki K. Marked stimulation of cell adhesion and motility by ladsin, a laminin-like scatter factor. J Biochem (Tokyo) 1994; 116:862-9.
52. Rabinovitz I, Nagle RB, Cress AE. Integrin alpha 6 expression in human prostate carcinoma cells is associated with a migratory and invasive phenotype in vitro and in vivo. Clin Exp Metastasis 1995; 13:481-91.
53. Raftopoulos I, Davaris P, Karatzas G, Karayannacos P, Kouraklis G. Level of a-catenin expression in colorectal cancer correlates with invasiveness, metastatic potential and survival. Journal of Surgical Oncology 1998; 68:92-99.
54. Gofuku J, Shiozaki H, Tsujinaka T, et al. Expression of E-cadherin and a-catenin in patients with colorectal carcinoma. Am J Clin Pathol 1999; 111:29-37.
55. Hiscox S, Jiang WG. Expression of E-Caderin, a, b and y-catenin in human colorectal cancer. Anticancer Research 1997; 17:1349-1354.
56. Benchimol S, Fuks A, Jothy S, Beauchemin N, Shirota K, Stanners CP. Carcinoembryonic antigen, a human tumor marker, functions as an intercellular adhesion molecule. Cell 1989; 57:327-34.
57. Jessup JM, Petrick AT, Toth CA, et al. Carcinoembryonic antigen: enhancement of liver colonisation through retention of human colorectal carcinoma cells. Br J Cancer 1993; 67:464-70.
58. Barbera-Guillem E, Smith I, Weiss L. Cancer-cell traffic in the liver. I. Growth kinetics of cancer cells after portal-vein delivery. Int J Cancer 1992; 52:974-7.
59. Tanabe KK, Ellis LM, Saya H. Expression of CD44R1 adhesion molecule in colon carcinomas and metastases. The Lancet 1993; 341:725-726.
60. Coulombe J, Pelletier G. Gangliosides and organ-specific metastatic colonization. Int J Cancer 1993; 53:104-9.
61. Irimura T, Nakamori S, Matsushita Y, et al. Colorectal cancer metastasis determined by carbohydrate-mediated cell adhesion: role of sialyl-Le^X antigens. Seminars in Cancer Biology 1993; 4:319-324.
62. Morris VL, Schmidt EE, MacDonald IC, Groom AC, Chambers AF. Sequential steps in hematogenous metastasis of cancer cells studied by in vivo videomicroscopy. Invasion Metastasis 1997; 17.
63. Sawada R, Tsuboi S, Fukuda M. Differential E-selectin-dependent adhesion efficiency in sublines of a human colon cancer exhibiting distinct metastatic potentials. Journal of Biological Chemistry 1994; 269:1425-1431.
64. To CTT, Tsao MS. The roles of hepatocyte growth factor/scatter factor and Met receptor in human cancers (review). Oncology Reports 1998; 5:1013-1024.

65. Hiscox SE, Hallett MB, Puntis MCA, Nakamura T, Jiang WG. Expression of the HGF/SF receptor, c-met, and its ligand in human colorectal cancers. Cancer Investigation 1997; 15:513-521.
66. Fujita S, Sugano K. Expression of c-met proto-oncogene in primary colorectal cancer and liver metastases. Jpn J Clin Oncol 1997; 27:378-383.
67. Di Renzo MF, Olivero M, Giacomini A, et al. Overexpression and amplification of the Met/HGF receptor gene during the progression of colorectal cancer. Clinical Cancer Research 1995; 1:147-154.
68. Hsu S, Huang F, Hafez M, Winawer S, Friedman E. Colon carcinoma cells switch their response to TGFb1 with tumor progression. Cell Growth Differ 1994; 5:267-275.
69. Huang F, Hsu S, Yan Z, Winawer S, Friedman E. The capacity for growth stimulation by TGFb1 seen only in advanced colon cancers cannot be ascribed to mutations in APC, DCC, p53 or ras. Oncogene 1994; 9:3701-3706.
70. Picon A, Gold LI, Wang J, Cohen A, Friedman E. A subset of metastatic human colon cancers expresses elevated levels of transforming growth factor b1[1]. Cancer Epidemiology Biomarkers & Prevention 1998; 7:497-504.
71. Reed, J.C. Mechanisms of apoptosis avoidance in cancer. Curr Opin Oncol 1999; 11:68-75.
72. Hetts WH. Apoptosis and its role in disease. JAMA 1998; 279:300-307.
73. Ambrosini G, Adida C, Altieri DC. A novel anti-apoptosis gene, survivin, expressed in cancer and lymphoma. Nat Med 1997; 3:917-21.
74. Irmler M, Thome M, Hahne M, et al. Inhibition of death receptor signals by cellular FLIP. Nature 1997; 388:190-5.
75. Bedi A, Pasricha PJ, Akhtar AJ, et al. Inhibition of apoptosis during development of colorectal cancer. Cancer Research 1995; 55:1811-1816.
76. Krajewska M, Moss SF, Krajewski S, Song K, Holt PR, Reed JC. Elevated expression of Bcl-X and reduced Bak in primary colorectal adenocarcinomas. Cancer Research 1996; 56:2422-2427.
77. Ouyang H, Furukawa T, Abe T, Kato Y, Horii A. The BAX gene, the promoter of apoptosis, is mutated in genetically unstable cancers of the colorectum, stomach, and endometrium. Clinical Cancer Research 1998; 4:1071-1074.
78. Glinsky GV, Glinsky VV, Ivanova AB, Hueser CJ. Apoptosis and metastasis: increased apoptosis resistance of metastatic cancer cells is associated with the profound deficiency of apoptosis execution mechanisms. Cancer Letters 1997; 115:185-193.
79. Takaoka A, Adachi M, Okuda H, et al. Anti-cell death activity promotes pulmonary metastatis of melanoma cells. Ocogene 1997; 14:2971-7.
80. Tatebe S, Ishida M, Kasagi N, Tsujitani S, Kaibara N, Ito H. Apoptosis occurs more frequently in metastatic foci than in primary lesions of human colorectal carcinomas: analysis by terminal-deoxynucleotidyl-transferase-mediated dUTP-biotin nick end labeling. Int J Cancer 1996; 65:173-177.

81. Termuhlen PM, Berman RS, Ellis LM, et al. Evidence for increased apoptosis in metastatic human colonic adenocarcinomas. American Journal of Pathology 1999.
82. Frisch SM, Francis H. Disruption of epithelial cell-matrix interactions induces apoptosis. J Cell Biol 1994; 124:619-26.
83. Bates RC, Buret A, van Helden DF, Horton MA, Burns GF. Apoptosis induced by inhibition of intercellular contact. Journal of Cell Biology 1994; 125:403-415.
84. Berman RS, Sweeney B, McConkey DJ. Metastatic colorectal cancer cells are resistant to anoikis, inducing Akt phosphorylation. Proceedings of 90th Annual Meeting of the American Association for Cancer Research 1999; 40:326 (A2162).
85. Tannapfel A, Katalinic A, Kockerling F, Wittekind C. The prediction of lymph node metastases in colorectal cancer by expression of the nucleoside diphosphate kinase/nm23-H1 and histopathological variables. American Journal of Gastroenterology 1997; 92:1182.
86. Yamaguchi A, al e. Inverse association of nm23-H1 expression by colorectal cancer with liver metastasis. British Journal of Cancer 1993; 68:1020-4.
87. Takaoka A, Hinoda Y, Satoh S, et al. Suppression of invasive properties of colon cancer cells by a metastasis suppressor KAI1 gene. Oncogene 1998; 16:1443-1453.
88. Cajot JF, Sordat I, Silvestre T, Sordat B. Differential display cloning identifies motility-related protein (MRP1/CD9) as highly expressed in primary compared to metastatic human colon carcinoma cells. Cancer Research 1997; 57:2593-2597.
89. Mori M, Mimori K, Shiraishi T, et al. Motility related protein 1 (MRP1/CD9) expression in colon cancer. Clinical Cancer Research 1998; 4:1507-1510.

11

RESULTS OF SURGICAL RESECTION FOR METASTATIC LIVER TUMORS

Stephen F. Sener, M.D.
Northwestern University Medical School, Chicago, IL

INTRODUCTION

According to the Surveillance, Epidemiology, and End Results (SEER) Program population-based registries, the age-adjusted colorectal cancer incidence rates have declined from a peak of 63 per 100,000 population in 1985 to 50 per 100,000 in 1995 (1). During 2000, there were approximately 130,000 newly diagnosed patients with colorectal cancer in the United States, and about 15-25% were estimated to have synchronous liver metastases (2,3).

After curative resections of primary colorectal cancer, about 5% of patients develop recurrent disease limited to the liver (4). There are currently approximately 6,500 patients per year in whom the liver is the only site of distant disease, and who are candidates for liver-directed treatment, including resection. Further, about 25% of those with liver metastases have disease limited to one lobe (5).

Natural history of patients with unresected liver metastases

The median survival time of patients with unresected liver metastases from colorectal cancer ranges from 5 to 24 months (6,7). The most important predictor of longer survival is the extent of liver disease at the time of diagnosis (8). Patients with solitary liver lesions have median survival time of 16-24 months, whereas those with bilobar metastases have median survival time of 5-10 months (7-10). It is important to establish that results after liver resection should be compared to those of patients who are resectable but unresected, and who are medically fit candidates for hepatectomy.

Performance status is a clinical predictor of longer survival time, whereas weight loss, anorexia, ascites, and abnormal liver functions are predictors of a shorter survival time (11, 12). Although 20% of patients with solitary lesions may live for three years, the five-year survival rates for unresected disease approach 0% regardless of the number of metastases or the method of non-surgical treatment

Preoperative Staging

The only absolute contraindications to resection are the presence of extrahepatic metastases and the inability to remove all hepatic disease. As the accuracy of preoperative imaging has improved over the years, the percentage of patients considered to have resectable liver metastases who were actually resected has increased from about 30% to about 60% (13-15). Recently, a study of 416 patients at Memorial Sloan-Kettering Cancer Center, using standard imaging techniques (Computerized Tomography (CT), CT portography, magnetic resonance imaging (MRI), and operative ultrasound), demonstrated that 87 (21%) of those with apparently resectable tumors had unresectable disease found at laparotomy (16). Patients who were unresectable were equally apportioned between extrahepatic disease (49%) and extensive bilobar liver metastases (51%). A scoring system was devised to stratify the risk of unresectable disease. Resectability decreased with increasing score, from 95% in those with a score of 0 (single, unilobar tumor) to 62% in those with a score of 3 (3 or more, bilobar tumors). Thus, the risk of finding unresectable disease at the time of laparotomy could be estimated by the conventional preoperative assessment of the extent of liver metastases.

The best method to identify occult disease prior to a major resection has yet to be determined. It has been suggested that laparoscopy with laparoscopic ultrasound or 2-^{18}F-fluoro-2-deoxyglucose (FDG) positron emission tomography (PET) may be used to identify additional disease not discovered by conventional imaging techniques. Laparoscopy with laparoscopic ultrasound has been shown to facilitate the evaluation of liver, subhepatic lymph nodes, and peritoneal cavity in patients with colorectal liver metastases, identifying criteria of unresectability in 31% to 48% of patients (17,18). Although there have been reports that PET scanning offers greater sensitivity than conventional imaging techniques in determining the extent of colorectal metastases, the accuracy, specificity, and tumor size resolution have yet to be determined in prospective, randomized clinical trials (19-21). PET scanning appears to be highly sensitive in identifying extrahepatic disease and would be a useful screening modality prior to resection (21). Since the risk of finding occult unresectable disease has been stratified by the extent of liver disease found by conventional imaging techniques, patients with three or more liver tumors and bilobar involvement might be the most appropriate candidates for further evaluation with laparoscopy or PET scanning prior to laparotomy.

Adjuncts to Exploration at Laparotomy

Ultrasound during laparotomy plays an important role in proper patient selection for resection. It is now routinely used to evaluate the extent of liver disease and proximity of tumor to vessels within the liver because the technique is significantly more sensitive than CT scanning and clinical staging (22-24). Previous authors have demonstrated that surgical management was altered in 19-52% of patients, based on intraoperative ultrasound findings in the liver.

Radioimmunoguided surgery (RIGS) was developed in 1983 to provide intraoperative information on the extent of disease and to assess the completeness of primary and metastatic tumor excision (25). This technique was used in 74 patients with metastatic colorectal cancer to the liver. After conventional radiographic staging failed to reveal extrahepatic metastases, patients were injected with a ^{125}I-radiolabeled monoclonal antibody to tumor-associated glycoprotein and explored with curative intent 21 to 24 days after injection (26).

Both standard and RIGS exploration identified extrahepatic tumor in 41 (55%) patients. In 12 (16%) additional patients, the RIGS technique identified lymph node metastases in gastrohepatic, celiac, and periarotic locations. Although the RIGS technique provided more accurate intraoperative staging of disease, it remains to be proven in randomized clinical trials whether complete excision of radiolabeled tissues confers a survival advantage compared to conventional resection techniques.

Results of Surgical Resection: Morbidity and Mortality

An essential step in providing meaningful five-year survival rates after liver resection is the minimization of morbidity and mortality rates from operation. Comparisons between publications are difficult because there are no standardized criteria for the definition of complications and perioperative death. Authors who have specifically reported morbidity and mortality rates have generally defined major morbidity as a complication which required invasive or intensive intervention such as reoperation, drainage of bile, pus, or fluid (pleural or peritoneal) collections, prolonged antibiotic therapy, parenteral nutrition, or hemodialysis (27).

Combining the results of selected papers in which large patient series and postoperative outcomes have been adequately described, revealed morbidity rates of about 35% (range, 11% to 59%) and mortality rates of about 5% (range 0% to 14%) (28-40). The most common major complication was intra-abdominal sepsis and the most common minor complication was pulmonary atelectasis or infection.

Sepsis occurred in about 15% of patients with postoperative complications. The etiologic factors for the development of sepsis that have been evaluated are: 1) the large residual cavity after resection and the subsequent formation of hematoma, biloma, or seroma; 2) loss of necrotic tissue at the line of liver transection; 3) contamination via drainage tubes; 4) extent of resection; 5) patient age; 6) operative time and blood loss; and (7) intestinal bacterial translocation (31-35). Sepsis has usually been managed by percutaneous drainage and has rarely been lethal.

Table 1. Risk factors after liver resection for metastatic colorectal cancer.

Risk of postoperative complications
Extent of liver resection
Operative blood loss

Determinants of survival
Margins of resection
Status of extrahepatic sites at laparotomy

Bile leak has been a frequent complication among those with morbidity, and has generally been self-limiting in the absence of a distal biliary stricture. It has usually been treated successfully by percutaneous drainage and temporary stent placement or balloon dilatation through endoscopic retrograde cholangiography. In attempts to prevent this complication, several authors have reported the use of dye injection through the cystic duct during liver resection, identifying leaks in the resected biliary tree prior to wound closure (27,46).

Bleeding has been the main source of life-threatening risk during liver resection and has resulted in organ failure, coagulation disorders, and other complications (27,29,38,40). Significant advances in surgical technique during the last two decades that have led to reductions in major operative blood loss are: the use of an ultrasonic dissector for transection of liver parenchyma; and control of hilar and suprahepatic blood vessels prior to liver resection. (The technical aspects of liver resection are described in Chapter 13.) Postoperative bleeding resulting in reoperation has been reported to occur in about 1% of patients (27).

Liver failure after resection of metastases has been uncommon because the operation usually has been done with an adequate amount of the healthy, residual liver. However, when it occurs, liver failure has resulted in death for about 70% of patients (46). Risk factors associated with this complication are major operative hemorrhage, extent of resection, use of chemotherapy prior to resection, and the presence of abnormal serum alkaline phosphatase or bilirubin prior to operation. (47). In series of liver resection for hepatocellular carcinoma, the incidence of liver failure for patients with cirrhosis has been reported to be about 15%, which emphasizes the importance of adequate preoperative liver function in the appropriate selection of patients for resection (48). Another source of postoperative liver failure has been thrombosis of the hepatic artery, occasionally related to the placement of arterial catheters for chemotherapy (49).

Multivariate analyses of the risk factors for postoperative complications have revealed that the extent of liver resection is a significant independent variable (Table 1) (27,38,40, 50). Univariate analyses have identified operative blood loss as a significant risk factor for complications, but this has not usually been confirmed by multivariate analyses (38,40,51). Nevertheless, blood loss reflects a combination of perioperative factors and should be considered an important element of risk for complications. In addition, it has been demonstrated that, as the operating team (surgeons, anesthesiologists, and nurses) gains more extensive experience, overall morbidity and mortality rates have decreased. (27,52).

Table 2. Results of liver resection for metastatic colorectal cancer		
	Number of	Five-year
Author, year (ref. #)	patients	survival (%)
Foster, 1978 (55)	168	20
Fortner et al., 1984 (13)	75	35
Adson et al., 1984 (7)	141	25
Butler et al., 1986 (34)	62	34
Hughes et al., 1986 (59)	607	33
Nordlinger et al., 1987 (37)	80	25
Doci et al., 1991 (61)	100	30
Scheele et al., 1991 (58)	219	39
Gayowski et al., 1994 (57)	204	32
Fong et al., 1997 (54)	456	38
Jamison et al., 1997 (65)	280	27
Jenkins et al., 1997 (62)	131	25
Bakalakos et al., 1998 (26)	301	29
Elias et al., 1998 (64)	151	28

Long-term Survival Results and Predictors of Outcome after Liver Resection

Over the last two decades, advances in surgical technique have lowered operative morbidity and mortality rates for resection at experienced centers. The five-year survival results of large series of liver resections are listed in Table 2. As previously described, non-surgical management of liver metastases resulted in five-year survival rates of 0%, regardless of the number of tumors or the type of medical therapy. Thus, liver resection represented a significant advance in the treatment of metastatic colorectal cancer. At this time, resection is considered to be safe, effective, and the only potentially curative treatment for colorectal cancer metastatic to the liver. As the screening modalities for occult unresectable disease become more accurate, patient selection criteria for liver resection will be refined to better identify those suitable for curative operation.

Many authors have evaluated the prognostic determinants of survival after resection, concentrating on the relative importance of the technical aspects of resection versus the biological features of metastatic disease. Biological factors that have been studied include carcinoembryonic antigen (CEA) level (53), number and size of liver metastases (53-57), node status of the primary colorectal cancer (7,27,30,34,58-60), and the disease-free interval between resection of the primary tumor and the detection of liver metastases (33,57,58,61). Cady et al. reported that there was significant correlation between the CEA level, the number of metastatic tumors, ploidy pattern on flow cytometry, and disease-free survival time (53). Others have not confirmed that CEA level or ploidy have prognostic significance (40, 54). Many of the referenced studies have demonstrated that the number (greater than four) and size (greater than 10 cm.) of liver metastases, the positive-node status of the primary tumor, and a short disease-free interval are predictive of poorer outcome. However, these factors should not be considered absolute contraindications to resection, since survival rates may be as high as 24% in the presence of these factors (54).

Positive resection margins (26,53,54,57-59,62-65) and identification of occult extrahepatic disease during laparotomy (35,53,54,58,59,64) have been demonstrated in many series to be the most important independent factors, which predicted an adverse outcome (Table 1). The importance of a 1-cm negative margin has been emphasized by some authors but not confirmed by others (53, 54, 58, 59, 63-65). Microscopic satellite lesions have been found within 1 cm. of metastatic tumors greater than 4 cm., increasing the risk of local recurrence after resection of larger tumors with narrow resection margins (63). In virtually all reports, a positive resection margin was highly predictive of a poor outcome.

Patterns of recurrence after liver resection

Recurrence following liver resection has occurred in 50% to 75% of patients and remains the most important problem confronting the surgeon and patient considering liver resection for metastatic disease (30,40,49,54,59,60,66,67). The sites of first recurrence after liver resection have been reported to be liver in 30% to 70% of patients, pulmonary parenchyma in about 20%, abdominal cavity (including loco regional primary tumor recurrence) in about 20%, and central nervous system in fewer than 10%. Of patients with recurrent liver metastases after resection, 20-30% had disease confined to the liver (59). Liver recurrence either alone or with extrahepatic disease has been more common when liver resection margins were positive and liver disease was bilobar (40). After unilateral wedge resection of metastatic disease, most patients with liver recurrence had disease in the contra lateral lobe (54). Thus, a more extensive operation at the time of the first resection would not have prevented the development of liver or extrahepatic recurrence (53,54).

NEUROENDOCRINE TUMORS

As liver resection for metastatic colorectal cancer has become a more familiar and increasingly safe operation, there has been more aggressive use of the procedure for other metastatic tumors to the liver, such as neuroendocrine malignancies. Although these tumors are malignant and the liver is the main site of metastatic disease, the rates of disease progression are slow and variable. Hence, liver resection may result in a long disease-free survival time, despite the high rate of recurrence after resection. In addition, the debilitating functional syndromes related to hormone production may justify palliative tumor resection.

Somatostatin receptor scintigraphy (SRS) may be used to define the extent of metastases in patients with neuroendocrine tumors. Frilling et al. reported that SRS confirmed the presence of disease in all 35 patients who had liver metastases identified by conventional imaging methods (68). In addition, 19 (54%) patients had extrahepatic tumors found by SRS but not detected by other imaging techniques. Thus, the effectiveness of SRS in identification of extrahepatic metastases may influence the selection of patients for liver resection.

Metastatic pheochromocytoma, carcinoid and islet cell tumors are most commonly reported in series of resections for non-colorectal hepatic metastases (69-71). Of 15 completely resected patients reported by Chen et al. (Johns

Hopkins), 10 recurred with a median time to recurrence of 21 months (69). Nine of the 10 recurrences were in the liver, and these were treated by repeat resection (four), cryoablation (one), and chemoembolization (one). The survival time of completely resected patients was compared to that of 23 patients who had a comparable burden of disease in the liver but who did not have resection. The five-year actuarial survival was 73% for those having resection and 29% for those treated medically (p=0.003). Que et al. (Mayo Clinic) reported a four-year median survival rate of 74% for 74 patients with carcinoid and islet cell tumors treated by curative resection (70). Dousset et al. reported a five-year median survival rate of 62% in patients treated by curative resection (71). Although a definitive trial proving the superiority of liver resection of neuroendocrine tumors over other forms of therapy will probably never be done, existing data suggest that liver resection for neuroendocrine metastases may prolong survival time.

OTHER PRIMARY TUMOR SITES

Isolated liver metastases most commonly occur from colorectal and neuroendocrine tumors, but may also be seen in gastrointestinal sarcoma, ocular melanoma, and occasionally in breast and other malignancies. Management of these tumors should be formulated after a complete evaluation of the extent of metastatic disease and based on the tempo and extent of the disease. In a report on an 11-year series of 140 liver resections for non-colorectal, non-neuroendocrine hepatic metastases, Lang et al. demonstrated a median survival of 32 months for patients who had negative margins of resection and were without extrahepatic tumor at the time of liver resection (72). Included in this series were patients with sarcoma (n=20), melanoma (n=9), as well as breast (n=34), pancreatic (n=16), renal (n=13), gastric (n=9), lung (n=6), and adrenal (n=6) cancers. Thus, resection of liver metastases from these diseases can provide long-term survivorship in a carefully selected group of patients.

REFERENCES

1. Centers for Disease Control and Prevention. National Center for Health Statistics. National Vital Statistics Reports. 1999;47(19):208.
2. Cancer Facts and Figures-1999. Atlanta, Ga. American Cancer Society, 1999.
3. Bengmark S, Hafstrom L. The natural history of primary and secondary malignant tumors of the liver: I. The prognosis for patients with hepatic metastases from colonic and rectal carcinoma treated by laparotomy. *Cancer* 1969;23:198.
4. Willett CG, Tepper JE, Cohen AM, Orlow E, Welch CE. Failure patterns following curative resection of colonic carcinoma. *Ann Surg* 1984;53:1354.
5. Wanebo HJ, Semoglou C, Attiyeh F, Stearns MJ Jr. Surgical management of patients with primary operable colorectal cancer and synchronous liver metastases. *Am J Surg* 1978;135:81.
6. Jaffe BM, Donegan WM, Watson F, Spratt JS. Factors influencing survival in patients with untreated hepatic metastases. *Surg Gynecol Obstet* 1968;127:1.

7. Adson MA, van Heerden JA, Adson MH, Wagner JS, Ilstrup DM. Resection of hepatic metastases from colorectal cancer. *Arch Surg* 1984;119:647.

8. Nagorney DM. Hepatic resection for metastases from colorectal cancer. *Prob General Surg* 1987;4:83.

9. Wood CB, Gillis CR, Blumgart LH. A retrospective study of the natural history of patients with liver metastases from colorectal cancer. *Clin Oncol* 1976;2:285.

10. Baden H, Anderson B. Survival of patients with untreated liver metastases from colorectal cancer. *Scand J Gastroenterol* 1975;10:221.

11. Goslin R, Steele G Jr, Zamcheck N, et al. Factors influencing survival in patients with hepatic metastases from adenocarcinoma of the colon and rectum. *Dis Colon Rectum* 1982;25:749.

12. Finan PJ, Marshall RJ, Cooper EH, Giles GR. Factors affecting survival in patients presenting with synchronous hepatic metastases from colorectal cancer: a clinical and computer analysis. *Br J Surg* 1985;72:373.

13. Fortner J, Silva JS, Golbey RB, et al. Multivariate analysis of a personal series of 247 consecutive patients with liver metastases from colorectal cancer: I. Treatment by hepatic resection. *Ann Surg* 1984;199:306.

14. Gibbs JF, Weber TK, Rodriguez-Bigas MA, et al. Intraoperative determinants of unresectability for patients with colorectal hepatic metastases. *Cancer* 1998;82:1244.

15. Steele G, Bleday R, Mayer RJ. A prospective evaluation of hepatic resection for colorectal carcinoma metastases to the liver: Gastrointestinal tumor study group protocol 6584. *J Clin Oncol* 1991;9:1105.

16. Jarnagin WR, Fong Y, Ky A, et al. Liver resection for metastatic colorectal cancer: assessing the risk of occult irresectable disease. *J Am Coll Surg* 1999;188(1):33.

17. Babineau T, Lewis D, Jenkins R, et al. Role of staging laparoscopy in the treatment of hepatic malignancy. *Am J Surg* 1994;167:151.

18. John TG, Greig JD, Crosbie JL, et al. Superior staging of liver tumors with laparoscopy and laparoscopic ultrasound. *Ann Surg* 1994;220:711.

19. Lai DTM, Fulham M, Stephen M, et al. The role of whole-body positron emission tomography with [18]fluorodeoxyglucose in identifying operable colorectal cancer metastases to the liver. *Arch Surg* 1996;131:703.

20. Vitola JV, Delbeke D, Sandler MP, et al. Positron emission tomography to stage unsuspected metastatic colorectal carcinoma to the liver. *Am J Surg* 1996;171:21.

21. Fong Y, Saldinger PF, Akhurst T, et al.. Utility of ^{18}F-FDG positron emission tomography scanning on selection of patients for resection of hepatic colorectal metastases. *Am J Surg* 1999;178:282.

22. Castaing D, Emond J, Bismuth H, et al. Utility of operative ultrasound in the surgical management of liver tumors. *Ann Surg* 1986; 204:600.

23. Machi I, Isomoto H, Yamashita Y, et al. Intraoperative ultrasound in screening for liver metastasis from colorectal cancer: comparative accuracy with traditional procedures. *Surgery* 1987;101:678.

24. Parker GA, Lawrence W, Horsley JS, et al. Intraoperative ultrasound of the liver affects operative decision making. *Ann Surg* 1989;209:569.

25. Aitken DR, Thurston MO, Hinkle GH, et al. Portable gamma probe for radioimmune localization of experimental colon tumor xenografts. 1983

Annual Meeting of the Association for Academic Surgery. Syracuse, NY. November 2-5, 1983. *J Surg Res* 1984;36:480.

26. Bakalakos EA, Young DC, Martin EW. Radioimmunoguided surgery for patients with liver metastases secondary to colorectal cancer. *Ann Surg Oncol* 1998;5(7):590.

27. Doci R, Gennari L, Montalto P, et al. Morbidity and mortality after hepatic resection of metastases from colorectal cancer. *Br J Surg* 1995;82:377.

28. Logan SE, Meier SJ, Ramming KP, Morton DL, longmire WP. Hepatic resection of metastatic colorectal carcinoma: a ten- year experience. *Arch Surg* 1982;117:25.

29. Bengmark S, Hafstrom L, Jeppsson B, Jonsson PE, Ryden S, Sunqvist K. Metastatic disease in the liver from colorectal cancer: an appraisal of liver surgery. *World J Surg* 1982;6:61.

30. Fortner JG. Recurrence of colorectal cancer after hepatic resection..*Am J Surg* 1988;155:378.

31. Nims TA. Resection of the liver for metastatic cancer. *Surg Gynecol Obstet* 1984;158:46.

32. Petrelli NJ, Nambisan RN, Herrera L, Mittelman A. Hepatic resection for isolated metastasis from colorectal carcinoma. *Am J Surg* 1985;149:205.

33. Cady B, McDermott WV. Major hepatic resection for metachronous metastases from colon cancer. *Ann Surg* 1985;201:204.

34. Butler J, Attiyeh FF, Daly JM. Hepatic resection for metastases of the colon and rectum. *Surg Gynecol Obstet* 1986;162:109.

35. Ekberg H, Tranberg KG, Andersson R, et al. Determinants of survival in liver resection for colorectal secondaries. *Br J Surg* 1986;73:727.

36. Bradpiece HA, Benjamin IS, Halevy A, Blumgart LH. Major hepatic resection for colorectal liver metastases. *Br J Surg* 1987;74:324.

37. Nordlinger B, Parc R, Delva E, Quilichini MA, Hannoun L, Huguet C. Hepatic resection for colorectal liver metastases. Influence on survival of preoperative factors and surgery for recurrences in 80 patients. *Ann Surg* 1987;205:256.

38. Holm A, Bradley E, Aldrete JS. Hepatic resection of metastasis from colorectal carcinoma. Morbidity, mortality, and pattern of recurrence. *Ann Surg* 1989;209:428.

39. Vogt P, Raab R, Ringe B, Pilchmayr R. Resection of synchronous liver metastases from colorectal cancer. *World J Surg* 1991;15:62.

40. Lind DS, Parker GA, Horsley JS III, et al. Formal hepatic resection of colorectal liver metastasis. Ploidy and prognosis. *Ann Surg* 1992;215:677.

41. Thompson HH, Tompkins RK, Longmire WP. Major hepatic resection. A 25-year experience. *Ann Surg* 1983;197:375.

42. Iwatsuki S, Shaw BW, Starzl TE. Experience with 150 liver resections. *Ann Surg* 1983;197:247.

43. Yanaga K, Kanematsu T, Takenaka K, Sugimachi K. Intraperitoneal septic complications after hepatectomy. *Ann Surg* 1986;203:148.

44. Pace RF, Blenkharn JI, Edwards WJ, Orloff M, Blumgart LH, Benjamin IS. Intra-abdominal sepsis after hepatic resection. *Ann Surg* 1989;209:302.

45. Wang X, Andersson R, Soltesz V, Guo W, Bengmark S. Water-soluble ethylhydroxyethyl cellulose prevents bacterial translocation induced by major liver resection in the rat. *Ann Surg* 1993;217:155.

46. Bismuth H, Houssin D, Ornowski J, Meriggi F. Liver resections in cirrhotic patients: a Western experience. *World J Surg* 1986;10:311.

47. Didolkar MS, Fitzpatrick JL, Elias EG, et al. Risk factors before hepatectomy, hepatic function after hepatectomy and computed tomographic changes as indicators of mortality from hepatic failure. *Surg Gynecol Obstet* 1989;169:17.
48. Choi TK, Edward CS, Fan ST, Wong J. Results of surgical resection for hepatocellular carcinoma. Hepatogastroenterology 1990;37:172.
49. Wanebo HJ, Quyen DC, Vezeredis MP, Soderberg C. Patient selection for hepatic resection of colorectal metastases. *Arch Surg* 1996;131:322.
50. Fong Y, Blumgart LH, Fortner JG, Brennan MF. Pancreatic or liver resection for malignancy is safe and effective for the elderly. *Ann Surg* 1995;222:426.
51. Mentha G, Huber O, Robert J, Klopfenstein C, Egeli R, Rohner A. Elective hepatic resection in the elderly. *Br J Surg* 1992;79:557.
52. Hughes K, Simon R, Songhorabodi S, et al. Resection of the liver for colorectal carcinoma metastases. A multi-institutional study of indications for resection. *Surgery* 1988;103:278.
53. Cady B, Stone MD, McDermott WV, et al. Technical and biological factors in disease-free survival after hepatic resection for colorectal cancer metastases. *Arch Surg* 1992;127:561.
54. Fong Y, Cohen AM, Fortner JG, et al.. Liver resection for colorectal metastases. *J Clin Oncol* 1997;15:938.
55. Foster JH. Survival after liver resection for secondary tumors. *Am J Surg* 1978;135:389.
56. Cobourn CS, Makowka L, Langer B, et al. Examination of patient selection and outcome for hepatic resection for metastatic disease. *Surg Gynecol Obstet* 1987;165:239.
57. Gayowski TJ, Iwatsuki S, Madariaga JR, et al. Experience in hepatic resection for metastatic colorectal cancer: analysis of clinical and pathologic risk factors. *Surgery* 1994;116:703.
58. Scheele J, Stangl R, Altendorf-Hofmann A, et al. Indicators of prognosis after hepatic resection for colorectal secondaries. *Surgery* 1991;110:13.
59. Hughes KS, Simons R, Songhorabodi S, et al. Resection of the liver for colorectal carcinoma metastases: a multi-institutional study of patterns of recurrence. *Surgery* 1986;100:278.
60. Iwatsuki S, Esquivel CO, Gordon RD, et al. Liver resection for metastatic colorectal cancer. *Surgery* 1986;100:804.
61. Doci R, Gennari L, Bignami P, et al. One hundred patients with hepatic metastases from colorectal cancer treated by resection. Analysis of prognostic determinants. *Br J Surg* 1991;78:797.
62. Jenkins LT, Millikan KW, Bines SD, Staren ED, Doolas A. Hepatic resection for metastatic colorectal cancer. *The American Surgeon* 1997;63:605.
63. Shirabe K, Takenaka K, Fujiwara Y, et al. Analysis of prognostic risk factors in hepatic resection for metastatic colorectal carcinoma with special reference to the surgical margin. *Br J Surg* 1997;84:1077.
64. Elias D, Cavalcanti A, Sabourin JC, et al. Resection of liver metastases from colorectal cancer: the real impact of the surgical margin. *Eu J Surg Oncol* 1998;24:174.
65. Jamison RL, Donohue JH, Nagorney DM, Rosen CB, Harmsen MS, Ilstrup DM. Hepatic resection for metastatic colorectal cancer results in cure for some patients. *Arch Surg* 1997;132:505.

66. Ekberg H, Tranberg KG, Andersson R, et al. Pattern of recurrence in liver resection for colorectal secondaries. *World J Surg* 1987;11:541.
67. Scheele J, Stangl R, Altendorf-Hofmann A. Hepatic metastases from colorectal carcinoma: impact of surgical resection on the natural history. *Br J Surg* 1990;77:124.
68. Frilling A, Malago M, Martin H, Broelsch CE. Use of somatostatin receptor scintigraphy to image extrahepatic metastases of neuroendocrine tumors. *Surgery* 1998;124:1000.
69. Chen H, Hardacre JM, Uzar A, Cameron JL, Choti MA. Isolated liver metastases from neuroendocrine tumors: does resection prolong survival? *J Am Coll Surg* 1998;187:88.
70. Que FG, Nagorney DM, Batts KP, et al. Hepatic resection for metastatic neuroendocrine carcinomas. *Am J Surg* 1995;169:36.
71. Dousset B, Saint-Marc O, Pitre J, et al. Metastatic endocrine tumors: medical treatment, surgical resection, or liver transplantation. *World J Surg* 1996;20:908.
72. Lang H, Nussbaum KT, Weimann A, Raab R. (Liver resection for non-colorectal, non-neuroendocrine hepatic metastases). (German) *Chirurg* 1999;70(4):439.

12

RESECTION FOR RECURRENT COLORECTAL LIVER METASTASES

Konstantine Avradopolous, M.D. and
Harold J. Wanebo, M.D.
Roger Williams Medical Center, Providence, RI
Sam G. Pappas, M.D.
Northwestern University Medical School, Chicago, IL

INTRODUCTION

Colorectal cancer is one of the most common gastrointestinal cancers worldwide. It is estimated that in the year 2001, 130,200 colorectal cases will be diagnosed in the United States. Also over the next year, 56,300 Americans will die of this disease. Colorectal cancer ranks third in estimated cancer deaths, behind lung and prostate cancer in men, and lung and breast cancer in women (1). The vast majority of these patients die of metastases (2,3). Among patients diagnosed with colorectal cancer, during the course of their illness, the liver will become involved in 40-70% of cases. It has been well documented that the treatment of choice, on first presentation of hepatic metastases, is surgical resection (4-7). Numerous series report 5-year survival rates of 22%-39%, with an average around 30% (4-7). Unfortunately, this means that 70% of patients will recur after hepatic resection for colorectal metastases. Among these patients, about 30% will present with liver only recurrences, and about one third to one half of these will be candidates for a second hepatic resection (2,3).

The natural history of liver metastases from colon carcinoma is well documented (8). Jaffe et al. studied 177 patients and found a median survival of five months with no five-year survivals. Multiple investigators have reported similar survival data (9,10,11). Patients with a solitary liver metastasis have a longer survival than patients with multiple lesions with the one-year survival rate being 5.7% for patients with widespread disease and 27% for disease localized to one segment, and as high as 60% for patients with a solitary metastasis (12). Bengtssongon showed a median survival of 6 months for less than 25% liver involvement, 6 months for 25-75% involvement and two months for >75% involvement (13). Depending on the extent of liver involvement, survival ranges from 6 months to a year, with chemotherapy adding little if any survival advantage. Five-year survivors are extremely rare.

Because surgery offers the only chance at extending survival, and surgeons have become more comfortable with extensive hepatic resections, numerous reports have addressed repeat hepatic resections over the last several years. These investigators have reported results of second hepatic resection for colorectal metastases raising questions concerning the applicability of this procedure, long-term benefits and ideal selection of patients for this aggressive approach.

PATTERNS OF RECURRENCE

It is imperative to understand the patterns of recurrence in this patient population before embarking on aggressive surgical approaches. As mentioned previously, 30% of patients will survive 5 years after resection of metastatic colorectal cancer. Seventy percent will recur (14). Using accumulated data from 2,533 patients in the literature, looking at recurrences after initial liver resections for colorectal metastases, patterns of recurrence were evaluated by Bismuth et al. (15). It was shown that 28% of the patients presented with liver only recurrences, and 21% with isolated extra-hepatic recurrence. The remainder (51%) developed both hepatic and extra-hepatic recurrences. Bismuth reports that a very select number of patients with hepatic recurrences, and even fewer with additional minimal resectable extrahepatic disease, were considered for re-resection. Despite the low number of candidates, because of the limited options available, he also reports increasing repeat resections with 6/105 before 1990 to 28% (49/177) in the last 5 years. It appears that patient selection is the key to successful repeat hepatic resections for colorectal metastases.

PATIENT SELECTION

A number of predictors of hepatic recurrence after initial resection of colorectal hepatic metastases have been described in the literature. These include number of liver metastases initially resected, (16,17,18) the size of the metastases, (19) the presence of extrahepatic disease, (17) the stage of the primary tumor, (18,20) the interval between colorectal and hepatic resection, (13) bilateral vs. unilateral lobar disease, (17,21,22) and resection margins of less than 1cm (14,15,17).

Recently, Adam et al. (23) reported results of 83 repeat hepatectomies. Sixty-four of these were second resections, 15 were third resections and 4 were fourth hepatectomies. Combined extrahepatic surgery was performed in 25% of these procedures. He specifically looked at factors of prognostic value. On univariate analysis, the curative nature of first and second hepatectomies (negative resection margins), interval between first and second resections greater than one year, the number of recurrent tumors, CEA levels and presence of extrahepatic disease were all statistically associated with prognosis. Specifically, patients with negative resection margins, one-year interval between resections, solitary lesions, normal CEA levels, and no extrahepatic disease had a better prognosis. Only the curative nature of the second resection, (i.e. 1 cm margins) and interval greater than one year were associated with survival upon multivariate analysis. This is consistent with data concerning initial hepatic resections.

Currently, we consider the following factors before embarking on second hepatic resections: number of initial lesions (<4), size of metastasis, adequacy of resection margins, presence of extrahepatic disease as well as stage of the primary tumor and disease free interval, bilateral vs. unilateral disease and anatomic resection.

Although it is difficult to give definitive recommendations on selection of patients for second hepatic resection, it makes sense to use the criteria for initial hepatic resections, mentioned above, to select candidates for repeat resections. Presently there is a trend toward aggressive surgical intervention in these patients, mainly because there is no other treatment that offers comparable survivals. Currently, in selecting patients for second resections we select patients who are good surgical candidates and have no medical contraindications. Also, in patients who have technically resectable liver disease we evaluate for unresectable extrahepatic disease. A thorough evaluation includes a CT scan of the abdomen and chest, tumor markers including CEA and CA 19-9, colonoscopy to rule out an anastomotic recurrence, angiography if hepatic artery catheter placement is considered and, finally, testing of the patient's liver function. Depending upon the clinical situation, selective patients with extrahepatic disease, specifically local-regional recurrences or lung metastases, may be considered for more extensive combined procedures.

TECHNICAL CONSIDERATIONS

Techniques of hepatic resection have been described in detail in the surgical literature (9). There are aspects of second hepatic surgery that should be considered before undertaking this challenge. It is the unique regenerative capacity of hepatic tissue that makes repeat liver resection a possibility. The normal liver tolerates a 70–80% resection safely with subsequent regeneration of the remnant (24).

On entering the peritoneal cavity, the first step is to carefully search for recurrent local disease, extrahepatic metastases or peritoneal seeding. There are usually multiple adhesions present and these must be taken down carefully. This includes adhesions along the length of the small bowel, the colon, and between the liver and abdominal wall. A complete examination of the liver must then be performed by palpation and intraoperative ultrasonography in order to confirm the number and size of metastases, define the relationships with intrahepatic vascular structures, and look for possible occult metastatic lesions. Repeat resections are often more difficult than first resections for a number of reasons. Re-exposure of the liver is complicated due to frequent adhesions of the cut surfaces of previous resections to adjacent organs.

Previous dissection of the hepatic pedicle and vena cava make vascular control more complicated. Liver tissue is often more fragile because of both liver regeneration, and chemotherapy which inevitably has been given preoperatively. Oftentimes, the operative time is increased compared to initial resections, and some surgeons have reported increased risk of bleeding on second resections (25). We use the CUSA (Cavitron ultrasonic aspirator) for parenchymal dissection of liver tissue in combination with direct vascular ligation and electrocautery as needed. Consideration of these technical factors is essential to successful results of second hepatic resections.

RESULTS OF SECOND HEPATIC RESECTIONS FOR METASTATIC COLORECTAL CARCINOMA

Tomas de la Vega performed the first repeat resection for metastatic colorectal disease in 1984 (26). Since that time multiple authors have reported numerous second hepatic resections. Fernandez-Trigo reviewed 170 patients from 20 different institutions throughout the world. These are included in the Repeat Hepatic Metastases Registry (27). In this series the mean age of the patients was 58 years and the mean follow-up was 22 months. Thirty-two percent of the patients presented with Duke's stage A or B and 58% presented with Duke's stage C. The majority of patients (75%) presented with colon cancer and 25% were rectal tumors. Ninety percent of the cases showed a histologic pattern of adenocarcinoma with moderate grade accounting for 72%. Mucinous adenocarcinoma was very unusual, accounting for 4% of the cases. After resection, adjuvant therapies were used in only 16% of the patients with 5-FU being the most common. Radiotherapy was rare, used in only 3%, and these were patients with rectal malignancies. Survival times were estimated using Kaplan-Meier curves. The overall 3 and 5-year survival rates projected were 37% and 26%, respectively. Median survival time was 30 months. Overall, this series shows 40% 3-year and 30% 5-year survival when patients are made disease-free by second resection. Residual disease left behind significantly decreases the 3 and 5-year survival rates to 28% and 11%, respectively.

Hugh et al. reviewed nine patients with second hepatic resection from a series of 70. He reported a perioperative mortality of 1 of 9 and morbidity in 2 out of 9. The interval between first and second resection was 17 months and the median survival after second resection was 17 months. In a more recent review, Gazzaniga reported 10, second hepatic resections (28). He reports a time interval between first and second hepatic resections of 15 months with an average follow-up of 27 months that corresponds with average survival. Only one out of ten patients, however, survived greater than 5 years. Bines retrospectively reviewed 131 patients and reported curative resection in 107 (29). These were initial hepatic resections. Thirty-one of these patients experienced recurrences confined to the liver. Thirteen of these 107 (12%) made up his study population. About 30% of the patients developed recurrence at the original resection site and 70% developed recurrences remote from the primary resection site. He reported a morbidity of 23% and a mortality of 8% among those submitted to second resections. Four of the 13 were dead of disease with a disease-free survival of 9.7 months. He reported a median survival for all patients of 24 months. Seven of the 13 had no evidence of disease with a follow-up of 34.9 months. He reported a five-year overall survival of 23% (3 of the 13) but an actual disease-free five-year survival of only 2 of 13 (15%). Pinson reported his results of hepatic surgery in 1996 (30). Pinson reviewed 95 patients undergoing initial resection and 10 patients who underwent a repeat operation for subsequent hepatic metastases. He reported an interval of 17 months between first hepatic resection and repeat resection and a mean follow-up of 33 months. There were no operative deaths. The 1-year and 3-year disease-free survival rates were 60% and 45%, respectively. One patient recurred in the liver only and 4 patients developed liver and extrahepatic metastases. One patient developed pulmonary metastases.

Tuttle reported 23-second hepatic resections in his review (31). His perioperative morbidity was 22% and perioperative mortality was 0%. Median survival in his study was 39.9 months with a 5-year actuarial survival of 32%. Three of 23 patients survived greater than five years, and 70% of the patients developed recurrent hepatic disease with a median time to recurrence of 11 months. In a recent report of 191 second liver resections, the median survival was 30 months with 26% 5-year survival (32). Disease-free interval greater than one year after resection of the colon primary was the best predictor of outcome. Adam et al. reported 64 patients from a group of 243 who were resected for recurrent colorectal liver metastases (33). Perioperative mortality, morbidity and hospital stay were comparable to first hepatectomies. The overall and disease-free survival was 41% and 26% respectively. Kin et al. reviewed 67 patients after first hepatic resection (34). There were 33 recurrences and 15 were selected for second resection. The median interval between the first hepatectomy and the second resection was 15 months. The median follow-up after the second resection was 16 months with a range of 2-66 months. The perioperative mortality was 0% with a cumulative survival at 5 years of 21%. Of the 15 second resections, 8 recurred after hepatectomy. These authors concluded that the procedure can be performed safely and provide long-term survival rates similar to first resections. Chiappa et al. reported their results of second hepatic resection (35). Chiappa reviewed 41 patients, all of whom had curative resections with negative margins and no evidence of extrahepatic disease. Twenty-six recurred (63%) and 16 of the 26 had disease confined to the liver and of these, 10 underwent a second resection. These ten patients all experienced recurrences at a median of 16 months. Six involved the resection line as well as a remote site, 3 involved a remote site and only one patient had involvement at the initial resection site. These authors estimated a 4-year specific survival of 44% and a disease-free survival at 4 years of 18%. They concluded that in carefully selected patients, hepatic resection is a worthwhile treatment and that mortality, morbidity and survival are similar to patients with an initial resection. Finally, Bradley et al. reported 134 patients with hepatic resections for colorectal cancer (36). Thirty-six developed hepatic only recurrences and 15 underwent second resection. The median time interval to recurrence was 15 months. Procedures included 9 wedge resections, three lobectomies, one lobe and wedge resection and two patients who were cryo-ablated. These authors reported a recurrence in 7 of 15 patients resected. Of these 7, two had a hepatic only recurrence, 4 developed hepatic and extrahepatic recurrence and one patient had an extrahepatic only recurrence. The estimated overall survival was 74% at 5 years with an estimated disease-free survival of 58% at 5 years. A summary of results of second hepatic resection is included in Table I.

Table 1- Results of Repeat Hepatic Resections

Author/Yr.	Resected	Mortality	Overall Median Survival (months)	Actual Overall 5 yr. Survival
De la Veta, '84	4	-	22*	-
Butler, '86	2	0/2	-	0
Joyeaux, '87	4	-	21*	-
Dagundi, '87	9	-	16*	-
Norlinger, '87	6	0/6	-	0
Fortner, '88	3	0/3	-	0
Lange, '89	9	0/9	15	0
Hohenberger, '90	6	0/6	23	-
Griffith, '90	9	1/9	23	1
Stone, '90	10	0/10	25	0
Huguet, '90	10	0/10	32*	0
Bozzeti, '92	10	1/10	23	0
Nakanurn, '92	6	0/6	28.5*	1
Goullat, '93	13	-	14	-
Vaillant, '93	16	1/16	33	2
Elias, '93	28	1/28	30	-
Fowler, '93	8	-	23*	0
Que, '94	21	1/21	40.8	1
Fong, '94	25	0/25	30.2	0
Chu, '95	9	1/9	17	1
Gazzaniga, '95	10	0/10	-	1
Pinson, '96	10	0/10	-	1
Tuttle, '96	23	0/23	29.9	3
Bines, '96	13	1/13	24	3
Jin, '98	15	0/15	16	1
Chiappa, '99	10	0/10	13	1
Totals	287	7/287=2.4%	23.8	16/287=5.6%

It should be noted that the majority of these papers are made up of small numbers of patients with a range of 2-28 patients and median of 10. An exception is Fernandez-Trigo's review, which includes 170 patients as described. This review was not included in the table because the survivals are estimated, and actual survivals are not available. On review of this table, between 1984 and 1999 there were 287 reported cases of second hepatic resections in the literature. The mortality rate was 7/287 or 2.4%. The overall median survival is 23.8 months. The overall 5-year survival is 16/287 or 5.6%. The morbidity (not included in the table) ranges between 20-50%. We can conclude from this data that second hepatic resections can be done safely, with reasonable morbidity and mortality rates. Also, survival is improved relative to historical controls, with an overall median survival of 23.8 months. Five-year survivals, however, do not compare well with initial hepatic resections. Survivals of 30% for second hepatic resections, which are noted in the literature (Fernandez-Trigo), are most likely secondary to excellent patient selection. These results emphasize the need for innovative approaches in treating hepatic metastases from colorectal carcinoma.

CONCLUSION

Hepatic metastasis due to colorectal carcinoma is common with 50 to 70% of all patients developing this during the course of their disease. Hepatic resection offers the best chance of cure with a 30% 5-year survival after initial resection. Unfortunately, 70% of patients will recur, and 28% of these will have hepatic only recurrences. Of this population, about a third to one half will be candidates for re-resection.

Presently, prognostic factors used to select patients for second hepatic resection include: curative nature of first and second hepatectomies, disease free interval of greater than 1 year between procedures, number of recurrent tumors, serum CEA levels, and the presence of extrahepatic disease. Criteria for initial hepatic resections may be used also. It is clear that repeat hepatic resections can be done with low morbidity and mortality in experienced hands. Furthermore, we know that systemic chemotherapy offers little survival advantage and a resection is the best treatment for hepatic metastasis.

Limited patient numbers compromise the majority of studies. Although some authors report survival rates of 30%, it should be noted that this is true only in highly selected patient populations and the vast majority of these patients will recur. Because the risk of recurrence is so high, additional therapy should be strongly considered. Also, innovative approaches including cryo-ablation, radio-ablation and hepatic artery infusion may play a role in the treatment of recurrent hepatic metastases of colorectal carcinoma.

REFERENCES

1. CA Journal 15(1):12-16 January/February 2000.
2. Nicolson GL. Generation of phenotypic diversity and progression in metastatic tumor cells. Cancer Metastases Rev 3:25-42, 1984.
3. Vezeridis MP. Biology of metastases, In: Wanebo HJ, editor. Colorectal Cancer. St Louis: Mosby-Year Book Inc. 26-105, 1993.
4. Foster JH, Lund J. Liver metastasis. Cur Prob Surg 18:158, 1981.
5. Welch JP, Donaldson GA. Clinical correlation of an autopsy study of recurrent colorectal cancer. Ann Surg 189:496-502, 1979.

6. Rosen CD, Gordy DM, Tasso HS, et al. Perioperative blood transfusion and determinants of survival after liver resection for metastatic colorectal carcinoma. Ann Surg 216:493-505, 1992.
7. Scheele J, Stengle R, Altendoor-Hoffman A, et al. Indicators of prognosis after hepatic resection for colorectal secondary. Surgery 110:15-29 1991.
8. Kemeny NM, Sugarbaker PH, Smith TJ, et al. A prospective analysis of laboratory tests and endocrine studies can detect hepatic lesions. Ann Surg 195:163-167, 1982.
9. Fong Y, Kemeny NM, Paty P, Blumgart LH, Cohen A. Treatment of colorectal cancer: hepatic metastasis. Sem Surg Onc 12:219-252, 1996.
10. Jaffe BN, Donnigen WL, Watson F. Factors influencing survival in patients with untreated hepatic metastasis. Surg Gyn Obstet 172:1-11, 1968.
11. Bengmark S, Hafstrom L. The natural history of primary and secondary malignant tumors of the liver: The Prognosis for cases of hepatic metastasis from colonic and rectal carcinoma at laparotomy. Cancer 23:198-202, 1969.
12. Goslin R, Steele D, Zantic ET, et al. Factors influencing survival in patients with hepatic metastasis from adenocarcinoma of the colon and rectum. Dis Colon Rectum 25:749-754, 1982.
13. Bengtssongon G, Carlsson G, Hasstrom L. Natural history of patients with untreated liver metastasis from colorectal cancer. Am J Surg 141:586-589, 1981.
14. Wood CB, Gillis CR, Blumgard LH. A retrospective study of the natural history of patients with global metastasis from colorectal cancer. Clin Onc 2:285-288, 1976.
15. Bismuth AH, Adam R, Nevarro S, Castaing D, et al. Re-resection for colorectal liver metastases. Surg Onc Clin North America 5(2)353-364, April 1996.
16. Cady B, McDermott WV. Major hepatic resection for metacrenous metastasis from colon cancer. Ann Surg 201:204-209, 1985.
17. Ekberg GH, Tranberg KJ, Anderson R, et al. Patterns of recurrence in liver resection for colorectal secondaries. World J Surg 11:541-547, 1987.
18. Fortner JG, Silva JS, Goby RB, et al. Multivariate analysis of a personal series of 247 consecutive cases of liver metastasis from colorectal cancer. Ann Surg 199:306-316, 1984.
19. Hughes KS, Simon R, Song RO, Body S, et al. Resection of the liver for colorectal carcinoma metastasis: A multi-institutional study of patterns of recurrence. Surgery 100:278-284, 1986.
20. Fortner JG. Recurrence of colorectal cancer after hepatic resection. Am J Surg 155:378-382, 1988.
21. Nagasue N, Yukaya H, Ogawa Y, et al. Human liver regeneration after major hepatic resection. Ann Surg 206:30-39, 1987.
22. Elias D, Lasser PH, Huang JM, et al. Repeat hepatectomy for cancer. Br J Surg 80:1557-1562, 1993.

23. Foster JH, Lundy J. Liver metastasis. Curr Probl Surg 18:(3)157-202, 1981.
24. August DA, Sugarbaker PH, Otto RT, et al. Hepatic resection for colorectal metastases: influence of clinical factors in adjuvant 5-FU administered through a catheter. Ann Surg 201:210-218, 1985.
25. Adam R, Bismuth H, Castaing D, Wauchter F, et al. Repeat hepatectomy for colorectal liver metastases. Ann Surg 225:51-62, 1997.
26. de la Vega T, Donahue E, Dulas A, et al. A ten-year experience with hepatic resection. Surg Gyn Obstet 159:223-228, 1985.
27. Trego VF, Shamsa F. Repeat resection for colorectal metastasis. In Hepatobility Cancer textbook. Kluwer Academic Publishers, Boston 1994.
28. Gazziniga GM, Ciferri E, Gazio S, Bagaloro C, Muni CO, et al. Repeated hepatic resections for repeat hepatic metastasis of colorectal cancer. Hepatic Gastroenterology 42:383-386, 1995.
29. Bines SD, Doolas A, Jenkins L, Millikan K, Roseman D. Survival after repeat hepatic resection for recurrent colorectal hepatic metastases. Surgery 120:(4) 591-596, 1996.
30. Pinson CW, Wright JK, Chapman WC, Girrard CL, et al. Repeat hepatic surgery to colorectal cancer metastasis to the liver. Ann Surg 223: (6)765-776, 1996.
31. Tuttle TM, Curley SA, Rao MS. Repeat hepatic resection as effective treatment of recurrent colorectal liver metastases. Ann Surg Onc 4:(2)125-130, 1997.
32. Neidleman N, Anderson R. Repeated liver resections for recurrent liver cancer. Br J Surg 83:893-901, 1996.
33. Adam R, Bismuth H, Castaing D, Waechter F, et al. Repeat hepatectomy for colorectal liver metastases. Ann Surg 225: (1)51-62, 1997.
34. Kin T, Nakajima Y, Kanehiro H, Hisanaga M, et al. Repeat hepatectomy for recurrent colorectal metastases. World J Surg 22:(10)1087-1091, 1998.
35. Chiappa A, Zbar AP, Biella FB, Staudacher C. Survival after repeat hepatic resection for recurrent colorectal metastases. Hepato-Gastroenterology 46:1065-1070, 1999.
36. Bradley A, Capman W, Wright JK, March JW, et al. Reporting a surgical experience with hepatic colorectal metastasis. The American Surgeon 65:560-567, 1999.

13

SURGICAL RESECTION OF HEPATIC TUMORS-PATIENT SELECTION AND TECHNICAL CONSIDERATIONS

George W. Daneker, Jr., M.D.
Georgia Surgical Associates, Atlanta, GA
Charles A. Staley, M.D.
Emory University, Atlanta, GA

INTRODUCTION

TECHNIQUES OF LIVER RESECTION

General Principles
Operative resection remains the principal curative treatment of patients with liver metastasis from colorectal carcinoma, pancreatic islet cell carcinoma, and primary hepatocellular carcinoma. The successful emergence of liver resection has resulted from improvements in imaging and tumor staging, a clearer understanding of hepatic anatomy and resulting surgical technique, and better management of concurrent medical problems. At present, the mortality for liver resection in patients with normal liver function should be below 5%.

Management of patients with liver malignancies demands an understanding of the biological behavior of the tumor, familiarity with the indications and limitations of surgical intervention, and a thorough knowledge of hepatic anatomy. In this chapter we will review hepatic anatomy, discuss patient selection for liver resection, and describe technical details for the major hepatic resections.

Anatomy
The liver is anatomically divided into lobes, sectors, and segments based on the arterial and portal venous blood supply, hepatic venous drainage, and biliary drainage (**Figure 1**). The proper hepatic artery, portal vein, and common bile duct divide into the major right and left branches, which then arborize throughout the ipsilateral lobe. The division between the lobes follows a plane running vertically, through the liver, connecting the anterior border of the gallbladder fossa to the left side of the inferior vena cava (IVC) posteriorly. This plane is known by an eponym as "Cantlie's line" and defines the right lobe, which contains 2/3 of the volume of the liver.

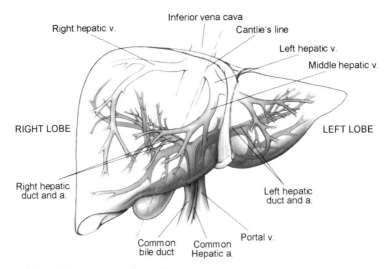

Figure 1 (above)-Functional hepatic anatomy.
Reprinted with permission from Wood WC, Skandalakis JE. Anatomic Basis of Tumor Surgery. St.Louis: Quality Medical Publishing, 1999.

The right and left lobes can be further subdivided into sectors based on the arborization of portal pedicles and hepatic veins (**Figure 2**). Using a plane of division along each of the three main hepatic veins, the liver is divided into four sectors, known as the right anterior, right posterior, left medial, and left lateral sectors. Each sector is supplied by a vascular and biliary pedicle comprised of the major lobar hepatic artery branch, portal vein branch, and bile duct branch. No clear topographic features or morphologic boundaries exist between the sectors in the right lobe. Within the left lobe, the umbilical fissure and falciform ligament define a plane of division between the medial and lateral sectors.

Figure 2 (below)- Sectoral hepatic anatomy.
Reprinted with permission from Wood WC, Skandalakis JE. Anatomic Basis of Tumor Surgery. St.Louis: Quality Medical Publishing, 1999.

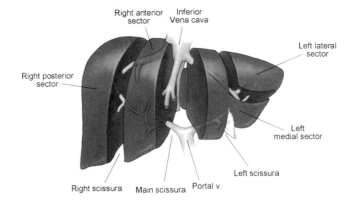

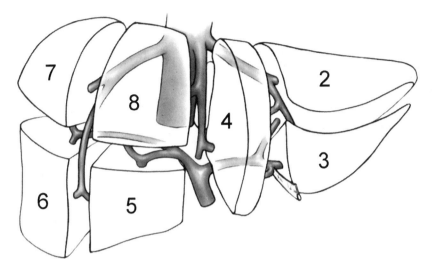

Figure 3-Segmental hepatic anatomy as described by Couinaud
Reprinted with permission from Wood WC, Skandalakis JE. Anatomic Basis of
Tumor Surgery. St.Louis: Quality Medical Publishing, 1999.

Each hepatic sector can be further subdivided into numbered segments as described
by Couinaud (**Figure 3**). This segmentation is one step further beyond the division
of liver into sectors and is based on the bifurcation of portal pedicles within the
sectors. The liver's segmental anatomy can be remembered as follows: in a
clockwise fashion beginning at the vena cava (12:00) are segments 2, 3, and 4, which
comprised the left lobe of liver. Segment 4, the portion of liver between the
falciform ligament and Cantlie's line, can be further divided into a superior half
(segment 4 a) and an inferior half (segment 4b). Continuing clockwise, the right
lobe is comprised of segments 5,6,7, and 8. No clear boundaries exist between the
segments of right lobe. The caudate lobe is assigned segment 1 by this system. The
caudate lobe is considered an autonomous segment from the standpoint of functional
anatomy. It receives branches from both hepatic arteries and portal veins, although
the majority of its blood supply comes from the left main portal pedicle. Venous
drainage of the caudate lobe is not into a hepatic vein but rather through a variable
number of bridging veins directly into the IVC.

The common bile duct branches into the main right and left hepatic ducts on the right
side of the liver hilum, anterior to the portal vein bifurcation, and overlying the
origin of the right main portal trunk. The right hepatic duct is short and ascends into
the parenchyma after the bifurcation. In 28% of cases, one of the main right
segmental ducts crosses to join the main left hepatic duct. Due to its length,
orientation, and the variable anatomy of the biliary tree, the right duct is more
vulnerable to injury then the more horizontally oriented left duct.

The hepatic veins arise from the IVC as it emerges from behind the liver immediately below the diaphragm. The suprahepatic IVC has a very short course before it passes through the diaphragm to join the right atrium. In a similar fashion, the hepatic veins have a short extrahepatic course before they enter the liver. The right hepatic main is usually single (61%) and drains the anterior and posterior sectors of right lobe. In 61% of patients there is an additional one or two large veins draining from the posterior or posterioinferior right lobe directly into the IVC. The middle hepatic vein runs along Cantlie's line and drains the right anterior and left medial sector. The left hepatic vein drains the left lateral sector and a small portion of the left medial sector. In 84% patients the left and middle hepatic veins arise from a common trunk. The bifurcation of this common trunk usually occurs near its origin from the vena cava and makes extrahepatic division of both the left and middle hepatic veins potentially hazardous.

PATIENT SELECTION

Colorectal Metastases

Each year there are about 150,000 new cases of colorectal cancer in the United States. Despite adjuvant chemotherapy, 50% of patients will develop tumor recurrence, many of which will have metastases in the liver. However, it is estimated that only 5-10% of patients with liver metastases will be candidates for hepatic resection (11). The issues currently debated regarding the role of surgery in the management of liver metastases include: 1) the potential benefits of hepatic resection compared with the natural history of the disease; 2) the risk of the operative procedure; 3) identification of those patients most likely to have a long term survival advantage from hepatic resection; and 4) the role of ablative techniques and adjuvant chemotherapy.

Prospective studies have demonstrated that serial serum CEA assays are the most effective screening test for the detection of subsequent hepatic metastases (12). Eighty-five to 90% of patients with hepatic metastases have an elevated CEA. Right upper quadrant pain and other symptoms do not usually occur until advanced metastatic disease is present. An elevated CEA, elevated liver function studies, or symptoms should precipitate further diagnostic studies including a detailed history and physical exam, chest x-ray, colonoscopy, and an abdominal and pelvic CT scan. Once hepatic metastases have been identified, further imaging studies are necessary to determine whether they are resectable lesions and are there associated extrahepatic disease. In a recent study at Emory, we have found that a biphasic helical abdominal CT scan or ferromagnetic contrast enhanced MR is equal in sensitivity and specificity for the detection of hepatic metastases compared to an expensive and invasive CT-angioportography. An extra benefit of the helical CT is the ability to identify the hepatic arterial anatomy noninvasively, which is helpful with operative planning and/ or intraarterial pump placement. A chest x-ray or a CT of the chest will screen for pulmonary metastases. To improve patient selection for hepatic resection, early reports have demonstrated a benefit of FDG-PET in detecting occult extrahepatic disease but further studies are necessary. At exploration, intraoperative ultrasound will identify another 10-20% of tumors not found on preoperative imaging and therefore change the intended operative strategy. (13).

The median survival of patients with liver metastases from colorectal cancer is generally less than 2 years with observation alone (11,14). Not surprisingly, the prognosis for patients with untreated hepatic metastases is closely related to the extent of liver replacement by tumor. Historical retrospective studies in the 1980s have demonstrated the benefit of hepatic resection compared to untreated patients (12,15). Surgical resection of metastatic colorectal cancer to the liver has traditionally yielded a 5-year survival rate of 25-35% (11,12,16,17).

With a better understanding of liver anatomy, the use of modern techniques of liver resection, and improved anesthesia and postoperative care, operative mortality has decreased to below 5% in most major centers (11). Liver failure, bleeding, abscess formation and other postoperative complications remain low in most studies.

The most difficult issue remains the selection of the patients most likely to benefit from surgical resection. In a multicenter retrospective review of 859 patients undergoing curative hepatic resection, Hughes et al reported a 5-year survival of 33%(12). With better imaging modalities including intraoperative ultrasound, improved operative technique and postoperative care, and better patient selection, 5-year survival ranges from 40-50%(18,19,20). Since over 90% of patients die of recurrent cancer, identifying important prognostic variables will help select those most likely to benefit long-term from hepatic resection. Reports examining the predictive value of age, gender, stage of primary disease, tumor size or CEA have been inconclusive.

As demonstrated by the Gastrointestinal Tumor Study Group and others, no benefit is obtained when metastatic disease involves the margin of resection (13). Every effort should be made to obtain a 1-cm margin of resection. Hepatic surgery should be avoided or abandoned if the resection will end in a positive margin. Historical data demonstrate an association between the number of metastases and survival when patients with four or less tumors are compared to patients with four or more tumors (11,12,16). With improvements in tumor ablative technology (cryosurgery and radiofrequency ablation), surgeons have begun to treat more than 4 lesions with a combination of resection and/or ablative therapy. However, no clear benefit of this approach has been reported with long-term follow-up. Extrahepatic disease in the portal or celiac nodes predicts a very poor prognosis and patients with nodal disease are not considered for hepatic resection. One exception to not resecting patients with extrahepatic disease is in the case of young patients with both liver and pulmonary metastases. In this select subset, staged liver and lung resection can result in a 20-40% 5-year survival (14). Outside of a clinical protocol, patients with 4 or less tumors with no extrahepatic disease and adequate liver reserve should be considered for potentially curative hepatic resection. Select non-colorectal hepatic tumors may benefit from hepatic resection if extrahepatic disease can be excluded. The overall five-year survival rate after resection of non-colorectal hepatic metastases is

20%(21). Though there is no clear benefit of adjuvant systemic chemotherapy after hepatic resection for colorectal cancer, recent studies have shown a benefit of adjuvant intraarterial chemotherapy.

Hepatocellular Carcinoma
The incidence of hepatocellular carcinoma (HCC) is increasing in many countries including the United States, mainly due to a steady increase in hepatitis C infections. Unfortunately, it now seems that hepatitis C virus (HCV) is more carcinogenic than Hepatitis B virus (HBV), judging from the frequency of HCC development among HBV- and HCV- induced cirrhosis (22). There have been numerous studies demonstrating changes in various oncogenes and tumor suppressor genes, but no consistent sequence of genetic changes has emerged similar to the adenoma-carcinoma sequence in colon cancer. Major risk factors for HCC include HBV and HCV-induced cirrhosis, alcoholic cirrhosis, aflatoxin exposure, and rare metabolic disorders. Most patients that present with symptoms of abdominal pain and weight loss have advanced disease with very few treatment options. An elevated serum alpha-fetoprotein (AFP) level above 500ng/ml is considered diagnostic for HCC, however mildly elevated levels from 20-400 ng/ml can be seen in cirrhotic patients without tumors.

Improvements in imaging have allowed noninvasive tests such as biphasic helical CT scan and dynamic MRI to replace invasive CT angioportography as the preoperative test of choice in both primary and metastatic liver cancer. Because of changes in the cirrhotic liver architecture due to fibrosis, necrosis, and numerous regenerative nodules, along with altered portal hemodynamics, the detection of HCC in the cirrhotic liver may involve several complementary imaging techniques (23).

In the United States, where HCC typically develops in the setting of well-established cirrhosis, fewer than 5-10% of patients meet the stringent criteria and are candidates for resection with acceptable risk. For patients without cirrhosis, surgical resection with partial hepatectomy is clearly the treatment of choice for HCC. In patients with well-compensated mild cirrhosis (Child's class A and B), partial hepatectomy should be considered. Functional liver tests including galactose elimination studies and indocyanine green dye retention studies can be helpful in determining hepatic reserve. The presence of extrahepatic disease, lack of sufficient hepatic reserve, satellite tumors, and main portal vein thrombosis are all contraindications to resection. Even when resection is possible, 70% of resected patients develop intrahepatic recurrence. The majority of these recurrences are de novo tumors and not recurrences at the surgical margin (24). In an attempt to make an impact on the high intrahepatic recurrence rate, numerous adjuvant chemotherapy trials have been completed with no clear benefit.

Because so few patients with HCC are candidates for resection and their survival is limited due to intrahepatic recurrence, many physicians favor orthotopic liver transplantation (OLT) for early HCC. Early series of OLT had disappointing results in terms of survival and tumor recurrence due to inappropriate patient selection criteria. More recently, with the restriction of OLT to patients with single tumors less than 5 cm or with 3 tumors less than 3 cm, 5-year survival improved to 60-70%(17,25). Furthermore, the rate of intrahepatic recurrence has decreased to 4-11%. For patients with these patient characteristics and end stage cirrhosis, OLT appears to be the best option. Although as waiting times for OLT grow longer, we may find that disease progression may disqualify them from OLT. With this concern, several institutions have started pre-transplant treatments with chemoembolization, percutaneous ethanol ablation, or percutaneous radiofrequency ablation. Preliminary results using these approaches in patients awaiting OLT increase the probability of transplantation and overall survival (26). However, OLT is still limited due to shortages in organ donation.

For those patients with resectable HCC with adequate liver reserve, hepatic resection is still the treatment of choice though tumor recurrence is still a major concern. If the encouraging improved survival and low tumor recurrence data matures and liver organ procurement increases, OLT may become the mainstay treatment for early hepatoma in the face of end stage cirrhosis. With improved technology, radiofrequency ablation (RFA) will most likely be the ablative method of choice for patients with unresectable disease since RFA can be performed percutaneously and at one sitting. Most importantly, improvements in the treatment of HCC will await novel systemic and regional chemotherapeutic regimens along with potential chemopreventive agents.

TYPES OF RESECTIONS

Liver resections are classified as either anatomic or nonanatomic. Anatomic resections follow defined anatomic landmarks and involve removal of a lobe, sector, or segment. The five major types of anatomic resections, in addition to resection of individual numbered segments, include: 1) right lobectomy; 2) left lobectomy; 3) resection of the right hepatic lobe and segment IV of the left lobe called a right trisegmentectomy; 4) resection of the left hepatic lobe and segments V and/or VIII of the right lobe called a left trisegmentectomy; and 5) resection of the lateral sector of the left lobe (segments II and III) called a lateral segmentectomy (**Figure 4**). Nonanatomic resections are based principally on tumor location and the parenchymal transection is not along anatomic landmarks. The identification of segmental boundaries, particularly in the right lobe, rarely impacts on nonanatomic resections. For these resections, tumors are rarely confined to within the single segment (other than the caudate lobe- Segment I) nor is formal segmental resection required to obtain a negative margin.

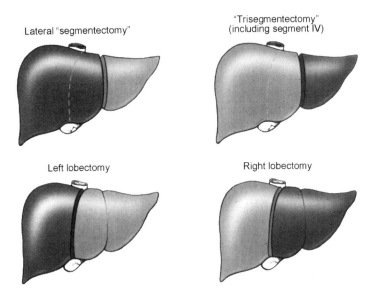

Lateral "segmentectomy"

"Trisegmentectomy" (including segment IV)

Left lobectomy

Right lobectomy

Figure 4-Anatomic liver resections
Reprinted with permission from Wood WC, Skandalakis JE. Anatomic Basis of Tumor Surgery. St.Louis: Quality Medical Publishing, 1999.

Right Hepatic Lobectomy
The right hepatic lobectomy is removal of liver segments V, VI, VII, and VIII, which comprise the right hemi-liver. Indications for this procedure include: (1) tumor(s) within the right lobe adjacent to the right main portal structures or portal structures and right hepatic vein, or (2) tumor(s) distributed within the right lobe that cannot be fully resected with a nonanatomic or segmental resection.

Right Hepatic Lobectomy-Incision and Exposure
Patient is placed the supine position with the arms extended perpendicular to the body. The full abdomen, out to the flank, and chest, up to the nipple line, is pepped and draped into the field. For the initial exploration, and incision two fingerbreadths below the costal margin is made from the midline to the mid-clavicular line. Through this incision exploration of the abdomen, including liver and porta, is conducted. Any portal lymphadenopathy is sampled and if positive for metastatic cancer by frozen section analysis, the procedure is aborted. If no extrahepatic tumor or more extensive intrahepatic tumor is detected, a bilateral subcostal incision is made. The right arm of the incision is extended towards the flank to the lateral peritoneal reflection. The left arm of the incision is extended lateral to the rectus sheath. For large bulky tumors, a midline paraxiphoid extension ("Mercedes-Benz") is useful for gaining access to the vena cava and hepatic veins. Although a thoracoabdominal incision is mentioned for large posterior right lobe tumors, this incision is morbid and rarely needed.

Once the final incision is made self-retaining retractors, which elevate the costal margin and give excellent exposure to the superior and posterior surfaces of the liver, are used to secure exposure. A second self-retaining retractor placed that the level of patient's hips is used to clear the operative field by providing downward traction on the abdominal viscera.

Right Hepatic Lobectomy-Hepatic Mobilization and Final Assessment of Resectability

The round ligament is divided as it courses from the umbilical fissure. The falciform ligament is divided halfway between the abdominal wall and the liver. While the assistant gently rotates the liver anterior and to the left, the triangular, right anterior, and right posterior coronary ligaments are divided medially to the level of the vena cava. As the liver is rotated off to the retroperitoneum, the right adrenal gland, bare area, and infrahepatic vena cava can be seen. If the diaphragm or adrenal gland are adherent to liver in the vicinity of the tumor, those structures should the resected en bloc with the lobe. Transverse division of the peritoneum over the suprahepatic vena cava is completed and the hepatic veins are identified. The dissection within the bare area is usually bloodless, although diaphragmatic fibrous investments around the vena cava and hepatic veins necessitate cautious sharp dissection.

Once fully mobilized, the liver is carefully inspected and examined by bimanual palpation. The liver is now examined by intraoperative ultrasound for identification of intrahepatic anatomy, assessment of tumor proximity to major vascular or biliary structures, and identification of occult tumors.

Right Hepatic Lobectomy-Posterior Dissection

The right lobe is then mobilized from the vena cava by division of 2-12 pairs of short hepatic veins extending directly from the anterior surface of the vena cava into the liver. These veins are fragile and best controlled by tying and clipping in continuity prior to transection. As noted in the anatomy section, one or two large veins extending from the vena cava into the liver, near the take-off of the right hepatic vein, are commonly encountered. Our preferred method of dividing these veins is by use of a 35mm endovascular GIA stapler with an articulating neck. Once the anxiety of using the stapler on a stout venous branch is overcome, this technique not only saves time, but also eliminates the aging experience of having a transected vessel slip out of the end of a vascular clamp. For the purist, or in those cases when the stapler cannot be positioned well, these veins can be carefully divided between vascular clamps and their ends oversewn with a running 3-0 or 4-0 Prolene suture.

The final barrier to the hepatic vein is a vascular/fibrotic ligament that spans the gap between segments VII and I (caudate lobe) over the vena cava. This ligament is divided using the stapler or between vascular clamps. Division of this structure is necessary for adequate visualization and mobilization of the right hepatic vein.

Extrahepatic division of the right hepatic vein prior to parenchymal transection is optimal, but not entirely necessary. In general, the mobility of the liver is greater and resection of pericaval parenchyma less challenging and safer if the hepatic vein is divided prior to parenchymal transection. The vein is cautiously freed from investing dense and areolar connective tissue extending from the retroperitoneum and diaphragm. The dissection alternates from the superior bare area, directed inferior and to the patient's right, to dissection underneath the liver and medial to the vein, directed superior and to the patient's left. The correct "angle of attack" for the dissection is 45-60% from the plane of the vein as it passes from the vena cava into the liver. The vein is freed from its take-off on the vena cava to its entrance into liver. The posterior dissection is completed at this point; however, the transection of the right hepatic vein is delayed until completion of the portal dissection. Transection is accomplished either with the stapler or between vascular clamps. If extrahepatic division of the vein is not possible, the vein should be encircled and controlled with an umbilical tape and red rubber catheter, known as a Rommel tourniquet. In this situation, the main right hepatic vein is divided within the parenchyma as or near the last step in the parenchymal transection.

Right Hepatic Lobectomy-Portal Dissection
Armed with the knowledge of portal arterial anatomy provided by the pre-operative angiogram (conventional bi-planar or CT reconstruction), the portal dissection is commenced. The peritoneum is divided vertically over the anteriorly situated hepatic artery. The proper hepatic artery is dissected up to and slightly beyond the lobar bifurcation where the cystic artery identified and divided as it courses to the right. The lateral leaf of portal peritoneum is then dissected to lateral edge of the porta. A cholecystectomy is then performed. The medial leaf of portal peritoneum is dissected, giving clear access to the common hepatic and proper hepatic arteries.

Attention is turned to the anterior surface of the common bile duct, which is dissected up to the liver. The hepatic plate, which envelopes the portal structures as they enter the liver parenchyma, is divided thereby allowing visualization of the proximal right and left hepatic duct as well as the portal venous bifurcation. Dissection of the bile duct bifurcation is kept laterally to the right in order to prevent injury to the proximal left duct and crossing segmental ducts. Since the common bile duct usually bifurcates at or above the hepatic plate, this step is usually the most tedious and technically difficult in the portal dissection. For this reason, intrahepatic division of the bile duct during parenchymal transection is an acceptable alternative. If division of the right main duct is possible, care is taken to identify segmental ducts passing from right to left. The right duct is doubly ligated clearly away from the bifurcation and divided.

After accurate identification of the arterial anatomy, the right hepatic artery is doubly ligated with a heavy suture and divided well away from the bifurcation. In the type III variant of arterial anatomy (11%), the right hepatic artery is identified and the divided in the posteriorlateral porta as it courses cephalad from the superior mesenteric artery.

The common duct is then gently retracted laterally giving access to the posteriorly situated portal vein. The portal bifurcation and right main portal trunk are dissected from the hepatic plate up to the first anterior sectoral branch. The right main portal trunk is then divided well away from the bifurcation using the stapler or between vascular clamps. After division of the portal vein a clear line of demarcation will be seen between the devascularized right lobe and perfused left lobe.

Right Hepatic Lobectomy-Parenchymal Transection
Extra-hepatic division or control of the right hepatic vein as described above is performed. The liver capsule is then scored with electrocautery at the line of demarcation between lobes. 1-0 chromic sutures, on a large blunt tipped needle, are then placed flanking the line of transection with a 2-cm margin on either side. These sutures are placed in a horizontal mattress fashion extending inward from the free liver edge for a distance of 6 to 8 cm. The liver parenchyma is then divided using the ultrasonic dissector (CUSA, Valley Labs, Inc.). Biliary and vascular structures smaller than 0.5mm are cauterized, structures 0.5 to 1.5 mm are controlled with clips, and structures larger than 1.5 mm are controlled with ligatures. Division of the parenchyma proceeds over a broad front with a steady, controlled pace.

The surgeon should be ever cognizant of intrahepatic anatomy, the edge of the tumor, and the relationship of the two. The edge of the tumor is usually difficult to precisely determine by palpation, even for well-circumscribed lesions. This frustrating fact is more relevant in nonanatomic resections and leads to a far too common incidence of "close margins". As a technical note, the annoying middle hepatic vein is present along Cantlie's line and the transection plane should be planned to cross the vein at one point. This is preferable to a transection adjacent to the vein that will meander into it at several points, with one harrowing point invariably near the junction of the vein with the IVC.

Vascular isolation via portal occlusion ("Pringle maneuver") is commonly, albeit not invariably used during parenchymal transection. In the right lobectomy, particularly with inflow and outflow control obtained by division of the vessels, there may be little bleeding from the transection margin. Inflow occlusion is more commonly used during lobar or nonanatomic resections when inflow and/or outflow control by formal vascular transection is not obtained. Although the liver will tolerate warm ischemia for over 60 minutes, our habit has been to occlude inflow for 15-20 minutes followed by a 4-5 minute perfusion or "rest" period. This practice may be more beneficial as a rest for the surgeon than for the liver, but we have had no episodes of hepatic dysfunction from ischemia and will likely continue it. Inflow occlusion is usually obtained using Rommell tourniquet. The common bile duct is usually excluded from the tourniquet.

Once parenchymal transection is complete, additional hemostasis is achieved with the argon beam coagulator. Major structures, particularly biliary, are examined for leaks and additional sutures are placed as needed. The resected surface is drained with a large sump drain adjacent to the edge of the liver extending into the porta. The omentum is mobilized and tacked over the resected edge of the liver. The falciform ligament is reconstructed to avoid torsion of the remaining liver. The abdominal wall is closed in one layer with heavy permanent suture.

Left Hepatic Lobectomy

The left hepatic lobectomy is removal of liver segments II, III and IV, which comprise the left hemi-liver. Indications for this procedure include: (1) tumor(s) within the left lobe adjacent to the left main portal structures or portal structures and left hepatic vein, or (2) tumor(s) distributed within the left lobe which cannot be fully resected with a nonanatomic or segmental resection.

Left Hepatic Lobectomy-Incision and Exposure

The incision and exposure are practically identical as described for the right hepatic lobectomy. The incision may not extend as far down the right but extend further down the left costal margin for left lobectomy.

Left Hepatic Lobectomy-Mobilization and Assessment of Resectability

The falciform ligament is divided posteriorly to the bare area of the liver. With gentle retraction by the assistant anterior and to the right, the left triangular and the commonly fused coronary ligaments are divided medially to the bare area and the IVC. As the dissection proceeds medially, care should be taken to prevent injury to the phrenic vein, which is ligated and divided where it joins the left hepatic vein. Division of the peritoneum overlying the suprahepatic IVC is completed and the left and middle hepatic veins are identified.

At this point, mobilization of the right lobe is begun if necessary. Mobilization of the right lobe and caudate lobes (Segment I) off of the IVC may be particularly helpful for simplifying a tricky transection plane through the deep left and caudate lobe, just above the IVC. This extensive mobilization is usually necessary for posterior left lobe tumor or tumor that lies close to the hepatic veins or IVC. The mobilization of right lobe has been described in the previous section. Mobilization of the caudate lobe is begun by division of the peritoneal layer extending from the caudate lobe onto the IVC **(Figure 5)**. Once the peritoneum has been divided, small branches extending correctly from the IVC into the caudate lobe are carefully ligated and divided. Although the caudate lobe mobilization is somewhat tedious and difficult, it is necessary if safe extrahepatic dissection and division of the left hepatic vein is to be achieved.

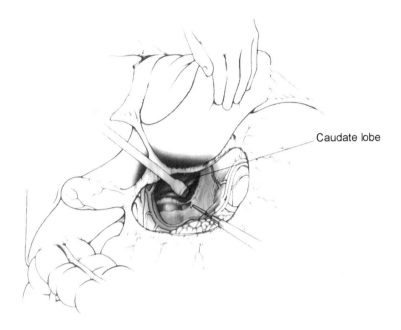

Caudate lobe

Figure 5-Exposure of the caudate lobe
Reprinted with permission from Wood WC, Skandalakis JE. Anatomic Basis of
Tumor Surgery. St.Louis: Quality Medical Publishing, 1999.

If the caudate lobe can be preserved, division of the fibrous attachments between the
caudate lobe and segments II and III of the left lobe improves access to the line of
parenchymal transection. The structures reached by opening the lesser omentum.
The liver is now carefully palpated and examined by ultrasound.

Left Hepatic Lobectomy-Posterior Dissection
The prelude to extrahepatic control of the left hepatic vein, mobilization of the
caudate lobe from the inferior vena cava, has been described above. Careful,
cautious sharp and blunt dissection above and below the liver is needed to dissect the
vein from the IVC. Dissection must proceed in the plane *between the caudate lobe
and the IVC.* Attempts to develop a plane between the caudate lobe and segments II
and III of the left lobe can result in torrential bleeding. Dissection of the left hepatic
vein is technically more difficult, when compared to the right, because: 1) the partial
visual obstruction of the junction between the vein and the IVC by the caudate lobe
and 2) the frequent presence of a very short common trunk leading to the left and
middle hepatic veins. Very careful dissection should allow encirclement of the left
vein or middle-left venous trunk with a Rommel tourniquet in most instances. If the
left hepatic vein is clearly identified and freed, then transection is accomplished
either with the stapler or between vascular clamps. The posterior dissection is
completed at this point; however, the transection is delayed until completion of the

portal dissection. If difficulty is encountered during the venous dissection, the left hepatic vein can be divided within the liver at the completion of the parenchymal transection.

Left Hepatic Lobectomy-Portal Dissection
The portal dissection is similar to that described for the right lobectomy with division of the left hepatic lobar artery, hepatic duct and portal vein branch. Dissection of the left-sided portal structures is usually technically easier than the right, since these structures normally assume a more horizontal course within the hepatic plate.

Left Hepatic Lobectomy-Parenchymal Transection
The technique of parenchymal transection is as described for the right lobectomy. Several technical notes about the left lobectomy are in order. First, the plane of transection will commonly run through a relatively "thick" part of the left lobe and constant orientation within the liver is especially necessary. Secondly, the plane of transection may involve some, all, or none of the caudate lobe. Resection of the caudate, if necessary, should be planned in the plane of transection. The aggravating presence of the middle hepatic vein should be dealt with by planning a transection plane across the vein at one point, rather than the plane adjacent to the vein that will meander into it at several points.

Resection of the Right Hepatic Lobe and Medial Segment (IV) of the Left Lobe (Right Trisegmentectomy)
The right trisegmentectomy is removal of liver segments IV, V, VI, VII, and VIII. Indications for this procedure include: (1) tumor(s) within the right lobe adjacent to the right main portal structures or portal structures and right hepatic vein with extension into segment IV of the left lobe, or (2) tumor(s) distributed within the right lobe and segment IV which cannot be fully resected with a nonanatomic or segmental resection. The right trisegmentectomy results in removal of up to 75% of the liver and should be reserved for healthy patients with normal liver function. The liver volume will be reconstituted over time by the remaining parenchymal mass.

Right Trisegmentectomy-Incision and Exposure
The incision and exposure is as described for the right lobectomy.

Right Trisegmentectomy-Mobilization and Assessment of Resectability
The liver is mobilized as for the right lobectomy. Tumor(s) that are posterior or extend well into Segment IV may also require mobilization of the left lobe.

Right Trisegmentectomy-Posterior Dissection
The posterior dissection for the right trisegmentectomy involves mobilization of the entire liver from the IVC. This dissection is a combination of the posterior dissections described for the right and left lobectomy. The right hepatic vein is usually divided outside the liver, however the middle hepatic vein is usually divided during the parenchymal transection, once unmistakably identified. Damage to the

left hepatic vein, can occur either during the usually difficult extrahepatic dissection or from accidental injury during parenchymal transection and is a potentially disastrous complication. If the left hepatic vein is compromised, a fatal acute Budd-Chiari syndrome will result.

Portal Dissection-Right Trisegmentectomy
The portal dissection is as described for the right lobectomy.

Parenchymal Transection- Right Trisegmentectomy
Transection is begun by division of the bridge of liver tissue spanning the gap between segments III and IV at the lower end of the umbilical fissure. Once this bridge is divided it is possible to identify and divide vessels passing to segment IV in the umbilical fissure. The line of transection then runs 0.5 to 1.0 cm to the right of the falciform ligament. The caudate lobe is left with the remaining liver, if possible. Other details are as described for the right lobectomy.

Resection of Segments II and III of the Left Lobe (Left "Lateral Segmentectomy")
The left lateral segmentectomy is removal of liver segments II and III. Indications for this procedure include: (1) tumor(s) within the left lobe adjacent to the sectoral portal pedicle or left hepatic vein, or (2) tumor(s) distributed within the left lobe which cannot be fully resected with a nonanatomic or segmental resection.

Left Lateral Segmentectomy-Incision and Exposure
The incision and exposure is as described for the left lobectomy. The incision extending down the right costal margin may stop at the lateral edge of the rectus sheath, if adequate access to the porta is obtained.

Left Lateral Segmentectomy-Mobilization and Assessment of Resectability
The liver is mobilized as for the left hepatic lobectomy. The gastrohepatic omentum is fully divided. The right lobe is not mobilized.

Left Lateral Segmentectomy-Posterior Dissection
The phrenic vein, left hepatic vein, and IVC are identified following dissection in the bare area. There usually is no need to obtain extrahepatic control of the left hepatic vein.

Left Lateral Segmentectomy-Portal Dissection
The gastrohepatic foramen is opened and a Rommel tourniquet is placed around the portal structures. If easily dissected from the porta, the common bile duct is excluded from the tourniquet. Inflow occlusion is usually needed during parenchymal transection.

Left Lateral Segmentectomy-Parenchymal Transection
Transection is begun by division of the bridge of liver tissue spanning the gap between segments III and IV at the lower end of the umbilical fissure. The line of

transection then runs 0.5 to 1.0 cm to the left of the falciform ligament and is scored on the liver. Heavy chromic sutures, on a large blunt tipped needle, are then placed flanking the line of transection with a 2-cm margin on either side. These sutures are placed in a horizontal mattress fashion extending inward from the anterior free liver edge as far as possible. The transection is then performed with the CUSA device. At the superior border of the transection the left hepatic vein or a major branch is identified and divided. The vascular stapler is quite useful for this purpose. Other technical details are as described previously.

Non-anatomic Resections
Indications for these procedures include: (1) tumor(s) where resection does not require sacrifice of a major portal branch or major portal branch and hepatic vein, or (2) a confined distribution of tumor(s) within the liver that can be fully resected with a nonanatomic or segmental resection.

Nonanatomic Resections -Incision and Exposure
The incision and exposure is as described for the right lobectomy.

Nonanatomic Resections –Mobilization and Assessment of Resectability
The size and location of the tumor dictates the extent of hepatic mobilization needed. In general, greater technical problems arise from inadequate mobilization than from over-mobilization. The details of mobilization are as described for right and left lobectomy.

Nonanatomic Resections –Posterior Dissection
Formal dissection or division of the hepatic veins is rarely needed. Exposure of the IVC and hepatic veins in the bare area of the liver is helpful when approaching posterior tumors. Identification and division of hepatic vein branches is accomplished during parenchymal transection.

Nonanatomic Resections –Portal Dissection
The gastrohepatic foramen is opened and a Rommel tourniquet is placed around the portal structures. If easily dissected from the porta, the common bile duct is excluded from the tourniquet. Inflow occlusion is almost always needed to minimize hemorrhage. Identification and division of portal branches is completed during parechymal transection.

Nonanatomic Resections –Parenchymal Transection
Peripheral lesions are managed by the inappropriately innocuous sounding "wedge" resection. A plane of transection, leaving a 2-cm margin, is scored on the liver. Overlapping 1-0 chromic horizontal mattress sutures are placed at least 1-cm back from the line of transection. These sutures are placed around the perimeter of the lesion or as deeply into the liver as can be done with ease. The parenchyma is then transected with the CUSA device. Vascular structures are controlled as described for previously. Inflow occlusion may not be needed for smaller wedge resections.

The technique of vascular control with chromic sutures is not useful for more centrally located tumors. A line of transection leaving a 1-2 cm margin is scored on the liver. The parenchyma is carefully transected using the CUSA device. The transection should progress in an even circumferential manner avoiding dissection "into a hole". The surgeon should constantly palpate the edge of the tumor to avoid compromising the margin, although an exact determination of the edge is usually difficult. Vascular inflow occlusion is routinely used. An encounter with a major vascular branch is common and usually occurs in the depths of the resection, particularly along the posterior margin. Patience and vascular isolation is needed to control troublesome bleeding. Blood loss from a large nonanatomic resection or resection near a major vascular trunk can exceed that of a lobectomy.

REFERENCES

1. Anson BJ, McVay CB. *Surgical Anatomy*. Philadelphia: WB Saunders, 1984, pp 616-629.
2. Bismuth H, Chiche L. Surgical anatomy and anatomic surgery of the liver. In Blumgart, LH, ed. *Surgery of the Liver and Biliary Tract*. Edinburgh: Curchill Livingstone, 1994, pp 3-9.
3. Daneker G. Liver. In Wood WC and Skandalakis JE, eds. *Anatomic Basis of Tumor Surgery*. St. Louis: Quality Medical Publishing, 1999, pp 505-545.
4. Makucchi M, Yamamoto J, Takayama T, et al. Extrahepatic division of the right hepatic vein in hepatectomy. *Hepatogastroenterol* 1991; 38:176.
5. Michels NA. Newer anatomy of the liver and its variant blood supply and collateral circulation. *Am J Surg* 1966; 112:337.
6. Mizumoto R, Suzuki H. Surgical anatomy of the hepatic hilum with special reference to the caudate lobe. *World J Surg* 1988; 12:2.
7. Nakamure S, Toshiharu T. Surgical anatomy of the hepatic veins and inferior vena cava. *Surg Gynecol Obstet* 1981; 152:43.
8. Skandalakis JE, Skandalakis PN, Skandalakis LJ. *Surgical Anatomy and Technique: A Pocket Manual*. New York: Springer-Verlag, 1995, p 471.
9. Smadja C, Blumgart LH. The biliary tract and the anatomy of biliary exposure. In Blumgart LH, ed. *Surgery of the Liver and Biliary Tract*. Edinburgh: Curchill Livingstone, 1994, pp 11-24.
10. VanDamme JP, Bonte J. *Vascular Anatomy in Abdominal Surgery*. New York: Thieme Medical Publishers, 1990.
11. Fong Y, Kemeny N, Blumgart LH, Cohen A: Treatment of colorectal cancer: hepatic metastasis. *Seminars in Surgical Oncology* 1996; 12:219.
12. Asbun HJ, Hughes KS: Management of recurrent and metastatic colorectal carcinoma. *Surg Clin N America* 1993; 73(1): 144.
13. Steele G Jr, Bleday R, Mayer RJ, et al: A prospective evaluation of hepatic resection for colorectal metastases to the liver: Gastrointestinal Tumor Study Group protocol 6584. *J Clin Oncol* 1991; 9:1105.
14. Kobayashi K, Kawamura M, Ishihara T: Surgical treatment for both pulmonary and hepatic metastases from colorectal cancer. *J Thor Cardiovascular Surg* 1999; 118(6): 1090.

15. Wagner JS, Adson MA, van Heerden JA, et al: The natural history of hepatic metastases from colorectal cancer: a comparison with resective treatment. *Ann Surg* 1994; 199:502.

16. Cady B, Stone M, McDermott WV, et al: Technical and biological factors in disease-free survival after hepatic resection for colorectal cancer metastases. *Arch Surg* 1992; 127:561.

17. Hughes KS, Simon R, Songhorabodi S, et al: Resection of the liver for colorectal metastases: A multi-institutional study of indications for resection. *Surgery* 1988; 103:278.

18. Figueras J, Jaurrieta E, Valls C et al: Resection or transplantation for hepatocellular carcinoma in cirrhotic patients: outcomes based on indicated treatment strategy. *J Am Coll Surg* 2000; 190:580.

19. Fuhrman GM, Curley SA, Hohn DC, Roh MS: Improved survival after resection of colorectal liver metastases. *Ann Surg Oncol* 1995; 2(6): 537.

20. Taylor M, Forster J, Langer B, et al: A study of prognostic factors for hepatic resection for colorectal metastases. *Am J Surg* 1997; 173:467.

21. Wolf RF, Goodnight JE, Krag DE, Schneider PD: Results of resection and proposed guidelines for patient selection in instances of noncolorectal hepatic metastases. *Surg Gynecol Obstet* 1991; 173:454.

22. Okuda K: Hepatocellular carcinoma. *J Hepatology* 2000; 32 (suppl. 1): 225.

23. Fernandez M Redvanly R: Primary hepatic malignant neoplasms. *Radiologic Clinics of North America* 1998; 36(2): 333.

24. Poon RT, Fan ST, Ng IO et al: Significance of resection margin in hepatectomy for hepatocellular carcinoma. *Ann Surg* 2000; 231(4): 544.

25. Llovet JM, Bruix J, Gores GJ: Surgical resection versus transplantation for early hepatocellular carcinoma: clues for the best strategy. *Hepatology* 2000; 31(4): 1019.

26. Llovet JM, Mas X, Aponte J et al: Radical treatment of hepatocellular carcinoma during the waiting list for orthotopic liver transplantation: a cost-effective analysis on an intention to treat basis. *Hepatology* 1999; 30(suppl): 223A.

27. Broelsch CE. *Atlas of Liver Surgery.* New York: Churchill Livingstone, 1993, pp1-118.

28. Cameron JL. Ed. *Atlas of Surgery*, vol. 1. Philadelphia: BC Decker, 1990, pp 152-205.

29. Meyers WC. Segmental hepatic resection. In Sabiston DC, ed. *Atlas of General Surgery*. Philadelphia, WB Saunders, 1994, pp 534-544.

30. Nagorney DM. Hepatic resections. In Chassin JL, ed. *Operative Strategy in General Surgery*. New York: Springer-Verlag, 1994, pp 585-598.

31. Roh MS. Liver resection. In Roh MS, Ames FC, eds. *Advanced Oncologic Surgery*, London: Wolfe, 1994, pp5.2-5.17.

32. Rosen CB, Donohue JH, Nagorney DM. Liver resection for metastatic colon and rectal carcinoma. In Cohen AM, Winawer SJ, eds. *Cancer of the Colon, Rectum, and Anus.* New York: McGraw-Hill, 1995, pp 805-821.

14

RADIOFREQUENCY ABLATION FOR PRIMARY AND METASTATIC LIVER TUMORS

Timothy M. Pawlik, M.D., M.P.H. and
Kenneth K. Tanabe, M.D.
Massachusetts General Hospital, Harvard Medical School, Boston, MA

INTRODUCTION

Due to the large number of patients with primary or metastatic hepatic malignancies who are not candidates for surgical resection, novel treatment approaches to control and potentially cure liver tumors have been explored. Percutaneous image-guided ablative therapies using direct intra-tumoral injection of compounds such as ethanol (1-3), hot saline (4), and acetic acid (5), as well as thermally mediated techniques such as cryotherapy (6), microwave therapy (7), interstitial laser photocoagulation (8), and radiofrequency ablation have all recently received much attention as minimally invasive strategies for the treatment of focal malignant diseases. The development of these new minimally invasive techniques has the potential to alter patient outcomes, since existing therapies often have either limited efficacy or are associated with significant morbidity and cost. Potential benefits of ablative therapies compared to surgical resection include the possibility of performing the procedure in the outpatient setting, decreased cost, reduced morbidity and mortality, and the ability to offer treatment to patients who would not be considered candidates for surgery due to age, disease extent, or co-existing morbidity. While the clinical efficacy of some ablative therapies has been established (ethanol injection) (1), the experience with other ablative therapeutic modalities is considerably more preliminary and requires additional assessment. One such ablative technique is radiofrequency tissue ablation. Still a relatively novel technique, radiofrequency ablation of both primary and secondary metastatic tumors of the liver has been investigated with increasing interest in recent years.

Although relatively uncommon in the Western Hemisphere, hepatocellular carcinoma (HCC) is the most common solid cancer worldwide, with an incidence estimated at greater than 1 million new cases per year (9, 10). Surgical resection and liver transplantation are the only effective therapies, however only 5% to 15% of newly diagnosed patients with HCC undergo a potentially curative resection (11, 12). Furthermore, patients with HCC often are not surgical candidates because of multifocal disease, proximity of tumor to key vascular or biliary structures that preclude negative surgical margins, or inadequate hepatic reserve because of underlying cirrhosis. With few curative treatment options, HCC is one of the most lethal malignancies, with greater than 90% of patients dying as a result of their HCC (13). Given the limitations of surgical resection, novel treatment methods such as radiofrequency ablation have been investigated for treatment of patients with HCC.

In addition to primary hepatic malignancies, the liver is the primary site for metastatic malignancies of the gastrointestinal tract. Hepatic metastases cause significant morbidity and mortality in patients with colorectal adenocarcinoma; of those who undergo a potentially curative operation for their primary tumor but subsequently recur, almost 80% will develop evidence of metastatic disease within the liver (14). Without resection the prognosis for patients with hepatic metastases from colorectal carcinoma is dismal, with 5-year survival reported to be less than 1% and median survival estimated at 9.6 months (15). Systemic chemotherapy has only modestly improved patient outcomes, leaving hepatic resection as the only widely available curative treatment for this patient population. Recent reports reveal that 5-year survival rates of 30% to 35% are observed following the resection of 4 or fewer hepatic metastases (16-19). Despite the promise offered by metastasectomy, it is associated with moderate morbidity and mortality (16, 20, 21). Size, location, and number of tumors, as well as vascular invasion, poor general health, and insufficient hepatic reserve, all may contribute to increase the difficulty of surgical resection (15, 22). There is a need for a simple and effective technique for treatment of unresectable metastatic disease in the liver. Radiofrequency ablation may provide such a tool.

INDUCTION OF COAGULATION NECROSIS

The principle aim of thermal tumor ablation therapy is to destroy an entire tumor by using heat to kill the malignant cells with minimal damage to adjacent vital structures. Ideally, the field of coagulation necrosis should include a 0.5 to 1.0 cm margin of normal tissue adjacent to the tumor in order to eliminate microscopic foci of disease and account for the uncertainty regarding the precise location of the tumor margin. Survival data from most surgical series has shown that those patients with colorectal carcinoma liver metastases with an adequate surgical margin (1 cm) on liver resection specimens have a greater overall survival rate as compared to patients with less than a 1 cm surgical margin (23). Given this, the goal of tumor eradication necessitates ablation of the entire tumor and at least a 0.5 to 1.0 cm peripheral margin of grossly normal tissue.

Mechanism of Thermal Destruction

Localized application of thermal energy destroys cells. Cellular homeostasis can be maintained with mild elevation of temperature to approximately 40°C, however when tumor cells are heated above 45°C to 50°C, intracellular proteins are denatured and cell membranes are destroyed through dissolution and melting of lipid bilayers (24, 25). Extracellular and intracellular water is driven out of the tissue, which results in the final destruction of the cells. In addition, when temperatures are increased to 45°C, tumor cells become more susceptible to damage by other agents such as chemotherapy and radiation (26, 27). Too much heat, however, is counter-productive. At extreme temperatures (> 100°C) the tissue undergoes vaporization and carbonization. This process is detrimental to the creation of a large volume of coagulative necrosis. The carbonized tissue and associated gas act as an insulator to radiation of energy into deeper tissues. This ultimately leads to a small necrotic core and preservation of the surrounding tissue. Therefore, in order to maximize the volume of tissue treated, thermal ablative therapies must achieve and maintain a 50°C to 100°C-temperature range throughout the entire target volume (28). This will ensure a more complete destruction of the target cell volume, rather than simply destroying only that tissue which is closest to the energy source.

RADIOFREQUENCY AS A SOURCE OF THERMAL ENERGY

Radiofrequency ablation is generally performed using thin (14 - 21 gauge), partially insulated electrodes that are placed under imaging guidance (ultrasound, MRI, or CT) into the tumor. This can be performed either intraoperatively as an open procedure or percutaneously as a closed, minimally invasive procedure. The electrodes are connected to a radiofrequency generator and a large grounding pad is placed on the patient's back or thigh. Current travels from the uninsulated portion of the active electrode towards ground (Figure 1). This current results in ion agitation in the tissue surrounding the electrode, which is converted by friction into heat and induces cellular death via coagulation necrosis (29). The tissue surrounding the electrode, rather than the electrode itself, is the primary source of heat (30). The geometry of the radiofrequency current pathway around the ablation electrode creates a relatively oblong zone of heat. Conduction of heat creates an expanding zone of ablated tissue. Although radiofrequency ablation can be performed using either monopolar or bipolar electrodes, currently monopolar is most commonly used. Bipolar electrode systems generate heat not only at the active electrode, but also between the two electrodes and adjacent to the ground needle. Although the resulting foci of coagulation are larger with bipolar current, the shape of the zone of coagulation necrosis resembles a "dumb-bell," thus decreasing its clinical utility, as most tumors are roughly spherical in shape (31).

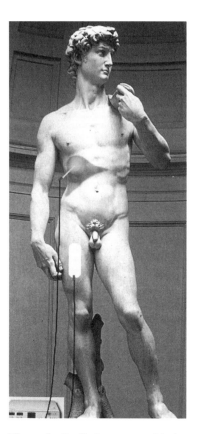

Figure 1. Radiofrequency ablation.

To coagulate tissues further from the electrode and thus adequately destroy an entire tumor mass, heat conduction through the tissue surrounding the electrode is required. Appropriate distribution of energy is required to maintain cytotoxic temperatures throughout a tumor. Multiple obstacles must be overcome to achieve effective energy distribution for whole tumor treatment. Perhaps the most significant problem to cope with is the heterogeneity of heat deposition throughout a given treated lesion. Heat deposition is greatest immediately surrounding the electrode with a corresponding fall-off of temperature at distances further from the electrode. This is due to a reduction in current flux at greater distances from the electrode and poor heat conduction through coagulated tissues. As noted above, a simple increase in heat output from the applicator cannot solve the problem, because temperatures greater than 100°C result in tissue boiling and vaporization with subsequent gas formation. This gas then acts as an insulator against both heat conduction and current flux. Given these limitations, radiofrequency ablation has traditionally been capable of producing coagulation zones extending only 8 mm away from an electrode (32, 33). This limitation sharply restricted the potential use of the radiofrequency ablation technique until recently when new methods for increasing the volume of tissue ablation have been characterized.

Increasing Radiofrequency Treatment Dimensions

Initial attempts at increasing the volume of coagulated tissue generated with radiofrequency ablation centered on increasing electrode tip length, increasing tip temperatures, and lengthening the duration of treatment. Although lesion diameter increases with electrode gauge and duration of treatment to a maximum of 6 min., lesions with mean diameters larger than 1.6 cm cannot be produced using a single electrode regardless of treatment time, tip temperature, or tip length (33). Longer electrode tip exposures produce greater volumes of necrosis but the cylindrical shape of the induced coagulation necrosis does not match the shape of most tumors. Furthermore, higher electrode tip temperatures and longer electrodes are associated with increased temperature variation along the electrode shaft. With exposed electrode tips exceeding 3 cm, a greater variability in coagulation uniformity is also observed, leading to unpredictable necrosis volumes. For all of these reasons, radiofrequency ablation with electrodes that have no greater than a 3 cm tip exposure which achieve temperatures of 90°C – 110°C have been most successful in yielding reproducible uniform, coagulative necrosis. These parameters produce a predictable shape of coagulation necrosis, but do not address the problem of small volumes of coagulation necrosis created by radiofrequency ablation. Several approaches have been developed to increase the diameter of coagulation necrosis achieved using conventional radiofrequency ablation techniques.

Multi-Electrode Arrays

An obvious method for increasing energy deposition throughout the tumor lesion is the repeated insertion of multiple radiofrequency electrodes into the tissue to increase the diameter of induced coagulation (34, 35). This approach, however, is not only time consuming but difficult to utilize in the clinical setting, as multiple positionings of electrodes is technically challenging. Initial studies by Goldberg et al. with multi-electrode arrays showed that simultaneous use of multiple electrodes permits destruction of more tissue in a single treatment session than is possible with multiple individual electrodes operating independently. In these studies, arrays with electrodes positioned at varying distances from one another were evaluated. Uniform tissue necrosis was observed with simultaneous radiofrequency application to three electrodes positioned 1.5 cm or less apart (Figure 2). Arrays of three electrodes positioned 1.5 cm apart produced spherical lesions approximately 3.0 cm in diameter, a diameter almost double that produced by a single electrode (35). Electrodes placed 2 cm or more apart, however, produced independent lesions 1.4 cm in diameter with incomplete necrosis between electrodes. In these same experiments, Goldberg et al. also investigated whether sequential rather than simultaneous application of current to the multiple electrodes could increase tissue necrosis. Greater necrosis was achieved when radiofrequency was applied simultaneously rather than sequentially. Based on these studies, Goldberg et al. recommended treatment with simultaneous application of radiofrequency energy to multiple electrodes spaced 1.5 cm or less apart.

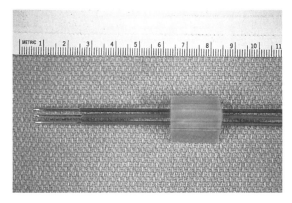

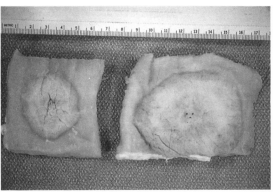

Figure 2. Multiple electrodes for radiofrequency ablation. (A) Three parallel electrodes are separated by a fixed distance for application of radiofrequency energy. (B) The volume of coagulation necrosis created by maximal radiofrequency energy deposition using either a single electrode (left) or a cluster of three electrodes (right). (Photos courtesy of S. Nahum Goldberg.)

Initially such a strategy was difficult to implement given the technical challenge of precisely positioning the probes at these distances. The development of self-contained multi-electrode arrays such as "umbrella" electrode arrays have overcome some of these problems and have produced larger zones of coagulation necrosis in clinical trials. These systems deploy an array of multiple curved stiff wires in the shape of an umbrella from a single 14 or 16 gauge cannula (Figure 3). Experiments using a 12-hook "umbrella" array *in vivo* in porcine liver have produced spherical regions of coagulation necrosis measuring up to 3.5 cm in diameter (36).

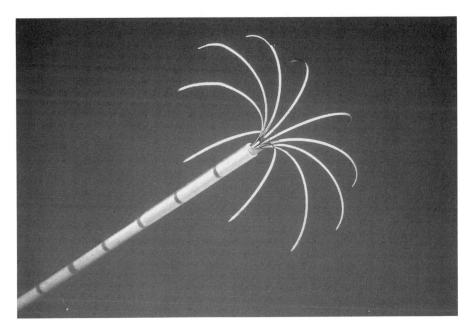

Figure 3. Multiple electrode array. Following introduction of a single needle, multiple electrodes can be simultaneously deployed in an "umbrella" configuration.

Injection during RF Ablation

The simultaneous injection of saline during radiofrequency ablation has also been used as a strategy to increase the volume of coagulation necrosis (37, 38). Normal saline is injected into the tumor through tiny holes at the distal end of the electrode during the radiofrequency ablation. Theoretically, the high local ion concentration produced by the normal saline increases the electrode's active surface area, thus increasing the extent of the coagulation necrosis. Trials using this technique, however, have been disappointing, with coagulation volume being unpredictable, irregularly shaped, and incomplete in some instances (38).

Internally Cooled Electrodes

Another tactic to increase coagulation volume has been the development of internally cooled radiofrequency electrodes. Within these electrodes are two hollow lumens that permit continuous internal cooling of the tip with a chilled perfusate (Figure 4a). Perfusion and irrigation of the electrode tip is established via water circulation through a closed circuit; the perfusate stays within the electrode and does not extravasate into the tumor or surrounding tissues. As a result, excessive heating of tissues nearest the electrode is reduced which prevents vaporization and carbonization. This permits more radiofrequency energy delivery and prevents excessive heating of tissue immediately surrounding the electrode (39). Thermometry studies have been performed to compare the relative heat distribution in *ex vivo* tissues surrounding 3 cm internally cooled electrodes with and without cooling. These studies revealed that without cooling a rapid decrease in temperature was observed from the electrode surface such that the cytotoxic temperature of 50°C was observed only 0.7 cm from the electrode. In contrast, when radiofrequency energy delivery was accompanied by internal cooling, a temperature of 50°C was observed 1.6 cm from the electrode (40) (Figure 4b).

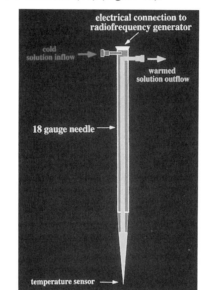

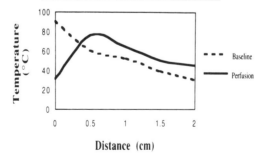

Distance (cm)

Figure 4. Internally cooled electrode. (A) Schematic diagram of an internally cooled electrode. (B) Maximum tissue temperatures achievable in *ex vivo* tissue using either a conventional (non-cooled) electrode or an internally cooled electrode plotted as a function of distance from the electrode. (Reproduced with permission from Goldberg, SN et al. Radiofrequency tissue ablation: increased lesion diameter with a perfusion electrode. *Acad Radiol* 1996; 3:636.)

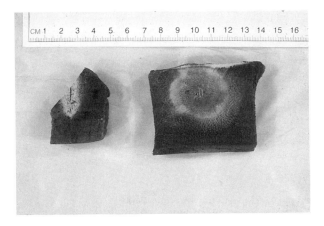

Figure 4C. The volume of coagulation necrosis observed following maximal radiofrequency energy deposition with an internally cooled electrode (right) is larger than with a conventional electrode (left) in *ex vivo* tissue. (Photos courtesy of S. Nahum Goldberg.)

Both *ex vivo* and *in vivo* studies have demonstrated the benefits of internally cooled electrodes. With internal electrode tip cooling, radiofrequency induced coagulation necrosis is greater than that achieved with non-cooled electrodes (39) (Figure 4c). Goldberg et al. compared an 18 gauge conventional electrode to an internally cooled electrode in *ex vivo* livers. With the internal electrode tip cooling, radiofrequency energy deposited into the tissue and resultant coagulation necrosis were significantly greater than that achieved without electrode cooling (40, 41). *In vivo* studies have been performed in swine muscle and liver (40). Although internally cooled electrodes uniformly produced coagulation necrosis with a greater diameter compared to conventional electrodes, the absolute measurements were significantly smaller than those observed in the *ex vivo* experiments (1.8 – 3.6 cm compared to 5.4 cm). Furthermore, with the use of internally cooled electrodes a longer treatment time was required. In *ex vivo* liver experiments, thermal equilibrium was not attained until after more than 30 minutes (41), which probably accounts for the increased duration of treatment needed to generate maximal ablation with internally cooled electrodes.

Limiting Vascular Inflow

The volume of coagulation necrosis observed following radiofrequency ablation of *ex vivo* calf livers has not been reproduced *in vivo* in experiments (40, 42). One major factor for this disparity is the presence of blood flow in the *in vivo* setting. Blood flow serves as a "heat sink," and is an important determinant of radiofrequency ablation efficacy. Tumors located in vascular environments are less susceptible to radiofrequency ablation as perfusion-mediated tissue cooling reduces the extent of coagulation necrosis. Furthermore, radiofrequency induced coagulation necrosis is often shaped *in vivo* by the surrounding hepatic vasculature (42, 43) (Figure 5a). There are important clinical implications of these observations. Theoretically, radiofrequency ablation may be more effective in tissues with reduced blood flow such as HCC and metastatic adenocarcinoma as compared to normal liver. In addition, radiologic or surgical manipulations to reduce hepatic blood flow during radioablation should augment therapy. In support of these theories, Goldberg et al. achieved greater coagulation *in vivo* in porcine livers when radiofrequency ablation was applied during balloon occlusion of the portal vein than when radiofrequency was applied during unaltered blood flow (44). In a separate *in vivo* porcine liver model, these results were confirmed with the coagulated focus created by radiofrequency during a Pringle maneuver being significantly larger in all three dimensions than coagulation without a Pringle maneuver (3.0 cm diameter vs. 1.2 cm diameter, respectively) (42). Furthermore, the pharmacologic modulation and attenuation of blood flow also has been shown to correlate with greater coagulation necrosis (45). Studies on the effects of mechanical occlusion on coagulation and heating during radiofrequency application have been performed in patients undergoing intraoperative radiofrequency therapy (44). The extent of coagulation was greater in each case with inflow occlusion (4.0 cm vs. 2.5 cm) (Figure 5b). Thus, it appears that intraoperative application of a Pringle maneuver may induce greater coagulation necrosis.

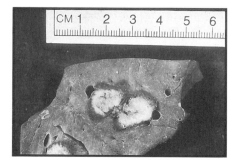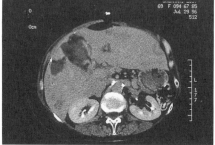

Figure 5. Heat sink effect. (A) The shape of zones of coagulation necrosis induced *in vivo* in pig livers is sculpted by blood flow in both hepatic veins and in portal triads. (Photos courtesy of S. Nahum Goldberg.) (B) Two colon carcinoma liver metastases of equivalent size were treated separately using the same amount of radiofrequency energy. The only difference between treatment parameters was that one of the lesions was treated during complete hepatic vascular inflow occlusion, and this produced a substantially larger zone of coagulation necrosis.

Cluster Radiofrequency

Early studies with multi-electrode arrays focused on the maximum distance which electrodes could be spaced while still ensuring contiguous coagulation necrosis between electrodes. More recent work has suggested that simultaneous application of radiofrequency current to a cluster of three closely spaced internally-cooled electrodes offers the potential of larger volumes of coagulation necrosis for ablation therapy (46) (Figure 6). Goldberg et al. showed that simultaneous radiofrequency application to arrays of three internally cooled electrodes spaced equidistantly at 0.5 cm or 1 cm apart produces a uniform circular cross-sectional area of coagulation necrosis measuring 4.1 cm in diameter. By comparison electrodes placed 1.5 cm – 2.5 cm apart produced a slightly larger ablation diameter (4.5 cm), but areas of non-necrosis were present within the treatment zone. Based on these and similar results, it appears that radiofrequency application to electrodes spaced no greater than 1 cm apart produces larger, more spherical regions of coagulation than otherwise identical radiofrequency application to three electrodes spaced 2 cm apart or greater. The reason for this is believed to be that the relatively closely spaced electrodes function as a single, large electrode.

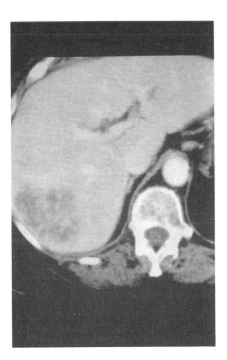 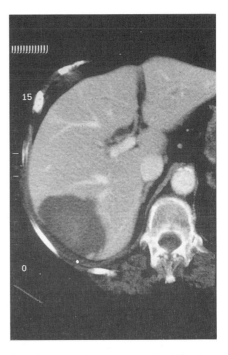

Figure 6.   Radiofrequency ablation using a 3-electrode array.   A CT scan demonstrating the liver tumor was obtained prior to (A) and immediately following (B) radiofrequency ablation. (Photos courtesy of S. Nahum Goldberg.)

Pulsed Radiofrequency Ablation

Another strategy to increase the extent of coagulation is the use of pulsed current instead of continuous currents. The concept is that by applying energy in a pulsed fashion, heat dissipation may occur between pulses thus allowing for a greater deposition of energy to tissues while preventing tissue vaporization or carbonization near the electrode. In an initial set of experiments performed by Goldberg et al. it was determined that increased coagulation necrosis could in fact be achieved with radiofrequency currents applied to internally-cooled electrodes in a pulsed fashion (47). Pulsed radiofrequency current was able to deposit a large amount of energy and heat while avoiding the rise in impedance seen in comparable continuous treatment applications. Furthermore, remote thermometry measurement revealed more rapid temperature increases and higher tissue temperatures when a pulsed technique was used, leading to overall greater energy and heat deposition and larger coagulation diameters (47). Thus, pulsed application of radiofrequency current allows greater energy deposition that results in a greater volume of tissue ablation.

CURRENT RECOMMENDATIONS

Complete ablation of the entire tumor mass requires the induction of a large volume of coagulation necrosis. In the past the small zone of coagulation necrosis achieved with radiofrequency energy has been the limiting factor in the clinical application of radiofrequency ablation. As noted above, however, numerous technologic advances have increased the zone of coagulation necrosis induced by radiofrequency ablation. Currently, pulsed-radiofrequency application to clusters of internally cooled electrodes enables the largest volume of tissue necrosis. On the other hand, many investigators prefer the non-cooled umbrella electrode. Undoubtedly, future advances in this rapidly growing field will continue to improve radiofrequency ablation application and technique.

IMAGING RADIOFREQUENCY ABLATION

Ultrasound

Ultrasound imaging is useful for optimal positioning of the electrode in the tumor (48). Ultrasonography as a follow-up imaging modality, however, has limited value (49). During radiofrequency ablation the treated tissue becomes hyperechoic (Figure 7). This increased echogenicity, which is caused by denatured proteins and a collection of microbubbles of gas, can obscure both the position of the electrode and the tumor mass itself. Thus, although ultrasound effectively guides initial electrode placement, monitoring of ablation is significantly hampered secondary to this hyper-echogenic area that develops during radiofrequency ablation.

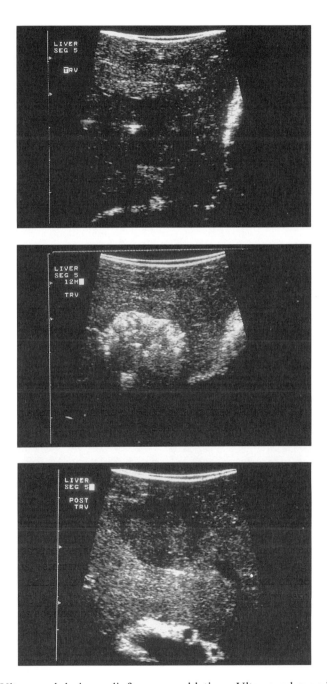

Figure 7. Ultrasound during radiofrequency ablation. Ultrasound examination of a liver tumor was performed prior to electrode insertion (A); during application of radiofrequency energy (B); and 15 minutes following removal of the electrode (C). The echogenicity that develops during radiofrequency ablation resolves within 15 minutes. (Photos courtesy of S. Nahum Goldberg.)

Similarly, ultrasound is only of marginal assistance in assessing the extent of tumor destruction following radiofrequency ablation. Changes in the tumor as seen on ultrasound can be highly variable ranging from no change to the presence of a peri-tumoral hyperechoic halo. This hyperechoic halo can make evaluation of the underlying malignancy difficult in the post-treatment setting. Given its variability and relatively inferior image quality, ultrasound is not useful for evaluation of the extent of radiofrequency ablation and its role should primarily be as a tool to guide initial electrode placement.

CT Scan

Both CT and MRI offer a much more reliable and unambiguous image of the post-radiofrequency ablated liver. Following radiofrequency ablation, contrast enhanced CT demonstrates regions of hypoattenuation (Figure 8). By 2 weeks following treatment these areas develop more distinct margins and can be differentiated from hyper-attenuating tumor on delayed opacification images. Short term (less than 1 month) correlation between radiologic and pathologic findings has demonstrated that CT scan accurately predicts the region of coagulation to within 2 mm (34, 38, 46).

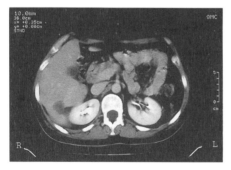 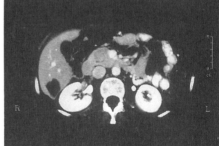

Figure 8. CT scan to assess the extent of tumor destruction. CT scan of a liver tumor was obtained prior to (A) and immediately following radiofrequency ablation (B). The absence of intravenous contrast in the ablated tumor results in hypoattenuation. (Photos courtesy of S. Nahum Goldberg.)

Although CT has been shown to be useful in confirming successful radioablation treatment 1 to 3 months following treatment, caution must be exercised when interpreting the results of these images. Goldberg et al. reported several cases where contrast enhanced CT scans at 3 months suggested complete ablation of the entire tumor, but later studies demonstrated peripheral tumor regrowth. Thus, although CT can accurately assess the completeness of ablation, it is unable to detect small volumes of residual viable tumor (Figure 9).

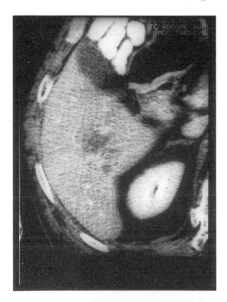
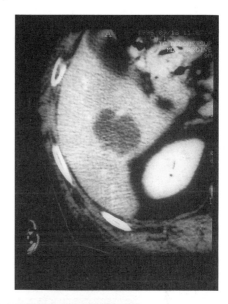
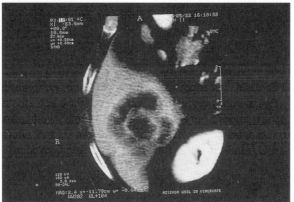

Figure 9. Liver tumor regrowth following radiofrequency ablation. CT scan of a liver tumor was obtained prior to (A) and immediately following (B) radiofrequency ablation appears to show complete tumor destruction. Careful inspection of the treated tumor shows that the area of hypoattenuation appears to be sculpted by a blood vessel. Tumor recurrence was detectable 6 months later (C).

MRI

Like CT imaging, MRI is useful in follow-up imaging of patients following radiofrequency ablation. However, unlike CT, MRI signal characteristics are more variable and can fluctuate more over time. Treated tumors may demonstrate foci of high, low, or heterogeneous T1 and T2 weighted signals (50, 51). Regions of the tumor that have been treated do not demonstrate enhancement following the intravenous administration of Gd-DTPA enhancement (50, 51). The signal characteristics can change over time with some completely ablated tumors demonstrating a densely enhancing peripheral rim of uniform thickness surrounding the region of coagulation necrosis. Although this peripheral rim is felt to be a normal inflammatory reaction to the radiofrequency-induced necrosis, any bulky or irregular peripheral enhancement should alert the clinician to the possibility of incompletely treated or recurrent cancer.

CLINICAL EXPERIENCE AND RESULTS OF RADIOFREQUENCY ABLATION OF PRIMARY AND METASTATIC MALIGNANCIES

In comparing clinical reports of radiofrequency ablation one must be aware of the different methods of radiofrequency ablation employed. As noted above, results of radiofrequency ablation may vary considerably depending on the technique used. Furthermore, radiofrequency ablation is still a relatively new therapeutic technique and the results of these studies must be viewed as preliminary. A brief summary of several clinical reports of radiofrequency ablation follows. Livraghi et al. reported using conventional (non-cooled, single electrode) radiofrequency electrodes with intratumoral saline injection to treat 14 patients with 24 hepatic malignancies and one patient with cholangiocarcinoma (38). In this particular study the lesions ranged in size from 1.2 to 4.5 cm in diameter. He reported a 52% rate of complete tumor necrosis 6 months following treatment. Of note, all successfully treated tumors were smaller than 3.5 cm in diameter. Similarly, Solbiati et al. reported complete treatment with the conventional technique (no saline injection) with no evidence of recurrence in 66% of patients treated with metastatic gastrointestinal carcinoma; again, all successfully treated lesions were less than 3 cm in diameter (49).

Curley et al. reported their results of radiofrequency ablation of unresectable primary and metastatic hepatic malignancies in 123 patients (52). In these patients, radiofrequency ablation was used to treat 169 tumors with a median diameter of 3.4 cm. Primary liver cancer was treated in 48 patients and metastatic liver tumors were treated in 75 patients. Percutaneous and intraoperative radioablation was performed in 31 patients and 92 patients, respectively. No treatment-related deaths occurred and the complication rate was only 2.4%. All treated tumors were completely necrotic on imaging studies after completion of the radiofrequency ablation treatments. With a median follow-up of 15 months, tumor had recurred in 3 of 169 treated lesions (1.8%), but metastatic disease had developed at other sites in 34 patients. Based on these results, these investigators concluded that radiofrequency ablation is a safe, well-tolerated, and effective treatment in patients with unresectable hepatic malignancies. Radiofrequency ablation may not cure most patients with primary or malignant metastatic disease -- as witnessed by the 34 patients with disease found at extra-hepatic sites -- but initial disease free follow-up rates of 20% to 50% justify aggressive treatment of isolated hepatic disease with a multi-modality approach including radiofrequency ablation.

CONCLUSION

Treatment of primary and secondary hepatic malignancies with radiofrequency ablation remains a relatively new strategy. Many patients with either HCC or secondary hepatic metastases are poor candidates for hepatic resection. However, given the proven efficacy of hepatic resection in these settings, a procedure such as radiofrequency ablation, which offers significantly less morbidity, may serve as an effective and safe technique to improve survival and quality of life in this patient population. To serve as an effective therapy the entire tumor and a 0.5 to 1.0 cm peripheral margin must be ablated. Traditionally, radiofrequency ablation has suffered from a limited size in the zone of tissue necrosis achievable. Several recent technical innovations, including internally cooled electrodes, the application of pulsed radiofrequency ablation, and use of cluster arrays have allowed increased energy deposition into tissues with a resultant increase in the volume of induced coagulation necrosis. The application of pulsed-radiofrequency current to clusters of internally cooled electrodes has produced coagulation necrosis zones of up to 3.5 cm. Although there have been numerous advances in the application of radiofrequency, imaging techniques for radiofrequency ablation remain imperfect. Ultrasound, CT, and MRI remain deficient and undoubtedly fail to detect residual tumors. Preliminary animal and clinical studies remain encouraging and have fueled optimism about radiofrequency ablation's future in the treatment of hepatic malignancies. Although radiofrequency ablation has not unseated surgical resection as the preferred treatment of hepatic neoplasms, at the current rate of progress it will very likely gain acceptance in the near future as an important tool to treat hepatic malignancies.

REFERENCES

1. Livraghi, T., Bolondi, L., Lazzaroni, S., et al. Percutaneous ethanol injection in the treatment of hepatocellular carcinoma in cirrhosis. A study on 207 patients. *Cancer* 1992;69:925.
2. Ebara, M., Ohto, M., Sugiura, N., et al. Percutaneous ethanol injection for the treatment of small hepatocellular carcinoma. Study of 95 patients. *J Gastroenterol Hepatol* 1990;5:616.
3. Lencioni, R., Bartolozzi, C., Caramella, D., et al. Treatment of small hepatocellular carcinoma with percutaneous ethanol injection. Analysis of prognostic factors in 105 Western patients. *Cancer* 1995;76:1737.

4.　Honda, N., Guo, Q., Uchida, H., et al. Percutaneous hot saline injection therapy for hepatic tumors: an alternative to percutaneous ethanol injection therapy [see comments]. *Radiology* 1994;190:53.

5.　Ohnishi, K., Yoshioka, H., Ito, S., et al. Prospective randomized controlled trial comparing percutaneous acetic acid injection and percutaneous ethanol injection for small hepatocellular carcinoma. *Hepatology* 1998;27:67.

6.　Wong, W. S., Patel, S. C., Cruz, F. S., et al. Cryosurgery as a treatment for advanced stage hepatocellular carcinoma: results, complications, and alcohol ablation. *Cancer* 1998;82:1268.

7.　Sato, M., Watanabe, Y., Ueda, S., et al. Microwave coagulation therapy for hepatocellular carcinoma. *Gastroenterology* 1996;110:1507.

8.　Pacella, C. M., Bizzarri, G., Ferrari, F. S., et al. [Interstitial photocoagulation with laser in the treatment of liver metastasis]. *Radiol Med (Torino)* 1996;92:438.

9.　Beasley, R. P. Hepatitis B virus. The major etiology of hepatocellular carcinoma. *Cancer* 1988;61:1942.

10.　Di Bisceglie, A. M. Hepatocellular carcinoma: molecular biology of its growth and relationship to hepatitis B virus infection. *Med Clin North Am* 1989;73:985.

11.　Tsuzuki, T., Sugioka, A., Ueda, M., et al. Hepatic resection for hepatocellular carcinoma. *Surgery* 1990;107:511.

12.　Nagorney, D. M., van Heerden, J. A., Ilstrup, D. M., et al. Primary hepatic malignancy: surgical management and determinants of survival. *Surgery* 1989;106:740.

13.　Rustgi, V. K. Epidemiology of hepatocellular carcinoma. *Gastroenterol Clin North Am* 1987;16:545.

14.　Cromheecke, M., de Jong, K. P., and Hoekstra, H. J. Current treatment for colorectal cancer metastatic to the liver. *Eur J Surg Oncol* 1999;25:451.

15.　Ballantyne, G. H. and Quin, J. Surgical treatment of liver metastases in patients with colorectal cancer. *Cancer* 1993;71:4252.

16.　Saenz, N. C., Cady, B., McDermott, W. V., Jr., et al. Experience with colorectal carcinoma metastatic to the liver. *Surg Clin North Am* 1989;69:361.

17.　Wagner, J. S., Adson, M. A., Van Heerden, J. A., et al. The natural history of hepatic metastases from colorectal cancer. A comparison with resective treatment. *Ann Surg* 1984;199:502.

18.　Gayowski, T. J., Iwatsuki, S., Madariaga, J. R., et al. Experience in hepatic resection for metastatic colorectal cancer: analysis of clinical and pathologic risk factors [see comments]. *Surgery* 1994;116:703.

19.　Iwatsuki, S., Esquivel, C. O., Gordon, R. D., et al. Liver resection for metastatic colorectal cancer. *Surgery* 1986;100:804.

20.　Hughes, K. S., Simon, R., Songhorabodi, S., et al. Resection of the liver for colorectal carcinoma metastases: a multi- institutional study of patterns of recurrence. *Surgery* 1986;100:278.

21.　Nakamura, S., Yokoi, Y., Suzuki, S., et al. Results of extensive surgery for liver metastases in colorectal carcinoma. *Br J Surg* 1992;79:35.

22. Steele, G., Jr., Bleday, R., Mayer, R. J., et al. A prospective evaluation of hepatic resection for colorectal carcinoma metastases to the liver: Gastrointestinal Tumor Study Group Protocol 6584 [see comments]. *J Clin Oncol* 1991;9:1105.

23. Jaeck, D., Bachellier, P., Guiguet, M., et al. Long-term survival following resection of colorectal hepatic metastases. Association Francaise de Chirurgie. *Br J Surg* 1997;84:977.

24. Rossi, S., Fornari, F., Pathies, C., et al. Thermal lesions induced by 480 KHz localized current field in guinea pig and pig liver. *Tumori* 1990;76:54.

25. McGahan, J. P., Browning, P. D., Brock, J. M., et al. Hepatic ablation using radiofrequency electrocautery. *Invest Radiol* 1990;25:267.

26. Seegenschmiedt, M. H., Brady, L. W., and Sauer, R. Interstitial thermoradiotherapy: review on technical and clinical aspects. *Am J Clin Oncol* 1990;13:352.

27. Overgaard, J. Hyperthermia as an adjuvant to radiotherapy. Review of the randomized multicenter studies of the European Society for Hyperthermic Oncology. *Strahlenther Onkol* 1987;163:453.

28. Goldberg, S. N., Gazelle, G. S., Halpern, E. F., et al. Radiofrequency tissue ablation: importance of local temperature along the electrode tip exposure in determining lesion shape and size. *Acad Radiol* 1996;3:212.

29. Cosman, E. R., Nashold, B. S., and Ovelman-Levitt, J. Theoretical aspects of radiofrequency lesions in the dorsal root entry zone. *Neurosurgery* 1984;15:945.

30. Organ, L. W. Electrophysiologic principles of radiofrequency lesion making. *Appl Neurophysiol* 1976;39:69.

31. Anfinsen, O. G., Kongsgaard, E., Foerster, A., et al. Bipolar radiofrequency catheter ablation creates confluent lesions at larger interelectrode spacing than does unipolar ablation from two electrodes in the porcine heart. *Eur Heart J* 1998;19:1075.

32. McGahan, J. P., Brock, J. M., Tesluk, H., et al. Hepatic ablation with use of radio-frequency electrocautery in the animal model. *J Vasc Interv Radiol* 1992;3:291.

33. Goldberg, S. N., Gazelle, G. S., Dawson, S. L., et al. Tissue ablation with radiofrequency: effect of probe size, gauge, duration, and temperature on lesion volume. *Acad Radiol* 1995;2:399.

34. Rossi, S., Buscarini, E., Garbagnati, F., et al. Percutaneous treatment of small hepatic tumors by an expandable RF needle electrode. *AJR Am J Roentgenol* 1998;170:1015.

35. Goldberg, S. N., Gazelle, G. S., Dawson, S. L., et al. Tissue ablation with radiofrequency using multiprobe arrays. *Acad Radiol* 1995;2:670.

36. Siperstein, A. E., Rogers, S. J., Hansen, P. D., et al. Laparoscopic thermal ablation of hepatic neuroendocrine tumor metastases. *Surgery* 1997;122:1147.

37. Mittleman, R. S., Huang, S. K., de Guzman, W. T., et al. Use of the saline infusion electrode catheter for improved energy delivery and increased lesion

size in radiofrequency catheter ablation. *Pacing Clin Electrophysiol* 1995;18:1022.

38. Livraghi, T., Goldberg, S. N., Monti, F., et al. Saline-enhanced radio-frequency tissue ablation in the treatment of liver metastases [see comments]. *Radiology* 1997;202:205.

39. Lorentzen, T. A cooled needle electrode for radiofrequency tissue ablation: thermodynamic aspects of improved performance compared with conventional needle design. *Acad Radiol* 1996;3:556.

40. Goldberg, S. N., Gazelle, G. S., Solbiati, L., et al. Radiofrequency tissue ablation: increased lesion diameter with a perfusion electrode. *Acad Radiol* 1996;3:636.

41. Goldberg, S. N., Gazelle, G. S., Solbiati, L., et al. Large volume radiofrequency tissue ablation: increased coagulation with cooled-tip electrodes. *Radiology* 1996;201:P387 (abstract).

42. Patterson, E. J., Scudamore, C. H., Owen, D. A., et al. Radiofrequency ablation of porcine liver in vivo: effects of blood flow and treatment time on lesion size. *Ann Surg* 1998;227:559.

43. Rossi, S., Garbagnati, F., De Francesco, I., et al. Relationship between the shape and size of radiofrequency induced thermal lesions and hepatic vascularization. *Tumori* 1999;85:128.

44. Goldberg, S. N., Hahn, P. F., Tanabe, K. K., et al. Percutaneous radiofrequency tissue ablation: does perfusion-mediated tissue cooling limit coagulation necrosis? *J Vasc Interv Radiol* 1998;9:101.

45. Goldberg, S. N., Hahn, P. F., Halpern, E. F., et al. Radio-frequency tissue ablation: effect of pharmacologic modulation of blood flow on coagulation diameter. *Radiology* 1998;209:761.

46. Goldberg, S. N., Solbiati, L., Hahn, P. F., et al. Large-volume tissue ablation with radio frequency by using a clustered, internally cooled electrode technique: laboratory and clinical experience in liver metastases. *Radiology* 1998;209:71.

47. Goldberg, S. N., Gazelle, G. S., Solbiati, L., et al. Large volume radiofrequency tissue ablation: increase coagulation with pulsed technique. *Radiology* 1997;205:P258 (abstract).

48. Bilchik, A. J., Rose, D. M., Allegra, D. P., et al. Radiofrequency ablation: a minimally invasive technique with multiple applications [see comments]. *Cancer J Sci Am* 1999;5:356.

49. Solbiati, L., Ierace, T., Goldberg, S. N., et al. Percutaneous US-guided radio-frequency tissue ablation of liver metastases: treatment and follow-up in 16 patients [see comments]. *Radiology* 1997;202:195.

50. Sironi, S., Livraghi, T., Meloni, F., et al. Small hepatocellular carcinoma treated with percutaneous RF ablation: MR imaging follow-up. *AJR Am J Roentgenol* 1999;173:1225.

51. Solbiati, L., Ierace, T., Goldberg, S. N., et al. Follow-up of liver metastases treated with percutaneous radiofrequency ablation: clinical outcome and survival rates. *Radiology* 1996;201:P268 (abstract).

52. Curley, S. A., Izzo, F., Delrio, P., et al. Radiofrequency ablation of unresectable primary and metastatic hepatic malignancies: results in 123 patients [see comments]. *Ann Surg* 1999;230:1.

15
CRYOSURGERY FOR PRIMARY AND METASTATIC LIVER TUMORS

James L. Peacock, M.D.
University of Rochester, Rochester, NY

INTRODUCTION

Cryosurgery is the application of extreme cold temperatures to achieve tumor cell death. Cryoablation, cryotherapy and cryosurgery are interchangeable terms which all apply to the process of tissue destruction using subzero temperatures. Topical application of cold substances to tumors was first reported in treatment of superficial tumors of skin, oropharynx and gynecologic systems. (1) The rationale for using extreme cold to treat tumors is the potential for *in situ* tumor destruction while sparing normal surrounding structures and without the complications of major surgical intervention. In 1963 Irving Cooper was the first to describe the feasibility of such an approach to the liver and other organs. (2) He devised a system of liquid nitrogen delivery through insulated cannulas that could be placed within the substance of the liver. Subsequently Andrew Gage and co-investigators performed in vivo studies of hepatic cryosurgery and described many of the physiologic responses to liver treatment. They showed that large areas of liver could be treated successfully and that large remnants of devitalized tissue did not produce toxic effects to the animal. (3)

Early attempts at freezing tumors were frustrated by inability to measure the treatment zone. Blind placement of thermocouples to measure actual tissue temperatures was an improvement, but still very crude devices for determining actual areas of tumor cell kill. Modern application of cryosurgery, however, awaited the development of intraoperative ultrasound to monitor effectively the zone of treatment. The combination of intraoperative ultrasound probes and cryogenic tissue probes for delivery of extreme cold have led toward a rapid expansion of clinical use in liver, kidney and prostate neoplasms. This chapter will discuss the scientific mechanisms, clinical applications and current results of cryosurgery as it relates to treatment of primary and metastatic tumors of the liver.

SCIENTIFIC MECHANISM

Exposure to temperatures below -20 C for longer than 1 minute is generally lethal to living cells. One must differentiate the use of extreme cold for cell kill from cell protection or so called cryopreservation. Cryopreservation is laboratory technique for storage and later retrieval of viable cells either in single cell suspension or small tissue masses. The success of subfreezing temperatures producing cell death rather than cell preservation depends somewhat on rates of freezing and thawing. Rapid freezing and gradual thawing, especially in repetitive cycles is much more likely to produce cell death as opposed to gradual freezing and rapid thaw.

The mechanisms by which tumor cells are killed are a combination of physical and biological events. Creation of ice crystals leads to cell lysis in two manners: first, physical properties of ice can damage the plasma membrane. Second, electrolytes and organic compounds are excluded from the ice and become hyperconcentrated in the extracellular space leading to migration of water from inside the cells and virtual cell dehydration. As more and more tissue freezes, the physical properties of ice crystals actually create a grinding effect that disrupts the tumor. During the subsequent thaw phase water passes back into cells and leads to increasing cell volume and bursting of cell membranes. (4) In addition to direct physical effects of ice on tumor tissue, cryotherapy has an effect on small arterioles and venules. Subfreezing temperatures obliterate these vessels and this leads to tumor destruction by devascularization. (5)

Tumor cells are not uniquely susceptible to damage by subzero freezing. Normal tissues such liver, kidney and prostate will also be destroyed by the same mechanisms. Bile ducts and the gallbladder wall are particularly vulnerable to freezing damage. The muscular wall of medium and larger arteries, on the other hand, is peculiarly resistant to cryodestruction. Even when completely frozen, muscular arteries will return to normal morphology and function after thawing. In vivo perfused organs will have protection of large vessels due to a heat sink phenomenon. (6) With constant flow of warm blood, external freezing probes are unable to completely freeze the endothelial layer. This phenomenon has clinical implications that will be discussed later.

EXPERIMENTAL RESULTS

The feasibility and effects of hepatic cryoablation have been studied in a variety of animal models. Early experiments by Gage et al. in dogs discovered problems with surface cracking as well as disturbances of clotting pathways. Necrosis of liver parenchyma was observed both grossly and histologically. Follow-up studies several months later showed dense fibrous tissue in the zone of cryotherapy. (3) Ravikumar extensively studied cryotherapy in a rat tumor model. Locally aggressive tumors were established in vivo in subcutaneously as well as within liver parenchyma of rats. Treatments with 1,2 or 3 cycles of freeze-thaw were evaluated for residual viable cancer cells. Occasional tumors with only 1 freeze-thaw cycle demonstrated residual viability compared to none of tumors treated with 2 or 3 cycles. These findings, as well as results from others have led to recommendations of multiple freeze-thaw cycles for best tumor kill. (7,8)

Other investigators have focused more on alterations of peritumoral blood flow as a mechanism by which cryotherapy causes tumor ablation. Brown et al performed hepatic cryotherapy on implanted fibrosarcoma tumors in rats and measured red cell flux using a laser doppler flowmeter. Their results show significant reduction of blood flow in the center and edges of the tumor immediately after cryotherapy as well as 8 hours post-treatment. They concluded that disruption of microcirculation in and around the tumor is a major factor in cryotherapy. (9)

Another postulated mechanism involved with hepatic cryotherapy, though less well proved, has been activation of immune factors. Bayjoo et al showed that circulating natural killer cells have increased cytotoxic potential as much as 11 days after delivery of cryotherapy. (10) Other studies have shown enhanced immunologic activity of regional lymph nodes after cryosurgery. (11)

Weber, Lee and associates addressed theoretical concerns of the heat sink phenomenon in porcine studies of liver cryosurgery. They showed complete necrosis of hepatic parenchyma around major vascular structures, suggesting that tumors adjacent to such vessels will not escape ablation due to a temperature sink. Additional evidence was provided that larger vessels due not fracture or thrombose with cryotherapy. Their studies also concluded that single freeze-thaw cycles were adequate to necrose liver tissue contrary to earlier reports. (12)

TECHNICAL ASPECTS

Equipment

Cryosurgical systems available today for treatment of liver tumors consist primarily of 3 components: a) cryogen storage unit, b) vacuum insulated conduction coils and c) cryoprobes, hollow metallic probes which come in a variety of sizes and shapes. The two most widely used systems are Cryotech (Candela Laser Corp., Wayland, Mass.) which uses liquid nitrogen as a cryogen, and Cryocare(EndoCare, Inc., Irvine, Calif.) which uses argon gas as a cryogen. Both systems effectively produce temperatures below -100 C at the probe tip. Advantages of the argon-based system are more rapid freezing rates, easier portability and cryoprobes that are less bulky since they do not require as much insulation. Multiple probes can be activated simultaneously with either system, which is quite helpful in treatment of larger lesions. Cylindrical cryoprobes are most often used for liver cryosurgery. Probes range in size from 3mm to 10mm diameter.

Choice of probes depends on the size of cryolesion desired. A 3mm probe will produce a cryolesion of approximately 3cm diameter; the 5mm probe, approximately a 4 to 5cm cryolesion; and the 10mm probe a 6cm or larger cryolesion. (13) Flat disc-like probes are available for treatment of tumors on the liver surface or resection margins. These probes produce a broad cryolesion approximately 1cm in depth.

The other critical piece of equipment is intraoperative ultrasound. A variety of intraoperative probes are produced for use in liver ultrasound. The most useful transducers are 5.0 or 7.5 MHz.

Operative technique

Patients are prepared for surgery with large bore intravenous access, foley catheter and arterial line. The Bair Hugger warming system is used to help prevent systemic hypothermia. Operative exposure is similar to liver resection. A generous right subcostal incision is made, occasionally with extension in the upper midline. Intra-abdominal adhesions are divided and a thorough examination of the peritoneal cavity is performed to rule out extrahepatic metastases. Biopsy of a portal lymph node with frozen section is important since this usually signifies disseminated disease. The liver is mobilized and carefully palpated bimanually. Intraoperative ultrasound of the liver is performed to identify size and location of all lesions. Ultrasound imaging is imperative to successful cryotherapy. Frequently IOUS will identify lesions not found with preoperative imaging. (14) Real time ultrasound is used to position the cryoprobe in the tumor and monitor the area of cryodestruction.

Towels are placed around the liver to prevent cooling of surrounding structures. The "fish" tissue protector commonly used for abdominal wound closure is also useful for insulation. An appropriate probe size is chosen based on the desired area of treatment. Ultrasound guides placement of the cryoprobe through the liver substance into the tumor. A 20 gauge spinal needle can be used as a probe simulator to help the surgeon determine the correct trajectory and depth for placement. Peel-away sheaths are also available to create a tract for cryoprobe placement using an adoptive Seldinger technique.

After probe placement the freezing process is begun. Generally 10-15 minutes of freezing will be necessary to obtain a suitable area of tissue destruction. The spherical volume of frozen tissue is called the iceball. Enlargement of the iceball is monitored by intraoperative ultrasound. The interface between frozen and normal tissue is seen by ultrasound as a hyperechoic rim called the freeze front. The freeze front should advance at least 1cm beyond the tumor edge for adequate treatment. When a 1 cm margin is reached freezing is discontinued and a passive thaw period occurs. The freeze front will regress spontaneously. When the tumor edge reappears, a second freeze cycle is begun, generally requiring only and additional 5 minutes. Active thawing can then facilitate probe removal. Actual removal of the probe from the iceball should not be attempted until the probe can rotate freely; otherwise liver cracking may occur. The probe tract then is packed with a hemostatic agent such as oxidized regenerated cellulose (Surgicel NuKnit). (15,16) Perihepatic drains are usually not required.

Mannitol is given intraoperatively to help protect against renal damage from myoglobinuria. Acute renal failure has been reported in some series, but generally is seen only with treatment of very large tumors. Also, platelet counts and coagulation profiles should be checked postoperatively since dissimenated intravascular coagulopathy has been reported. These complications can be avoided by confining treatment to tumors <6cm in diameter and no more than 50% cumulative volume of the liver. Generally, patients recovery smoothly and can be discharged an average of 5 days later. CT scan performed at one week after treatment will show an area of necrosis, the cryolesion, which commonly has residual gas bubbles, not to be confused with infection. Follow-up scans at 3 months and 6 months will show metamorphosis of the necrotic cryolesion into a rounded area of fibrous scar. Their enlargement over time identifies local recurrences in the liver, whereas cryolesions without residual tumor will remain the same or actually shrink with time.

Other technical considerations include the use of vascular inflow occlusion (Pringle maneuver) during cryotherapy. Vascular inflow occlusion theoretically enhances the effect of tissue freezing by removing the so-called heat sink phenomenon. Some authors have reported, however, that greater risk of hemorrhage occurs with inflow occlusion. We recommend inflow occlusion if intraoperative ultrasound shows areas of tumor abutting major intrahepatic vessels.

Complications of hepatic cryosurgery include hemorrhage from surface cracking. Such problems are usually apparent early following the thaw phase. Surgeons must be prepared to perform tractotomy and ligation, or major hepatic resection in unusual cases of post treatment hemorrhage. Delayed hemorrhage has been reported in less than 1% of cases. Bile leak has also been reported, but was manageable non-operatively. Other less commonly seen complications included myoglobinuria and DIC. Freezing very large tumors (>5cm diameter) increases the possibility of myoglobinuria or coagulopathy. (17) Right pleural effusion is very common but rarely symptomatic.

Current Applications

Cryotherapy has been reported for almost all solid malignancies of the liver, both primary and metastatic. In general this technique has been applied in situations where liver resection is contraindicated, such as bilobar metastases, tumors adjacent to major vessels, and patients with significant comorbidities and high surgical risk. Most authors have not proposed cryotherapy as a replacement of standard liver resection. Polk et al have reported a unique application of cryotherapy using cryo-assisted resection. After creating the iceball surrounding the tumor these authors proceeded with segmental liver resection using the probe and iceball as fixture for excising the tumor with a sufficient margin. (18) Others have reported using cryotherapy in combination with hepatic artery infusion.

CLINICAL RESULTS

Hepatocellular carcinoma

Hepatocellular carcinoma usually occurs in the setting of liver cirrhosis and frequently is multicentric. In addition these cancers commonly present as large tumors with invasion of portal or hepatic veins. These factors make cryoablation a more attractive approach for treatment. The largest experience with such an approach to primary liver cancer comes from the Liver Cancer Institute in Shanghai, China. In 1996 Zhou and others reported on 167 patients with pathologically proven primary liver cancer treated by cryosurgery. Some of these patients also had hepatic artery infusion. In this series there were no reported deaths or serious complications from hemorrhage or bile leakage. The group of patients with tumors <5cm had 1, 3, and 5-year survival rates of 92.2%, 72.5%, and 47.8% respectively. Patients with tumors greater than 5cm had survival rates of 66.1%, 35.4% and 24.5% at 1, 3, and 5 years. (19) Smaller series of patients from Australia and the U.S. have shown the feasibility and safety of using cryosurgery in the cirrhotic patient, but do not reveal any meaningful survival information. (20,21)

Colorectal Metastases

By far the widest application of hepatic cryosurgery in North America has been treatment of metastatic colorectal cancer. Although resection is the current standard for colorectal metastases, fewer than 20% of patients are candidates. Currently most experts recommend resection for patients with 3 or fewer metastases and disease confined to one lobe of the liver. Cryotherapy can treat as many as eight or ten lesions in the liver with bilobar distribution. Colorectal metastases tend to be hyperdense by ultrasound compared to normal liver parenchyma making them well suited for localization and treatment with intraoperative ultrasound. While there have not been any randomized prospective studies in cryotherapy of colorectal liver disease, numerous institutions have reported their results with follow-up ranging from 12 to 40 months. In 1991 Ravikumar, Steele and associates reported results on 24 patients with colorectal metastases. All but two patients had elevation of CEA levels preoperatively. Median follow-up was 2 years. Nine patients (37%) died of recurrent disease and another eight patients (33%) are living with recurrence. Seven patients (29%) are alive and disease free. Only two patients (8%) developed recurrence at the site of cryotherapy. (7) Later, Weaver and coauthors reported a large experience with treatment specifically of colorectal metastases. Forty-seven patients were treated using cryoablation with an average of 3 lesions treated per patient. At the completion of treatment all patients were disease-free. Median follow-up was 26 months. Sixty-two percent of patients treated were alive at 24 months. There were no documented recurrences at the site of cryosurgery. (22)

Other results in metastatic colon cancer come from Australia where Morris et al have extensive experience with liver cryosurgery. Their most recent report includes 116 patients treated over a 7-year period. The mean diameter of tumors treated was 4.4cm and the mean number of metastases was 3.9. Over 80% of patients had tumors distributed in both hepatic lobes. In addition to cryotherapy, however, 90% of patients received at least one cycle of intraarterial chemotherapy. Perioperative mortality was 0.9% and total perioperative morbidity was 27%. Median survival was 26 months, with 1, 2, 3, and 5-year survival rates of 82.4%, 55.7%, 32.3%, and 13.4%, respectively. Factors which independently correlated with disease relapse included preoperative CEA level > 100 ng/ml, diameter of cryotreated metastasis greater than 5.0cm, presence of extrahepatic disease, poor differentiation of the primary tumor, and incomplete treatment of all metastases. (23)

Virtually all the available data on outcome of cryotherapy for colorectal metastases is derived from retrospective studies of single institution experiences. A genuine assessment of treatment benefit is hampered by the absence of prospectively designed guidelines on patient inclusion. A reasonable consensus, however, is that cryoablation of hepatic metastases is safe, with perioperative mortality rates less than 1%, and that patients who undergo complete treatment of all lesions can expect a 50% chance of 2 year survival. The optimistic side of these studies is that very few recurrences in the local treatment zone are reported. Nearly all relapses are found in other areas of the liver, or extrahepatic sites.

An important benefit of cryosurgery for the treatment of colorectal metastases is as an adjunct to liver resection. Cryoablation is an attractive means for treatment of a close surgical margin, especially in situations where additional resection would jeopardize major vessels or sacrifice too much liver parenchyma. The flat cryoprobe placed on the resection surface can ablate the margin to approximately 1cm depth. Wallace et al showed in their experience that addition of cryotherapy to resection puts patients into a much better survival group compared to incomplete or "non-curative" resections. (24)

Other metastatic tumors

Cryoablation has been utilized for a variety of other metastatic diseases. Essentially any metastatic tumor that is contemplated for resection can be treated with cryotherapy. Success of treatment, to a large degree, depends on visibility with intraoperative ultrasound for localization and monitoring of treatment zone. Also the biology of the tumor has an important role in treatment success. Neuroendocrine tumors metastatic to liver are particularly well suited for cryotherapy. These tumors tend to occur in multiple lobes and are usually slowly progressive. Reduction of tumor burden in these cases can provide significant palliation for patients. Morris and others have shown long-term relief from symptoms by treatment with cryoablation. (25)

FUTURE APPLICATIONS

Techniques for laparoscopic cryotherapy and percutaneous cryotherapy of the liver are already under development. Laparoscopic ultrasound probes are available for treatment monitoring. Widespread results with these new technologies are not available yet. The feasibility of combining cryotherapy with liver resection and/or hepatic artery chemotherapy has been shown and awaits further clinical results. The safety of cryotherapy and its effectiveness in killing solid tumor nodules has been well established. We need more clinical trials with stricter prospective treatment guidelines before the true role of this device in cancer care will be known. In the meantime cryotherapy certainly serves as a valuable adjunctive tool for the surgical oncologist who treats primary and metastatic disease of the liver.

REFERENCES

1. Shephard J, Dawber RPR: The historical and scientific basis of cryosurgery. Clin Exp Dermatol 1982; 7:321
2. Cooper IS: Cryogenic surgery. New Engl J Med 1963;268:743
3. Dutta P, Montes , Gage AA. Experimental Hepatic Cryosurgery. Cryobiology 1977;14:598
4. Ravikumar TX, Sotomayor R, Goel R Cryosurgery in the Treatment of liver Metastasis From Colorectal Cancer 1997 J Gastrointestinal Surg 1: 426
5. Kane RA. Ultrasound-Guided Hepatic Cryosurgery for Tumor Ablation 1993 Sem Interventional Radiol. 10:132
6. Steele G. Cryoablation in hepatic surgery. Semin Liv Dis 1994;14:120
7. Ravikumar TS, Steele,Jr G, Kane R, King V. Experimental and clinical observations on hepatic cryosurgery for colorectal metastases. Cancer Res 1991;51:6323
8. Neel HB, Ketcham AS, Hammond WG. Requisites for successful cryogenic surgery of cancer. Arch Surg 1971;102:45
9. Brown NJ, Bayjoo P, Reed MWR. Effect of cryosurgery on liver blood flow. Br J Cancer 1993;68:10
10. Bayjoo P, Rees RC, Goepel JR, Jacob G. The effect of cryosurgery of liver tumour on natural killer cell activity in the rat. Int J Immunopath Pharm 1991;4:187
11. Miya K, Saji B, Morita T, et al. Immunological response of regional lymph nodes after tumor cryosurgery: experimental study in rats. Cryobiology, 1986; 23:290
12. Weber SM, Lee, Jr. FT, Chinn DO, Warner T, Chosy SG, Mahvi DM. Perivascular and intralesional tissue necrosis after hepatic cryoablation: results in a porcine model. Surgery 1997; 122:742
13. Kane RA. Ultrasound-guided Hepatic cryosurgery for tumor ablation. Sem Interventional Radiol. 1993;10:132

14. Kane RA, Hughes LA, Cua EJ, Steele,Jr. GD, Jenkins RL, Cady B. The impact of intraoperative ultrasonography on surgery for liver neoplasms. J Ultrasound Med 1994;13:1

15. Madura JA, Mulligan DC. Probe tract hemostasis using oxidized regenerated cellulose in hepatic cryosurgery. Contemp Surg 1998;52:251

16. Ravikumar TS. Interstitial therapies for liver tumors. In Surg Onc Clin NA. 1996;5:365

17. McCarty T, Kuhn JA. Cryotherapy for liver tumors. Oncology 1998; 12(7): 979

18. Polk W, Fong Y, Karpeh M, Blumgart LH. A technique for the use of cryosurgery to assist hepatic resection. J Am Coll Surg 1995;180:171

19. Zhou X, Tang Z, Yu Y: Ablative approach for primary liver cancer, in Cady B, Ravikumar T(eds): Surg Onc Clin NA 1996; 5:379 Philadelphia, WB Saunders

20. Morris DL, Ross WB: Australian experience of cryoablation of liver tumors in Cady B, Ravikumar T(eds): Surg Onc Clin NA 1996; 5:391, Philadelphia, WB Saunders

21. Wren SM, Coburn MM, Tan M, Daniels JR, Yassa N, Carpenter CL, Stain SC: Is cryosurgical ablation appropriate for treating hepatocellular cancer?: Arch Surg 1997; 132:599

22. Weaver LM, Atkinson D, Zemel R. Hepatic cryosurgery in treating colorectal metastases. Cancer 1995;76:210

23. Seifert JK, Morris DL. Prognostic factors after cryotherapy for hepatic metastases from colorectal cancer. Annals of Surgery 1998:228:201

24. Wallace JR, Christians KK, Pitt HA, Quebbeman EJ. Cryotherapy extends the indications for treatment of colorectal liver metastases. Surgery 1999;126:766

25. Cozzi PJ, Englund R, Morris DL: Cryotherapy treatment of patients with hepatic metastases from neuroendocrine tumours. Cancer 1995;76:501

16

HEPATIC ARTERY INFUSIONAL CHEMOTHERAPY FOR COLORECTAL LIVER METASTASES

Aaron R. Sasson, M.D., James C. Watson, M.D. and Elin R. Sigurdson, M.D., Ph.D.

Fox Chase Cancer Center, Philadelphia, PA

INTRODUCTION

Colorectal cancer is diagnosed in 130,000 patients annually, and is the second leading cause of cancer related deaths (1). A significant percentage of patients with colorectal cancer will develop metastases, and the liver is the predominant site in nearly 60% of patients. Of these patients, one quarter will have disease isolated to the liver and only a minority of patients will be candidates for surgical resection. Even with complete tumor removal the five-year survival is less than 40% and recurrences are common (2,3). Administration of systemic chemotherapy for metastatic colorectal cancer provides a response rate less than 30%, and results in a median survival only 12 months.

The limited benefit of systemic chemotherapy for the treatment of colorectal hepatic metastases has prompted investigation of alternative approaches such as regional therapy. The ability to administer high concentrations of anticancer drugs to the liver is the principle which regional therapy, hepatic arterial infusion (HAI), is based upon. Chemotherapy administered by HAI could expose the metastases to high drug concentrations with minimal systemic effects. The development of a totally implantable infusion pump has allowed for the safe administration of hepatic arterial chemotherapy in the outpatient setting (4). Patients with metastatic colorectal cancer isolated to the liver are excellent candidates for regional chemotherapy delivered via the hepatic artery. This chapter will cover the (1) rationale for the use of hepatic arterial chemotherapy for the treatment of colorectal liver metastases, (2) the results of studies evaluating its efficacy in resectable and unresectable liver metastases, (3) the technical aspects of HAI catheter placement, (4) complications associated with pump insertion, and (5) toxicities associated with intrahepatic therapy.

RATIONALE

Anatomical basis

The liver is an organ with a rich blood supply, with both the portal vein and hepatic artery providing nutrients. Venous drainage of the colon and rectum is through the portal vein and it is believed that this is how gastrointestinal malignancies spread to the liver. The liver derives most of its blood supply from the portal vein. In contrast, liver metastases (>3mm in size) are perfused almost exclusively by the hepatic artery (5,6). Injection of the hepatic artery or portal vein with tritiated floxuridine (^{3}H-FUDR) results in similar mean concentrations of the drug in the liver (7). However, the mean FUDR level measured in the tumor was significantly increased (15-fold) when the drug was injected via the hepatic artery as compared to the portal vein. A small-randomized study, in patients with colorectal metastases to the liver, compared FUDR given by either portal vein infusion or HAI (8). None of the patients treated with portal vein infusion responded, whereas 50% of the patients with HAI demonstrated a response. Furthermore, several patients in the portal vein infusion group who subsequently received HAI had a 30% response rate. Metastatic liver tumor's dependence on blood supply from the hepatic artery allows for the selective delivery of anticancer drugs to the tumor.

Pharmacological basis

The ideal agent for use in HAI is one that is highly extracted by the liver during the first pass with a short systemic half-life. The higher the extraction by the liver the lower the systemic concentration of the drug, which limits the systemic toxicity. Ensminger and associates have demonstrated that >the liver extracts 94% of FUDR during the first pass (9). In comparison, the first pass extraction of 5-fluorouracil (5-FU) ranges from 19-55%. Drug levels of FUDR, administered intra-arterially, were 400 times higher in hepatic tissue than in extrahepatic tissue. This allows the infusion of FUDR via HAI while limiting exposure of FUDR in the systemic circulation. Since systemic exposure of drugs administered by HAI is low, drugs with a steep dose response curve can be utilized more efficaciously. Large doses, which result in greater tumor response, can be given with minimal systemic toxicity, but is limited by hepatotoxicity.

Another rationale for hepatic arterial chemotherapy, especially for patients with metastatic colorectal cancer, is the concept of a step-wise pattern of metastatic progression (10,11). This theory states that hematogenous spread occurs first via the portal vein to the liver, then from the liver to the lungs, and other distant sites. Thus, aggressive treatment of metastases confined to the liver (i.e., either resection or hepatic infusion) will yield prolonged survival for some patients.

EFFICACY OF HAI THERAPY

Treatment of unresectable liver metastases

The liver is the most common site of dissemination with up to 70% of patients developing liver metastases during the course of their disease (12). The effect of chemotherapy on patients with isolated unresectable liver metastases is not well known. Fluorouracil is the primary agent used in the treatment of metastatic colorectal carcinoma. Unfortunately response to systemic therapy is low and prolonged survival is rare. A meta-analysis comparing 5-FU vs. 5-FU with leucovorin (LV) demonstrated response rates of 11% and 23% respectively (13). Most trials include patients with widely metastatic disease, making it difficult to analyze the effect of therapy on isolated liver metastases.

Regional therapy was investigated as an effort to improve response rate. Early trails with HAI using implantable pumps and continuos FUDR resulted in response rates ranging from 29% to 83% (14-16). These encouraging results have prompted prospective randomized trials comparing systemic therapy vs. HAI in patients with isolated unresectable colorectal metastases to the liver (17-23). The trials are listed in Table 16.1.

Table 16.1. Randomized Trials of HAI Vs Systemic Chemotherapy for Treatment of Isolated Unresectable Colorectal Liver Metastases.

Group (ref. no.)	No. patients*	HAI		Systemic		P value
		Regimen	Response Rate	Regimen	Response Rate	
MSKCC (19)	99	FUDR	52%	FUDR	20%	0.001
NCOG (18)	117	FUDR	42%	FUDR	10%	0.0001
NCI (20)	50	FUDR	62%	FUDR	17%	0.003
Mayo (21)	61	FUDR	45%	5-FU	21%	0.02
France (22)	163	FUDR	49%	5-FU[1]	14%	-
London (17)	100	FUDR	50%	5-FU[2]	0%	0.001
German (23)[3]	148	FUDR	43%	5-FU	20%	<.02
		5-FU	45%			

MSKCC - Memorial Sloan Kettering Cancer Center, NCOG-Northern California Oncology Group, NCI-National Cancer Institute, HAI-Hepatic arterial infusion, FUDR- Floxuridine, 5-FU – 5-Fluorouracil
*Refers to number of patients receiving treatment
(-) No p value reported

[1] Less than 50% of patients received systemic chemotherapy
[2] Less than 25% of patients received systemic chemotherapy
[3] Three-arm trial comparing HAI FUDR, HAI 5-FU, and systemic 5-FU

Table 16.2. Comparison of trials with adjuvant HAI following liver resection.

Group (ref. no.)	No. patients	Regimen	5 yrs.
MSKCC (35)	156	HAI (FUDR) + IV (5-FU/LV)	61%*
		Control: IV (5-FU/LV)	49%
German Cooperative (36)	226	HAI (5-FU/LV)	N/A
		Control: Observation	N/A
Intergroup (37)	109	HAI (FUDR) + IV (5-FU)	63%
		Control: Observation	32%

Abbreviations: MSKCC - Memorial Sloan Kettering Cancer Center, HAI – Hepatic arterial infusion, FUDR- Floxuridine, IV – intravenous (systemic), 5-FU – 5-Fluorouracil
* Denotes statistical significance

When interpreting these trials, study design, chemotherapy regimens, and patient characteristics need to be considered. Investigators have demonstrated the influence of liver tumor burden on survival. Patients with less than 20% involvement have a median survival of 20 months, while for patients with greater that 60% involvement the median survival is only 6 months (24). Serum levels of lactate dehydrogenase (LDH) and carcinoembryonic antigen (CEA) have been shown to be prognostic factors (25). In several studies, patients with portal lymph node involvement were included (18,19,21,22). This subgroup of patients perhaps has a worse prognosis, and they do not receive optimal therapy from HAI since these nodes are not treated when HAI is utilized. Crossover between the systemic therapy group and HAI group were allowed in two large studies, making survival analysis between the two treatment arms difficult (18,19).

In the seven prospective randomized trials, HAI therapy using an implantable pump consisted of FUDR administered continuously for 14 days in 28-day cycles. In the majority of these studies, the FUDR dose was 0.3 mg/kg/day (19-22). The study from the Northern California Oncology Group (NCOG) reduced the dose to 0.2 mg/kg/day due to increased toxicity (18). Two European studies used a FUDR dose of 0.2 mg/kg/day (17,23). In studies from Memorial Sloan-Kettering Cancer Center (MSKCC), NCOG, and National Cancer Institute (NCI) systemic FUDR (dose ranging from .075 mg/kg/day to 0.15mg/kg/day) was administered in the control group (18,19,20). In the remaining studies, 5-FU based therapy served as the control group (17,21-23). However, in a study from London and France, only a minority of the patients in the control group received any chemotherapy (17,22).

In all studies, tumor response rates from HAI (FUDR) therapy (43% to 62%) were significantly greater than the control group (9% to 21%). In the majority of trials, hepatic arterial based therapy also resulted in a longer median survival. However, this was not statistically significant, with the exception of the London and France trials (17,22). The trials conducted by MSKCC and NCOG allowed patients who failed systemic therapy to cross over and receive HAI, obscuring the ability to detect a difference in survival (18,19). In the MSKCC trial, 60% of the patients randomized to systemic therapy crossed over to HAI after tumor progression. Of these patients, 25% went on to a partial response after the crossover, and 60% had a decrease in serum CEA levels. Those who did not cross over had a median survival of only 8 months, compared with 18 months for those patients who crossed over to hepatic infusion, p=0.04 (19).

Another factor making interpretation of survival data difficult is the inclusion of patients who had extrahepatic diseases (18,20-22). This subgroup of patients is unlikely to receive any benefit from HAI therapy since drug levels at extrahepatic sites are inadequate. In the study by the NCI, 38% of the HAI group had positive portal lymph nodes. Subset analysis of patients without extrahepatic disease revealed a significant improvement in the two year survival from 47% in the HAI group vs 13% in the systemic group, p= 0.03 (20). In a report from the Mayo Clinic, 19% of patients receiving HAI therapy had extrahepatic disease, the presence of which adversely impacts survival, p=0.04 (21). This has led many investigators to conclude that the use of HAI therapy, as the sole treatment, is a relative contraindication in patients with extrahepatic disease.

A prospective randomized trial conducted by the German Cooperative Group on Liver Metastases was recently reported (23). This trial compared two different HAI regimens against systemic therapy with 5-FU (800 mg/m^2/day) and LV (200 mg/ m^2/day). The HAI regimens used were 5-FU (1000 mg/ m^2/day) and LV (200 mg/ m^2/day), and FUDR (0.2mg/kg/day). The tumor response rates utilizing HAI administered therapies were significantly higher than for the systemic regimen. Response rates for the different groups were, 45% HAI (5-FU/LV), 43% HAI (FUDR), and 20% systemic 5-FU/LV. Although there was no statistical difference in survival, the group with HAI (FUDR) did have a lower median survival than the other two treatment groups. This could be explained by the increase in extrahepatic progression in the HIA (FUDR) group compared with the HAI (5-FU/LV) group, 41% vs 13%, respectively. Since the extraction of FUDR by the liver is so great, there is limited systemic exposure; in contrast, the extraction of 5-FU by the liver is no greater than 55% (9). This would account also for the increased number of adverse events (toxicity) in the HAI (5-FU/LV) group.

Two meta-analyses of prospective randomized trials comparing regional therapy (HAI) vs systemic therapy for the treatment of colorectal metastases confined to the liver have been done (26,27). The Meta-Analysis Group in Cancer confirmed a statistically significant increase in the tumor response rate from HAI therapy (41%) compared to systemic therapy (14%) (26). Patterns of failure from the different regimens were also evaluated, and liver as the site of first failure was decreased by an absolute value of 25% for HAI therapy. However, as show in other trials, extrahepatic disease progression was greater using regional therapy (45%) compared to systemic treatment (8%). The ability to detect a survival advantage from HAI has been hampered by small number of patients in individual trials and crossover of patients to regional therapy. However, the meta-analyses demonstrated a modest increase in survival for HAI therapy and identified it as an independent prognostic variable (26,27).

Adjuvant treatment following liver resection
Surgical resection is the most effective therapy for liver metastases from colorectal carcinoma (2,3). Despite complete surgical resection, tumor recurrence in the remaining liver occurs in nearly 50% of patients (28). The role of adjuvant therapy following surgery has not been well defined. Preliminary data regarding the use of adjuvant treatment, particularly regional therapy, suggests a benefit in improving disease free and overall survival (29-32). City of Hope investigators reported their results of a prospective randomized trial of adjuvant HAI following liver resection (33,34). Patients with solitary liver metastasis were randomized to resection plus HAI or resection alone. Time to disease progression was significantly increased form 9 months (resection alone) to 31 months (resection plus HAI) (33). Additionally, no patients treated with adjuvant HAI therapy developed any liver recurrences, however the number of patients in this group was small. Patients with multiple resectable liver metastases were randomized to resection and HAI or HAI alone. Improvements in survival and subsequent hepatic disease progression were seen in the group with resection and HAI.

Recently, reports from three large (n>100) prospective randomized trails of adjuvant HAI following resection have been reported, Table 16.2 (35-37). The Intergroup (Eastern Cooperative Oncology Group (ECOG) and Southwestern Oncology Group (SWOG) trial randomized 109 patients to receive either surgery alone or surgery followed by HAI (FUDR) and systemic therapy (5-FU) (37). Only patients with three or fewer metastatic lesions were eligible. A significant benefit in disease free survival and time to liver recurrence was seen in the group that received adjuvant treatment. Overall 5-year survival for resection plus adjuvant HAI and systemic therapy (63%) was greater than for resection alone (32%), (p=NS), with a mean follow-up time of only 33 months. A trial by the German Cooperative on Liver Metastases randomized patients (n=226) to surgery alone vs surgery plus adjuvant HAI (5-FU/LV) (36). Although no difference in overall survival was detected, both disease free survival and median time to liver recurrence were increased in the surgery plus HAI group.

A recent study from MSKCC compared liver resection followed by either combined therapy (HAI and systemic) or monotherapy (systemic) (35). The combined therapy group received HAI (FUDR, 0.25 mg/kg/day) and systemic (5-FU, 325 mg/ m^2/day and LV, 200 mg/ m^2/day), whereas the monotherapy group received only systemic (5-FU, 370 mg/ m^2/day and LV, 200 mg/ m^2/day). A significant improvement in the actuarial overall survival at two years was observed in the combined therapy group (86%) compared to the monotherapy group (72%). Additionally, the five-year rates of hepatic free progression were 74% in the group with HAI and systemic therapy and 44% in the group with systemic therapy only. Multivariate analysis identified treatment with combined therapy to be a significant factor in improving the risk ratio for death, hepatic progression and overall progression. These improvements occurred despite the need for FUDR dose reduction (due to toxicity). This implies that the benefit from regional therapy maybe the result from a high initial dose of FUDR. These recent studies provide encouraging results in the use of regional therapy in the adjuvant setting following curative resection of hepatic colorectal metastases.

TECHNICAL ASPECTS

Pump design
Medtronic (Minneapolis, Minnesota) and Arrow International (Walpole, Massachusetts) currently manufacture fixed flow rate pumps. Both companies manufacture single catheter pumps, dual catheter pumps are not available at this time. The implantable infusion devices store drugs in a collapsible titanium reservoir, in which delivery of drug is controlled by pressure generated as a propellant expands at body temperature. A small gauge needle inserted in to the center septum fills the pump reservoir (20-60 cc). Direct access to the catheter is also available through a separate access port. This port allows direct arterial injection for flushing, imaging studies, and drug boluses.

Preoperative evaluation
Proper patient selection is facilitated by a multidisciplinary approach, involving the surgeon, medical oncologist and radiologist. Patients being considered for HAI chemotherapy should have a complete staging workup including colonoscopy, chest x-ray, and computed tomographic (CT) scan of the abdomen and pelvis to exclude the presence of extrahepatic disease. Patients with extensive (>70%) liver replacement should not be selected for pump placement if hepatic reserve is not sufficient to withstand laparotomy. Patients should also undergo a preoperative visceral angiogram to define the superior mesenteric artery (SMA) and celiac arterial anatomy. Variations in hepatic arterial anatomy occur in approximately 25-40% of patients, Figure 16.1 (38-40). The most common variations involve the presence of accessory and/or replaced arteries. When a left or right hepatic artery arises from an abnormal location, typically the superior mesenteric artery or left gastric artery, respectively, this represents an accessory or replaced variant. If a right or left hepatic artery from the common hepatic artery is present, then the aberrant vessel is termed an accessory artery. If the right or left hepatic artery from the common hepatic artery is absent, then the aberrant vessel is termed a replaced artery. Additionally, the arteriogram also confirms patency of the portal vein. Patients with portal vein occlusion are excluded because should the hepatic artery occlude during surgery or while receiving chemotherapy the liver may infarct.

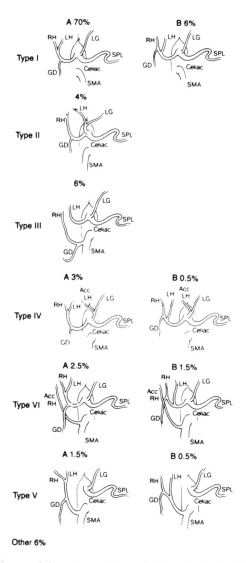

Figure 16.1 Hepatic arterial anatomy. Normal (Type I A). Trifurcation (Type I B). Replaced left hepatic artery (Type II). Replaced right hepatic artery (Type III). Accessory left hepatic artery (Type IV). Accessory right hepatic artery (Type VI). Hepatic artery arising from superior mesenteric artery (Type V). LH = left hepatic artery; RH = right hepatic artery; GD = gastroduodenal artery; LG = left gastric artery; SPL = splenic artery; SMA = superior mesenteric artery. Reproduced with permission (40).

Surgical technique
A midline incision provides excellent exposure of the vessels and allows for easy abdominal exploration and for colectomy for synchronous disease. The operation is conducted with the utmost attention to detail in order to minimize the risk of complications, some of which will preclude subsequent use of the pump (40). The surgeon's goal is to achieve proper catheter placement so that drug perfusion is precisely targeted to the liver and arterial/catheter complications are avoided. Despite the variability in the arterial anatomy, a pump with a single catheter will be adequate to provide access to the entire hepatic arterial inflow, in the majority of cases. The catheter should not be placed directly into the hepatic artery as this may result in thrombosis of the vessel. Instead, the catheter is placed into an accessible side branch, typically the gastroduodenal artery (GDA).

At operation, a thorough examination of the abdomen is performed to look for extrahepatic disease. The lymphatic drainage of the liver (the portal and celiac nodes) should be examined and biopsied if suspicious for metastasis. The extent of liver involvement, which is a prognostic indicator, is then determined. The extent of liver involvement is assessed by assuming that the right lobe of the liver is approximately 60% of the total liver volume, the left medial segment 25%, and the left lateral segment 15%, and estimates the portion of each segment involved. While crude, this technique correlates well with the percentage of liver involvement estimated by the radiologist from the CT scan.

Next the hepatic artery and its branches are dissected. The common hepatic artery (CHA) and the GDA are palpable superior to the first portion of the duodenum. The GDA is medial to the common bile duct, and awareness of this anatomical relationship will help minimize the risk of injury to the bile duct. The right gastric artery is ligated and divided. The distal CHA, the entire GDA, and the proximal proper hepatic artery are dissected away their retroperitoneal attachments. It is important to mobilize the full length of the GDA circumferentially, to the first portion of the duodenum. This will allow for easier access when inserting and securing the catheter. Several small suprapyloric side branches will be encountered and should be ligated. Frequently, branches to the pancreas and duodenum will arise from the posterior aspect of the GDA. It is essential to identify and divide these branches to avoid perfusion of the pancreas and duodenum. The common hepatic artery is mobilized 1 cm proximally, and the proper hepatic artery about 2 cm distally in order to identify any branches to the stomach or duodenum. The GDA is temporarily occluded to confirm the presence of antegrade flow through the hepatic artery. Absence of flow indicates a proximal stenosis and alternate cannulation technique will be required. No attempt is made to dissect the common bile duct, as this may disrupt the blood supply and lead to stricture formation. To prevent chemical cholecystitis the gallbladder is removed in all cases (41).

The pump pocket should be created in the lower abdomen so the pump lies below the waist and away form the liver where it may interfere with CT scans. The pump should be handled carefully, avoiding contact with the patient's skin. The catheter is tunneled into the abdominal cavity, and the pump is secured to the abdominal fascia with nonabsorbable sutures. The catheter should be positioned deep to the pump to prevent injury by a needle. The pump pocket is irrigated with a solution of Bacitracin and then closed to minimize contamination. The GDA is ligated with a non-absorbable tie at the level of the first portion of the duodenum, and vascular control of the common and proper hepatic arteries is achieved with vascular clamps or vessel loops. An arteriotomy is made distally in the GDA, and the catheter inserted up to but not beyond the junction with the hepatic artery. If the catheter protrudes into the common hepatic artery turbulence of blood flow can lead to thrombosis of the vessel. On the other hand, failure to pass the catheter to the arterial junction leaves a short segment of the GDA exposed to full concentrations of chemotherapy (without the diluting effect of blood flow), and this may result in sclerosis, thrombosis, or late dislodgment. Once accurately positioned, the catheter should be secured 2 or 3 times with non-absorbable ties behind the tying rings on the catheter. Infusing 5 cc of half strength fluorescein into the catheter, through the bolus port and examining the liver, stomach, and duodenum with a Wood's lamp confirm perfusion of both lobes of the liver. Following the fluorescein test, the catheter is flushed with heparin containing solution. Antibiotic coverage should be maintained for 48 hours. Any sign of erythema indicative of a wound infection postoperatively should be treated immediately and aggressively with intravenous antibiotics.

Management of aberrant hepatic arterial anatomy
Trifurcation of the hepatic artery is frequently seen and is managed in the same manner as the GDA arising from the right or the left hepatic artery, Figure 16.1. There are three surgical options, each of which poses additional risks compared to the technique for standard arterial anatomy. First, the hepatic arterial tree may be accessed through the splenic artery just to the left of the celiac axis. Both the GDA and the right gastric arteries are ligated. The catheter is placed in the splenic artery and passed across the celiac axis to lie freely in the hepatic artery, ending proximal to the bifurcation. The catheter is secured in the splenic artery. Disadvantages of the splenic artery technique are that it requires considerably more dissection, there can be difficulty passing the catheter across the celiac axis in some patients, and there may be an increased risk of arterial thrombosis when the hepatic artery is of small caliber. A second option is retrograde cannulation of the common hepatic artery through the GDA into the CHA. This requires the attachment of a short, stiff, small gauge catheter onto the end of the silastic catheter so that when placed retrograde into the CHA the catheter tip will not kink and cause thrombosis. The technique is simple but frequently results in arterial dissection and thrombosis. A third option is to place the catheter in the GDA and ligate the left hepatic artery. Ligation of the left hepatic artery assures mixing of drug with all blood flowing through the remaining right hepatic artery into the liver. However, there is a small risk of incomplete crossover perfusion to the left liver. Choice of technique is based upon the surgeon's experience and preference.

An accessory left hepatic artery arises from the left gastric artery, crosses the gastrohepatic ligament, and enters the liver at the base of the umbilical fissure, Figure 16.1. The native left hepatic artery, which arises from the CHA, also supplies the left liver. The simplest surgical option is to ligate the accessory left hepatic artery and place the pump catheter in the GDA. Cross-perfusion is highly reliable, although it has not been proven that adequate, or equal, blood flow develops in the partially devascularized left liver. Use of two catheters, one in the GDA and one in a branch of the left gastric artery eliminates the concern about the adequacy of cross perfusion; however, two separate infusion pumps are required.

An accessory right hepatic artery originates from the SMA and supplies the posterior portion of the right lobe of the liver, while the main right hepatic artery supplies the anterior portion of the right lobe, Figure 16.1. Accessory or replaced right hepatic arteries rarely have side branches adequate for cannulation. The most common procedure is to ligate the accessory vessel and cannulate the GDA.

A replaced left hepatic artery generally arises from the left gastric artery and supplies the left liver, Figure 16.1. There is no native left hepatic artery. The surgeon may ligate the replaced left hepatic artery and place the pump catheter in the GDA. However, in this setting there is a risk of incomplete cross perfusion of up to 40% (42). Patients with bulky disease in the left liver may be better served by placing catheters in both the GDA and the replaced left hepatic artery.

The replaced right hepatic artery originates from the SMA and supplies the right lobe of the liver; the native left hepatic artery, which may be accessed using the GDA, Figure 16.1, supplies the left lobe. If the surgeon ligates the replaced right hepatic artery, cross perfusion from the left hepatic artery will occur in over 90% of cases (42). Alternatively, a second pump and catheter may be used to cannulate the vessel directly through a small arteriotomy. The catheter is cut flush at one of the rings, and the catheter placed so the ring lies just inside the vessel. The arteriotomy is closed with simple nylon sutures. A more technically difficult technique, but very effective is to use the saphenous vein to patch to the right hepatic artery and secure the catheter.

Celiac axis stenosis is occasionally seen and can be determined intra-operatively by the loss of blood flow through the hepatic artery when the GDA is clamped. Careful review of the angiogram pre-operatively is essential in identifying stenotic lesions. Cannulation of the GDA in this situation would lead to sever hepatic ischemia. The technique required in these cases involves cannulating the common hepatic artery (proximally) and placing the tip of the catheter at the junction of the GDA and the hepatic artery.

Postoperative assessment
Following surgery and prior to administering chemotherapy, the distribution of arterial perfusion is assessed by a radionuclide pump study. A baseline technetium

sulfur-colloid scan is obtained to identify the liver outline. Pump perfusion is then assessed by infusing 3-5 mCi of technetium labeled macro-aggregated albumin (MAA) through the bolus port of the pump (43). When the MAA scan produces an image that matches the sulfur-colloid liver scan, the pump is perfusing the entire liver as intended. Perfusion of extrahepatic tissues will produce technetium signals outside of the liver image, Figure 16.2. Incomplete perfusion of the liver will produce an incomplete image of the liver on MAA scan. The incidence of misperfusion is 5-7% and can often be corrected by surgical or angiographic intervention (39,44).

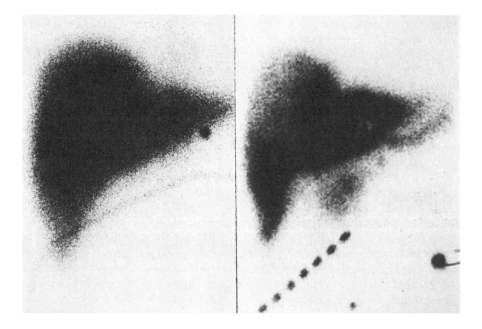

Figure 16.2 Extrahepatic perfusion. A technetium sulfur-colloid scan outlining the liver is shown in the left panel. A MAA scan through the pump side-port demonstrates extrahepatic perfusion (right panel).

Small branches of the hepatic artery to the stomach, duodenum and pancreas are often not seen on preoperative digital subtraction angiography. If these small vessels are not divided and ligated, perfusion of the bowel with FUDR will produce severe pain, gastrointestinal ulceration and, if the pancreas is perfused, severe pancreatitis. These complications are potentially lethal, and if identified prior to onset of chemotherapy, must be corrected prior to initiating HAI therapy. If extrahepatic perfusion is seen on the ^{99m}Tc MAA scan, the next step is to perform an angiogram by bolus injection through the pump sideport. This will usually demonstrate the unligated vessel that is the cause of extrahepatic perfusion. Occasionally, this is unsuccessful, and a transfemoral celiac or SMA study will be needed to identify the problem. Extrahepatic perfusion identified by the post-operative MAA scan occurred in <2% of cases (39,44). The cause can be identified by arteriogram and corrected using angiographic embolization in 40% of cases (39,44). In the remaining cases re-operation was required.

Incomplete perfusion occurs in a small minority of patients, and typically involves aberrant anatomy. Identification of the cause can be accomplished by an angiogram through the bolus port. The causes included failure to ligate a replaced or accessory hepatic artery or failure to achieve cross perfusion after ligation of a replaced or accessory artery. If an accessory or replaced artery was ligated, the development of cross perfusion may be delayed. A delayed MAA scan (4 weeks) will confirm complete liver perfusion in the majority of cases (39,44). Incomplete perfusion due to an accessory or replaced vessel that was not ligated can be corrected by angiographic embolization.

COMPLICATIONS WITH HEPATIC ARTERY INFUSION PUMP PLACEMENT

Surgical and technical complications of pump placement do occur, and the spectrum and frequency of these complications need to be understood by the surgeon, the medical oncologist, and the patient. Operative mortality following pump placement is less than 1% (39,44). In one series, two patients succumbed to hepatic failure post-operatively (44). This underscores the importance of careful patient selection. Technical complications may occur in the immediate postoperative period in a small minority of patients (<10%) of cases.

Acute and chronic gastroduodenal complications
Acute gastric or duodenal ulcers can develop after chemotherapy administration (44). Patients typically present with severe epigastric pain after their first course of chemotherapy. Despite the presence of ulcers in the stomach and duodenum, these patients due not respond to standard ulcer medications. Angiography will demonstrate extrahepatic perfusion, and treatment requires re-operation or embolization. Once the ulcer has healed, chemotherapy can be restarted. A small minority of patients may develop gastritis or duodenitis without any evidence of extrahepatic perfusion (39). These patients typically respond to acid suppression medication and HAI therapy can resume after treatment. If a patient develops unexplained epigastric pain during infusional chemotherapy, the pump should be immediately emptied and refilled with heparin containing solution saline until the etiology of the pain can be elucidated.

Arterial or catheter thrombosis
Catheter or hepatic artery thrombosis occurs in as many as 10% of patients (44). Continuos infusion of through the pump can minimize the incidence of catheter thrombosis (39). Additionally avoiding back bleeding into the catheter during

sideport manipulation and refilling the pump in a timely fashion will reduce the risk of thrombosis. Hepatic artery thrombosis may be the result of technical problems or chemotherapy induced vasculitis. The mean time to arterial thrombosis from vasculitis is 10 months (44). Arterial or catheter thrombosis should be suspected when during refilling the pump the volume in the reservoir is more than expected. Additionally, arterial thrombosis may present as extrahepatic perfusion, Figure 16.3. Although hepatic artery thrombosis may not be salvageable, catheter thrombosis can occasionally be treated with thrombolytic agents (39).

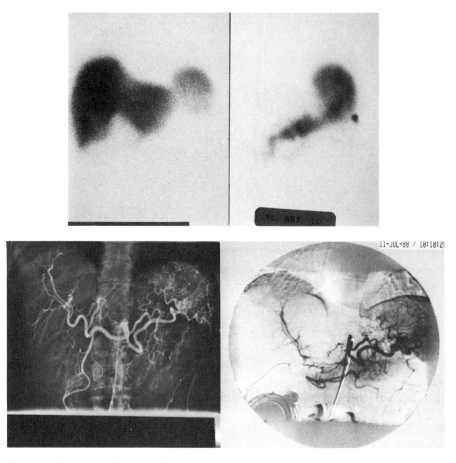

Figure 16.3   Hepatic arterial thrombosis chemotherapy sclerosis. A technetium sulfur-colloid scan outlining the liver is shown in the top left panel. An MAA scan through the pump sideport demonstrates retrograde flow through the celiac axis with perfusion of the spleen and stomach (top right panel). A celiac angiogram of the same patient, bottom right panel, confirms thrombosis of the hepatic artery. The pre-operative angiogram is shown in the bottom left panel for comparison.

Septic Complications

If meticulous aseptic technique is utilized, infectious complications can be reduced. Any sign of pump pocket redness is treated aggressively with parenteral antibiotics. Purulent drainage from the pump pocket necessitates pump removal. We have not seen an increased incidence of infectious complications in patients undergoing concurrent pump insertion and colectomy. However, it is important to place the pump first, close the pump pocket, exclude the catheter from the rest of the procedure, and then proceed with the colectomy. This way, contact with potentially contaminated instruments is minimized. Because this violates the principle of treating the primary problem first, the surgeon may mobilize the bowel initially. In this manner, the colectomy can be performed rapidly and safely should the patient have difficulty on the operating table.

Hemorrhagic Complications

Although the incidence of postoperative intraabdominal bleeding is less than 1%, this is a potentially life threatening complication (39,44). If intraabdominal hemorrhage is suspected, prompt return to the operating room is indicated. The cause is typically dislodgment of the catheter from the artery. When the catheter is placed in the GDA, placing suture ties on both sides of the catheter beads will help prevent catheter migration

TOXICITY

Systemic side effects from regional chemotherapy are minimal, provided that there is no extrahepatic perfusion and the liver avidly extracts the agent being administered. As a result, hepatic arterial delivery of FUDR does not produce myelosupression (45). Nausea, vomiting, or diarrhea, following HAI of FUDR is infrequent and very mild. Severe symptoms should prompt investigation for possible extrahepatic perfusion (46). The most serious complication of HAI therapy is biliary sclerosis, and can occur in as many as 20% of patients (20,22). Similar to liver metastases, the bile ducts derive their blood supply almost exclusively from the hepatic artery, and are exposed to chemotherapy when HAI is utilized (47). Although the specific cause has no been identified, the ischemic and inflammatory effect of chemotherapy is suspected (46,48).

Biliary toxicity is heralded by elevation of serum aspartate aminotransferase (AST), alkaline phosphatase and total bilirubin. The earliest biochemical indicator of toxicity is a rising AST, whereas elevation of alkaline phosphatase and bilirubin levels signal more severe toxicity. Monitoring liver enzymes during therapy is paramount in preventing the sequela of biliary sclerosis. If detected in the early stages, the biliary toxicity is reversible, and the liver enzyme levels will return to baseline. If AST elevation occurs, HAI therapy should be discontinued until the patient recovers and the chemotherapy dose reduced if HAI is reinitiated. Persistent jaundice after treatment should raise the concern of biliary toxicity. Endoscopic retrograde cholangiography will confirm the diagnosis, and demonstrate multiple ductal strictures without intrahepatic ductal dilatation (41). CT scan of the abdomen should be performed to exclude extrinsic tumor compression from portal lymphadenopathy.

Decreasing hepatic toxicity

The addition of an anti-inflammatory agent, dexamethasone, may decrease biliary toxicity. A prospective randomized study conducted at MSKCC compared intrahepatic FUDR with dexamethasone versus FUDR alone (49). Patients treated with dexamethasone and FUDR received higher FUDR doses and had a decreased incidence of elevated bilirubin level, although the differences were not statistically significant. Of interest, is the observation that patients treated with dexamethasone and FUDR had a markedly improved tumor response rate.

An interesting approach decrease hepatic toxicity by using circadian modification of HAI was studied at the University of Minnesota (50). They compared constant infusion versus circadian modified hepatic arterial FUDR infusion. The group with circadian modification received two-thirds of the daily dose between 3 P.M. and 9 P.M. Circadian modification resulted in a decreased incidence of biliary toxicity, however tumor response rates were not reported.

Another approach at decreasing toxicity from HAI involves alternating HAI FUDR with HAI 5-FU. This regimen has been shown to produce limited hepatobiliary side effects (51,52). Furthermore, the tumor response rates were over 50%. New studies are underway to assess CPT-11 and oxaliplatin in conjunction with FUDR.

CONCLUSION

A significant percentage of patients with colorectal carcinoma will develop liver metastases. The use of systemic chemotherapy based on 5-FU produce tumor response rates ranging from 10% to 20% (13). The dependence of liver tumors on the hepatic arterial blood supply and the ability to deliver high doses of chemotherapy agents to the liver are the rationale for HAI therapy. Hepatic delivered FUDR has been shown to produce tumor response rates over 40% (26). For patients with liver metastases, surgical resection is the only curative treatment, however liver recurrence is common (2,3). In an attempt to reduce the risk of hepatic recurrence, the use of HAI in the adjuvant setting seems promising (35-37). Severe toxicity may occur with either intrahepatic or systemic therapy. Intrahepatic therapy may produce gastrointestinal or hepatobiliary toxicity, particularly biliary sclerosis. The toxicity of intrahepatic therapy may be minimized with precise surgical technique and close monitoring of serum liver enzymes. Further studies are needed to determine the optimal dosing schedule, ideal chemotherapy drug regimens, and methods to decrease extrahepatic disease progression.

REFERENCES

1. Greenlee RT, Murray T, Bolden S, Wingo PA. Cancer statistics, 2000. *CA Cancer J Clin* 2000;50(1):7.
2. Iwatsuki S, Dvorchik I, Madariaga JR, et al. Hepatic resection for metastatic colorectal adenocarcinoma: A proposal of a prognostic scoring system. *J Am Coll Surg* 1999;189:291.
3. Fong Y, Fortner J, Sun RL, Brennan MF, Blumgart LH. Clinical score for predicting recurrence after hepatic resection for metastatic colorectal cancer: Analysis of 1001 consecutive cases. *Ann Surg* 1999;230:309.
4. Blackshear PJ, Dorman FD, Blackshear PJ Jr, et al. The design and initial testing of an implantable infusion pump. *Surg Gynecol Obstet* 1972;134:51.
5. Ackerman NB. The blood supply of experimental liver metastases. IV. Changes in vascularity with increasing tumor growth. *Surgery* 1974;75:589.
6. 6. Breedis C, Young C. The blood supply of neoplasms in the liver. *Am J Pathol* 1954;30: 969.
7. Sigurdson ER, Ridge JA, Kemeny N, Daly JM. Tumor and liver drug uptake following hepatic artery and portal vein infusion. *J Clin Oncol* 1987;5:1936.
8. Daly JM, Kemeny N, Sigurdson E, Oderman P, Thom A. Regional infusion for colorectal hepatic metastases: A randomized trial comparing the hepatic artery with the portal vein. *Arch Surg* 1987;122:1273.
9. Ensminger WD, Rosowsky A, Raso V. A clinical pharmacological evaluation of hepatic arterial infusions of 5-fluoro-2-deoxyuridine and 5-fluorouracil. *Cancer Res* 1978;38:3784.
10. Weiss L, Grundmann E, Torhorst J, et al. Hematogenous metastatic patterns in colonic carcinoma: An analysis of 1541 necropsies. *J Pathol* 1986;150:195.
11. Weiss L. Metastatic inefficiency and regional therapy for liver metastases from colorectal carcinoma. *Reg Cancer Treat* 1989;2:77.
12. Daly J, Kemeny N. The therapy of colorectal hepatic metastases. In: DeVita VT, Hellman S, Rosenberg S (eds.), Important Advances in Oncology. J.B. Lippincott, New York 1986;251.
13. Modulation of fluorouracil by leucovorin in patients with advanced colorectal cancer: Evidence in terms of response rate. Advanced Colorectal Cancer Meta-Analysis Project. *J Clin Oncol* 1992;10:896.
14. Balch CM, Urist MM, Soong SJ, McGregor M. A prospective phase II clinical trial of continuous FUDR regional chemotherapy for colorectal metastases to the liver using a totally implantable drug infusion pump. *Ann Surg* 1983;198:567.
15. Niederhuber JE, Ensminger W, Gyves J, et al. Regional chemotherapy of colorectal cancer metastatic to the liver. *Cancer* 1984;53:1336.
16. Weiss GR, Garnick MB, Osteen RT, et al. Long-term arterial infusion of 5-fluorodeoxyuridine for liver metastases using an implantable infusion pump. *J Clin Oncol* 1983;1:337.
17. Allen-Mersh TG, Earkam S, Fordy C, Abrams K, Houghton J: Quality of life and survival with continuous hepatic artery floxuridine infusion for colorectal liver metastases. *Lancet* 1994;344:1255.

18. Hohn DC, Stagg RJ, Friedman MA, et al. A randomized trial of continuous intravenous versus hepatic intraarterial floxuridine in patients with colorectal cancer metastatic to the liver: the Northern California Oncology Group trial. *J Clin Oncol* 1989;7:1646.
19. Kemeny N, Daly J, Reichman B, Geller N, Botet J, Oderman P. Intrahepatic or systemic infusion of fluorodeoxyuridine in patients with liver metastases from colorectal carcinoma – A randomized trial. *Ann Int Med* 1987;107:459.
20. Chang AE, Schneider PD, Sugerbaker PH, Simpson C, Culnane M, Steinberg SM. A prospective randomized trial of regional versus systemic continuous 5-fluorodeoxyuridine chemotherapy in the treatment of colorectal liver metastases. *Ann Surg* 1987;206:685.
21. Martin JK Jr, O'Connell MJ, Wieand HS, et al. Intra-arterial floxuridine vs systemic fluorouracil for hepatic metastases from colorectal cancer: a randomized trial. *Arch Surg* 1990;125:1022.
22. Rougier P, Laplanche A, Huguier M, et al. Hepatic arterial infusion of floxuridine in patients with liver metastases from colorectal carcinoma: long-term results of a prospective randomized trial. *J Clin Oncol* 1992;10:1112.
23. Lorenz M, Muller HH. Randomized, multicenter trial of fluorouracil plus leucovorin administered either via hepatic arterial or intravenous infusion versus fluorodeoxyuridine administered via hepatic arterial infusion in patients with nonresectable liver metastases from colorectal carcinoma. *J Clin Oncol* 2000;2:243.
24. Kemeny N, Daly J, Oderman P, Niedzwiecki D, Shurgot B. Prognostic variables in patients with hepatic metastases from colorectal cancer: Importance of medical assessment of liver involvement. *Cancer* 1989;63:742.
25. Kemeny N, Braun DW. Prognostic factors in advanced colorectal carcinoma:The importance of lactic dehydrogenase, performance status, and white blood cell count. *Am J Med* 1983;74:786.
26. Reappraisal of hepatic arterial infusion in the treatment of nonresectable liver metastases from colorectal cancer. Meta-Analysis Group in Cancer. *J Natl Cancer Inst* 1996;88:252.
27. 27.Harmantas A, Rotstein LE, Langer B. Regional versus systemic chemotherapy in the treatment of colorectal carcinoma metastatic to the liver. Is there a survival difference? Meta-analysis of the published literature. *Cancer* 1996;78:1639.
28. Fong Y, Cohen AM, Fortner JG, et al. Liver resection for colorectal metastases *J Clin Oncol* 1997;15:938.
29. Curley SA, Roh MS, Chase JL, Hohn DC. Adjuvant hepatic arterial infusion chemotherapy after curative resection of colorectal liver metastases. *Am J Surg* 1993;166:743.
30. Moriya Y, Sugihara K, Hojo K, Makuuchi M. Adjuvant hepatic intra-arterial chemotherapy after potentially curative hepatectomy for liver metastases from colorectal cancer: A pilot study. *Eur J Surg Oncol* 1991;17:519.
31. Kemeny N, Conti JA, Sigurdson E, et al. A pilot study of hepatic artery floxuridine combined with systemic 5-fluorouracil and leucovorin. A potential

adjuvant program after resection of colorectal hepatic metastases. *Cancer* 1993;71:1964.

32. Kokudo N, Seki M, Ohta H, et al. Effects of systemic and regional chemotherapy after hepatic resection for colorectal metastases. *Ann Surg Oncol* 1998;5:706.

33. Wagman LD, Kemeny MM, Leong L, et al. A prospective randomized evaluation of the treatment of colorectal cancer metastatic to the liver. *J Clin Oncol* 1990;8:1885.

34. Kemeny MM, Goldberg D, Beatty JD, et al. Results of a prospective randomized trials of continuous regional chemotherapy and hepatic resection as treatment of hepatic metastases from colorectal primaries. *Cancer* 1986;57: 492.

35. Kemeny N, Huang Y, Cohen AM, et al. Hepatic arterial infusion of chemotherapy after resection of hepatic metastases from colorectal cancer. *N Engl J Med* 1999;341:2039.

36. Lorenz M, Muller HH, Schramm H, et al. Randomized trial of surgery versus surgery followed by adjuvant hepatic arterial infusion with 5-fluorouracil and folinic acid for liver metastases of colorectal cancer. German Cooperative on Liver Metastases. *Ann Surg* 1998;228:756.

37. Kemeny MM, Adak S, Lipsitz S, Gray B, MacDonald J, Benson III AB. Results of the intergroup [Eastern Cooperative Oncology Group (ECOG) and Southwest Oncology Group (SWOG)] prospective randomized study of surgery alone versus continuous cepatic artery infusion of FUDR and continuous systemic infusion of 5FU after hepatic resection for colorectal liver metastases. *Proc Am Soc Clin Oncol* 1999;18:1012. (abstract)

38. Hiatt JR; Gabbay J; Busuttil RW. Surgical anatomy of the hepatic arteries in 1000 cases. *Ann Surg* 1994;220:50.

39. Curley SA, Chase JL, Roh MS, Hohn DC. Technical considerations and complications associated with the placement of 180 implantable hepatic arterial infusion devices. *Surgery* 1993;114:928.

40. Daly J, Kemeny N, Oderman P, Botet J. Long-term hepatic arterial infusion chemotherapy. *Arch Surg* 1984;119:936.

41. Kemeny M, Battifora H, Blayney D, et al. Sclerosing cholangitis after continuous hepatic artery infusion of FUDR. *Ann Surg* 1985;202:176.

42. Cohen AM, Higgins J, Waltman AC. Effect of ligation of variant hepatic arterial structures on the completeness of regional chemotherapy infusion. *Am J Surg* 1987;153:378.

43. Kaplan WD, D'Orsi CJ, Ensminger WD, Smith EH, Levin DC. Intra-arterial radionuclide infusion: a new technique to assess chemotherapy perfusion patterns. *Cancer Treat Rep* 1978;62:699.

44. Campbell KA, Burns RC, Sitzmann JV, Lipsett PA, Grochow LB, Niederhuber JE. Regional chemotherapy devices: effect of experience and anatomy on complications. *J Clin Oncol* 1993;11:822.

45. Kemeny N, Daly J, Oderman P, et al. Hepatic artery pump infusion toxicity and results in patients with metastatic colorectal carcinoma. *J Clin Oncol* 1984;2:595.

46. Pettavel J, Gardiol D, Bergier N, et al. Necrosis of main bile ducts caused by hepatic artery infusion of 5-fluoro-2-deoxyuridine. *Reg Cancer Treat* 1988;1:83.

47. Northover JM, Terblanche J. A new look at the arterial supply of the bile duct in man and its surgical implications. *Br J Surg* 1979;66:379.

48. Doria MI Jr, Shepard KV, Levin B, et al. Liver pathology following hepatic arterial infusion chemotherapy. *Cancer* 1986;58:855.

49. Kemeny N, Seiter K, Niedzwiecki D, et al. A randomized trial of intrahepatic infusion of fluorodeoxyuridine with dexamethasone versus fluorodeoxyuridine alone in the treatment of metastatic colorectal cancer. *Cancer* 1992;69:327.

50. Hrushesky W, von Roemelling R, Lanning R, Rabatini J. Circadian-shaped infusions of floxuridine for progressive metastatic renal cell carcinoma. *J Clin Oncol* 1990;8:1504.

51. Davidson BS, Izzo F, Chase JL, et al. Alternating floxuridine and 5-fluorouracil hepatic arterial chemotherapy for colorectal liver metastases minimizes biliary toxicity. *Am J Surg* 1996;172:244.

52. Stagg R, Venook A, Chase J, et al. Alternating hepatic intra-arterial floxuridine and fluorouracil: A less toxic regimen for treatment of liver metastases from colorectal cancer. *J Natl Cancer Inst* 1991;83:423.

17

PEDIATRIC LIVER TUMORS

Marleta Reynolds, M.D.
Children's Memorial Hospital, Chicago, IL

INTRODUCTION

In children, 70% of primary hepatic neoplasms are malignant. The liver is the 3rd most common site of intraabdominal malignancy following Wilms' tumor and neuroblastoma. Malignant hepatic neoplasms are the 10th most common pediatric malignancy affecting 1.6 per million in the United States. (0.9 per million children with hepatoblastoma and 0.7 per million children with hepatocellular carcinoma) (1). Secondary hepatic malignancies are most common in children with Wilms' tumor, neuroblastoma and leukemia. Benign liver tumors are rare and most occur in infants [Table I].

Table I Primary Liver Tumors

Benign	Malignant
Hemangioendothelioma	Hepatoblastoma
Hemangioma	Hepatocellular Carcinoma
Mesenchymal Hamartoma	Sarcoma
Focal Nodular Hyperplasia	Rhabdomyosarcoma
Adenoma	Angiosarcoma
Teratoma	Leiomyosarcoma
	Cholangiocarcinoma

BENIGN LIVER TUMORS

Hemangioendothelioma

Hemangioendothelioma is the most common benign vascular hepatic tumor in childhood and usually presents as a large intraabdominal mass by 6 months of age. Girls are affected more commonly than boys with a ratio of 4.3:1 to 2:1(2). Skin hemangiomas are present in 11% and have also been found in the brain and other organs (3). Over one-third of infants develop signs and symptoms related to the tumor. High output cardiac failure might develop in up to 50% of infants if the tumor creates a relative arteriovenous fistula. Platelet trapping (Kasabach-Merritt syndrome), anemia, consumptive coagulopathy, obstructive jaundice, and intraperitoneal hemorrhage from rupture have also been reported (3).

When an infant presents with a large abdominal mass, abdominal ultrasound and computed tomography (CT) or magnetic resonance imaging (MRI) can be useful in making a diagnosis.   Ultrasound findings of hemangioendothelioma include a complex liver mass with large hepatic veins.   There may also be a dilated proximal aorta (4, 5).   On CT imaging multiple well-encapsulated homogeneous masses with lower attenuation coefficients are identified on pre-contrast studies.   After contrast injection the rounded lesions enhance early and on delayed images the lesions become isodense to normal liver (6). (Figure 1)

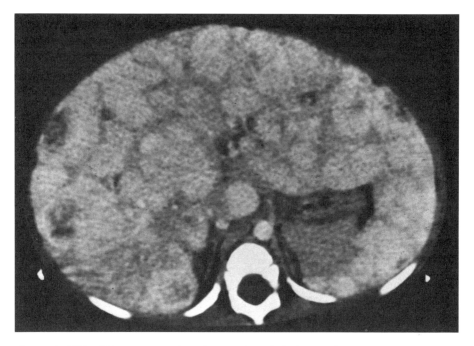

Figure 1. This CT scan reveals a hemangioendothelioma that involves the entire liver.   This child did not respond to therapy and was scheduled for liver transplantation.   She expired during the operation.

Review of the imaging studies can usually differentiate a hemangioendothelioma from hemangioma.   If the imaging studies are equivocal a biopsy may be required to confirm the diagnosis (7).   Laboratory values are non-specific and may include a low hemoglobin, elevated bilirubin and transaminase, and low platelet count.   Alpha feto-protein levels may also be elevated.

Two types represent the histology of hemangioendothelioma.   Both can be identified in the same specimen and histology does not predict outcome (2, 8).   Type I consists of dilated vascular spaces lined by immature endothelial cells separated by fibrous stoma.   In type 2 the vascular channels are irregularly branched and are lined by pleomorphic endothelial cells with papillary budding into the vessels (8).   There is no mitotic activity.

The infant with an asymptomatic hemangioendothelioma should be followed with abdominal ultrasound and close clinical observation until spontaneous involution occurs. The infant who presents with symptoms must be rapidly evaluated and treatment initiated. High doses of prednisolone (4 to 5 mg/kg per day for 28 days and tapered over 3-5 weeks) have been useful in some infants (9). Diuretics and digitalis can be used to treat congestive heart failure. Antineoplastic drugs have also been used alone or in combination with steroids with response in some infants (8). More recently alpha interferon has been used to encourage involution (10, 11)

The hemangioendothelioma that does not respond to medical therapy and consists of a single nodule or involves a single lobe of the liver can be treated with selective hepatic arterial embolization or surgical resection. With bilobar disease embolization may play a role in stabilizing the infant prior to transplantation. Orthotopic liver transplantation has been recommended in those infants in whom no therapy has proved successful. Only isolated case reports of orthotopic liver transplantation to treat hepatic hemangioendothelioma have been published (12). Our recent experience with this tumor has resulted in two intraoperative deaths, one for a right hepatic lobectomy and one during orthotopic liver transplantation. Regardless of new treatment strategies mortality rates still approach 90%.

Cavernous Hemangioma

Cavernous hemangioma is a benign neoplasm that varies in size and is usually identified by 6 months of age. Infants often present with an enlarged liver and most are asymptomatic. A large hemangioma may produce platelet trapping (Kasabach-Merritt syndrome) or congestive heart failure from excessive blood flow through the tumor. Spontaneous rupture has also been reported (2).

Diagnostic studies useful in differentiating a cavernous hemangioma from other hepatic pathology include abdominal ultrasound, computed tomography, magnetic resonance imaging and occasionally angiography. Biopsy is seldom indicated.

Most hemangiomas of the liver will involute spontaneously. If symptoms develop or if the size is so great that rupture is feared arterial embolization can be useful in reducing flow and thus the size and threat of the tumor (Figures 2a,b). Surgery is seldom indicated but preoperative embolization may reduce operative morbidity.

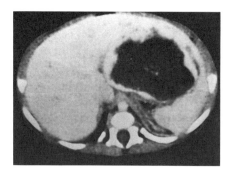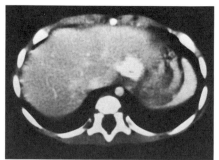

Figure 2a. *(Left panel)* A CT scan of the liver in this 4 month-old infant reveals a large hemangioma. The infant developed thrombocytopenia and underwent selective hepatic embolization. 2b. *(Right panel)* One year later follow-up CT reveals near complete resolution of the lesion.

Mesenchymal Hamartoma

A mesenchymal hamartoma is a rare benign liver tumor that is discovered as an asymptomatic abdominal mass in an infant or young child. It is more common in males, involves the right lobe of the liver 75% of the time, and may be pedunculated in up to 30% (14). Ultrasound and or CT is usually diagnostic (Figure 3).

Histology reveals cystic areas, biliary epithelium, hepatocytes and mesenchymal elements. Surgical resection is curative. Pedunculated lesions are easily removed. Formal hepatic lobectomy is seldom indicated, because these tumors can usually be shelled out with minimal blood loss and operative morbidity.

Focal Nodular Hyperplasia

Focal nodular hyperplasia usually affects adolescent females and is often found incidentally. Abdominal ultrasound or CT imaging demonstrates a characteristic central scar with branching in small non-encapsulated singles or multiple masses. Resection is recommended to prevent spontaneous rupture and hemorrhage (15).

Adenoma

Hepatic adenomas are rare in children. They can occur at any age and have been reported with increased frequency in teenagers taking oral contraceptives (13). Many times the lesion is found when the liver is imaged for a different reason or at exploratory laparotomy. Resection is diagnostic and therapeutic.

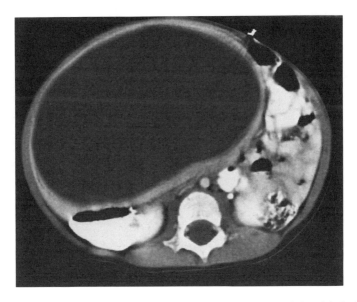

Figure 3. A 1 year-old infant presented with an enlarging right sided abdominal mass. He was asymptomatic. This CT reveals a large mesenchymal hamartoma of the liver that was successfully resected.

MALIGNANT TUMORS

Hepatoblastoma

The most common hepatic malignancy in children is hepatoblastoma. The child is usually less than three years of age and presents with an abdominal mass and anemia. Boys are more frequently affected in a ratio of 1.5 to 1. Hepatoblastoma occurs with increased frequency in children with Beckwith-Wiedeman syndrome (deletion of chromosome 11), hemihypertrophy or with a family history of adenomatous polyposis (16, 17). Anomalies associated with hepatoblastoma include renal anomalies, diaphragmatic and umbilical hernia, Meckel's diverticulum and others (18). (Table II)

Over the past three decades there has been an increased incidence of hepatoblastoma reported in premature infants with birth weights less than 1500 gms (19).

There are four histologic subtypes of hepatoblastoma; pure fetal, epithelial – mesenchymal, small cell undifferentiated (anaplastic) and macrotrabecular. Pure fetal histology is associated with a better prognosis and anaplastic a worse prognosis (20, 21).

Nuclear DNA analyzed by flow cytometry may be useful in predicting outcome. Diploidy, found most frequently in tumors with pure fetal histology, correlates with a good prognosis. Aneuploidy is associated with poor outcome (22).

TABLE II. Conditions Associated with Hepatoblastoma*

Absence of right adrenal gland
Alcohol embryopathy
Beckwith-Wiedemann syndrome
Beckwith-Wiedemann syndrome with opsoclonus, myoclonus
Bilateral talipes
Cleft palate, macroglossia, dysplasia of ear lobes
Cystathioninuria
Down's syndrome, malrotation of colon, Meckel's diverticulum, pectus
    excavatum, intrathoracic kidney, single coronary artery
Duplicated ureters
Fetal hydrops
Goldenhar syndrome—oculo-auriculovertebral dysplasia, absence of portal vein
Hemihypertrophy
Heterotopic lung tissue
Heterozygous alpha-1 -antitrypsin deficiency
HIV positive, hepatitis-B-virus positive
Horseshoe kidney
Hypoglycemia
Inguinal hernia
Isosexual precocity
Maternal clomiphene citrate and Pergonal maternal oral contraceptive
Meckel's diverticulum
Osteoporosis
Patient on oral contraceptive`
Persistent ductus arteriosus
Polyposis coli families
Prader-Willi syndrome
Renal dysplasia
Right diaphragmatic hernia
Synchronous Wilms' tumor
Umbilical Hernia
Reprinted with permission [18] from W. B. Saunders

Although most infants and children with hepatoblastoma present with an asymptomatic abdominal mass, some exhibit pain, fever, and anorexia and weight loss. Laboratory studies may reveal anemia, thrombocytopenia, leukocytosis and in 70% an elevated alpha feto protein concentration.

Abdominal ultrasound provides rapid screening of abdominal masses in children. When localized to the liver, the ultrasound may identify single or multiple lesions, and the number of lobes involved. Doppler evaluation of the patency and/or involvement of the inferior vena cava and hepatic veins is useful when considering resection. CT or MRI is helpful in identifying pulmonary metastases and compliments ultrasound in evaluating resectability. (Figure 4)

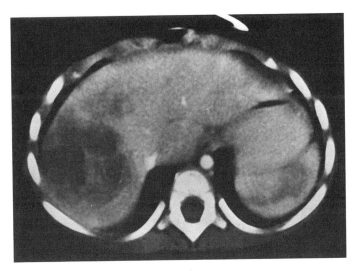

Figure 4. This CT scan reveals a mass in the right lobe of the liver. A right hepatectomy was done to remove a hepatoblastoma. Chemotherapy was administered postoperatively.

Invasion of hepatic veins, inferior vena cava or portal vein preclude initial resection and may be impossible to identify without laparotomy. (23, 24, 25)

The staging system for hepatoblastoma adopted recently by the two large pediatric oncology groups is that developed by the International Society of Pediatric Oncology (26). The liver is divided into four sectors. Specific classification depends on the number of unaffected sectors. (Figure 5)

Extrahepatic growth is considered separately. (Reprinted from 26 with permission of Harcourt Brace & Co., Ltd.)

Long-term survival of children with hepatoblastoma is only possible with complete surgical resection of the tumor. In Stage I, II and some Stage III tumors, surgical resection can be accomplished as the primary treatment strategy with chemotherapy administered postoperatively. In over 50% of the children, the tumor is determined to be unresectable and preoperative chemotherapy is administered. In the majority of children (70%) a significant reduction in tumor size will permit surgical resection.(27) Some centers treat every child with hepatoblastoma with initial chemotherapy followed by surgical resection.(28)

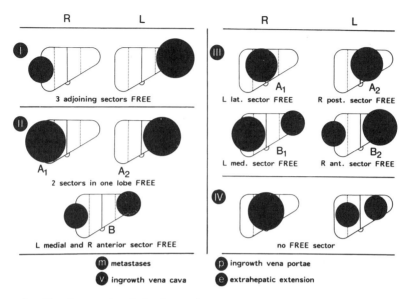

Figure 5.   The International Society of Pediatric Oncology Preoperative Staging System (SIOPEL I).   The liver is divided into four sectors.   Classification (Stage I, II, III, IV) depends on the number of unaffected sectors (FREE from tumor). Current drugs used to treat hepatoblastoma include Cisplatin, vincristine, 5-fluorouracil (5FU), and doxirubicin (1). The Pediatric Intergroup Hepatoma Study comparing these drugs found the doxirubicin-containing regimen to be more toxic and have equal efficacy (29). New agents, including carboplatin and etoposide are included in current study of advanced stage disease.(Personal communication)

Transcatheter arterial chemoembolization using cisplatin and doxorubicin has been effective in reducing tumor size with minimal morbidity in a small group of patients (30). A large controlled study will be needed to compare this modality to systemic chemotherapy. Peripheral blood stem cell transplantation has been recommended in those patients in who resection is incomplete and microscopic residual tumor can be identified. (31)

Serum alpha feto protein (AFP) is an excellent tumor marker to follow response to treatment and recurrence. The German Cooperative Pediatric Liver Tumor Study demonstrated a correlation between initial serum AFP and survival (21). In another study population, a high initial AFP and a 2-log decrease in AFP by the end of therapy were predictive of improved survival. Tumor growth patterns were also predictive of outcome.   Poor outcome was predicted by vascular invasion, multiplicity of tumor nodules and disseminated tumor. Histology, tumor volume and presence of local infiltration were not predictive of outcome (32).

In the past decade, reports from several large series have concluded that preoperative chemotherapy can alter tumor dimension enough to allow complete resection in the majority of patients. Children in whom complete tumor resection was possible with or without preoperative chemotherapy have a predicted 2-year survival of between 85 and 92% (27,21,29).

Following surgery and pre-op and/or postoperative chemotherapy, hepatoblastoma may recur locally or with distant metastatic disease. Aggressive surgical resection of pulmonary metastases can yield extended disease free intervals (33,34,35). This is especially true if the disease free interval initially exceeds 6 months, the surgical resection occurs shortly after the AFP begins to rise and is complete (33). In some children, chemotherapy will not convert a tumor to one that is respectable. (Figures 6a,b)

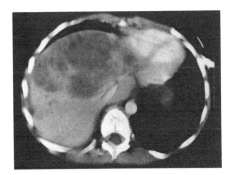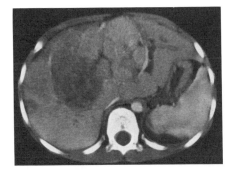

Figures 6a,b. Two images of this CT scan in a child with hepatoblastoma show the mass to extend to the confluence of hepatic veins and inferior vena cava and extending to and possibly beyond the falciform ligament. Chemotherapy reduced tumor size but did not provide enough resolution to allow complete resection. This child is now two years post transplant and doing well.

Orthotopic liver transplantation may be considered in these children. Survival ranges from 50 – 80% (36,37,38). Extrahepatic disease and multifocal tumors are associated with a worse prognosis. In over 30% recurrent tumor developed in spite of post-transplant chemotherapy (39).

Congenital Hepatoblastoma

Congenital hepatoblastoma has been identified by fetal ultrasound. It can be associated with polyhydramnios and fetal non-immune hydrops or rupture during vaginal delivery. Fetal histology is typically represented and distant metastases are more frequent at diagnosis. Metastatic work-up should preceed therapy and surgical resection planned. The use of chemotherapy in congenital hepatoblastoma as a preoperative and/or postoperative therapy is controversial (40).

Hepatocellular Carcinoma

Hepatocellular carcinoma does not usually develop in children under 5 and most children are over 10 years. Boys are affected more commonly than girls. Although hepatocellular carcinoma can occur in children without underlying hepatic conditions, it is more likely to develop in children with hepatic fibrosis and cirrhosis secondary to metabolic liver disease, viral hepatitis, extrahepatic biliary atresia, total parenteral nutrition, and chemotherapy induced fibrosis (15).

As with other hepatic malignancies, children with hepatocellular carcinoma present with an enlarging abdominal mass, weight loss, fever and anorexia. In over one-half of the children, the serum alpha feto protein may be elevated. Serum transaminase may also be elevated (41). The right lobe of the liver is involved more frequently than the left, and metastases develop in the lymph nodes and lung.

Surgical resection of the involved liver is the only curative treatment for hepatocellular carcinoma. This tumor seldom responds to preoperative chemotherapy although Vincristine, 5FU, and doxorubicin have been used in the preoperative and post-operative setting. Survival for up to 13% of children with hepatocellular carcinoma has only been reported in those in whom complete surgical resection was possible (42).

UNCOMMON HEPATIC MALIGNANCIES

Angiosarcoma occurs more commonly in girls and has been reported in less than 30 children. The children are usually between 3 and 5 years of age and present with an enlarging abdominal mass. Bilobar and/or metastatic disease at presentation are not uncommon. Angiosarcoma has been described in children treated for hemangioendothelioma. Complete resection can be curative (43).

Malignant mesenchymal tumors represent 6% of primary hepatic tumors in children. Mean age at presentation is 7 years. The child develops an enlarging abdominal mass that may be painful (Figure 7).

Histologic evaluation usually reveals embryonal sarcoma. Like hepatoblastoma, the resectable lesion is removed and the unresectable treated with preoperative chemotherapy. Vincristine, Actinomycin D, cyclophamide and doxorubicin have been used. With complete surgical resection, 2-year survival is 50% (Babin).

Occasionally, an embryonal rhabdomyosarcoma will develop within the liver rather than in the extrahepatic biliary tree.

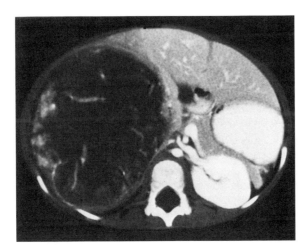

Figure 7. A 7 year-old female child presented with an abdominal mass. The CT scan demonstrates a large right hepatic mass. A right hepatectomy was done and embryonal sarcoma diagnosed. She is disease free 2 years following resection.

Malignant tumor with rhabdoid features (MTR) was originally described in the kidney but has since been found in many other organs including the liver. It usually presents in infancy and the infant will be suspected of having hepatoblastoma. The alpha feto protein will be normal. Biopsy will yield typical histologic and cytologic features. Immunohistochemistry expression of vimentin and epithelial markers will be present (45). This malignancy seldom responds to chemotherapy and is universally fatal (Figure 8).

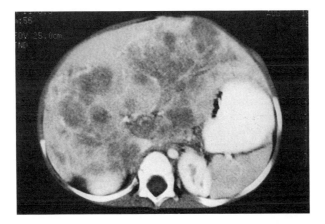

Figure 8. A 17 month-old male infant presented with a painful enlarging abdominal mass. This CT shows a multifocal hepatic tumor. Biopsy revealed rhabdoid tumor of the liver.

Fibrosarcoma, leiomyosarcoma, and malignant fibrous histiocytoma are other rare mesenchymal tumors that may arise in the liver. Chemotherapy is usually ineffective and surgery seldom possible (44).

Cholangiocarcinoma can also involve the intrahepatic biliary systems, especially in children with biliary atresia, Caroli's disease, cystic fibrosis and sclerosing cholangitis. A rising bilirubin in an otherwise stable patient should lead to further evaluation. Carcinoembryonic antigens (CEA) values may be elevated. Surgical resection is only possible if the proximal biliary tree is uninvolved. Liver transplant is not recommended for these patients (1). Chemotherapy is ineffective.

Lastly, both benign and malignant germ cell tumors may arise in the liver. Surgical resection is indicated for both and is curative.

REFERENCES

1.   Bowman LC, Riely CA. Management of pediatric liver tumors (Review). Surg Oncol Clin North Am 1996; 5:451-459.
2.   Selby DM, Stocker JT,Waclawiw MA et al: Infantile hemangioendothelioma of the liver. Hepatology 1994; 20:39-45.
3.   Daller JA, Bueno J, Gutierrez J, et al. Hepatic hemangioendothelioma: clinical experience and management strategy. J Pediatr Surg 1999; 34(1): 98-106.
4.   Abramson SJ, Lack EE, Teele RL. Benign vascular tumors of the liver in infants: Sonographic appearance. AJR 1982; 138:629-632.
5.   Smith WL, Franken EA, Mitros WJ. Liver tumors in children. Semin Roentgenol 1983;18:136-148.
6.   Lucaya J, Enriquez G, Amat L,. et al. Computed tomography of infantile hemangioendothelioma. AJR 1977; 144:821-826.
7.   von Schweinitz D, Gluer S, Mildenberger H. Liver tumors in neonates and very young infants: diagnostic pitfalls and therapeutic problems. Eur J Pediatr Surg 1995; 5:72-76.
8.   Davenport M, Hansen L, Heaton ND, Howard ER. Hemangioendothelioma of the liver in infants. J Pediatr Surg 1995;30:44-48.
9.   Samuel M, Spitz L. Infantile hepatic hemangio-endothelioma: the role of surgery. J Pediatr Surg 1995;30:1425-1429.
10.   Woltering MD, Robben S, Egeler RM. Hepatic hemangioendothelioma of infancy: treatment with interferon alpha. J Pediatr Gastroenterol Nutr 1997;24:348-351.
11.   Fok TF, Chan MS, Metreweli C, et al. Hepatic hemangioendothelioma presenting with early heart failure in a newborn: treatment with hepatic artery embolization and interferon. Acta Paediatr 1996;85:1373-1375.
12.   Achilleos OS, Buist LJ, Kelly DA, et al. Unresectable hepatic tumors in childhood and the role of liver transplantation. J Pediatr Surg 1996;31:1563-1567.

13. Weinberg AG, Finegold MJ. Primary hepatic tumors in childhood [Review]. Human Pathol 1983;14:512-537.
14. Craig JR, Peters RL, Edmondson HA. Tumors of the liver and extrahepatic bile ducts. AFIP, Bethesda, MD., pp. 63-64, 190-197, 1989.
15. Williams RA, Ferrell LD. Pediatric liver tumors. Pathology 1993;2:23-42.
16. Mann JR, Kasthuri N, Raafat F, et al. Malignant hepatic tumors in children: incidence, clinical features and etiology. Paediatr Perinat Epidemiol 1990;4:276-289.
17. Giardiello FM, Offerhaus JA, Krush AJ, et al. Risk of hepatoblastoma in familial adenomatous polyposis. J Pediatr 1991;119:766-768.
18. Stocker JT. Hepatoblastoma. Semin Diagn Pathol 1994;11:136-143.
19. Tanimira M, Matsui I, Abe J, et al. Increased risk of hepatoblastoma among immature children with a lower birth weight. Cancer Research 1998;58:3032-3035.
20. Raney B. Hepatoblastoma in children: a review. J Pediatr Hematol Oncol 1997;19:418-422.
21. von Schweinitz D, Hecker H, Harms D, et al. Complete resection before development of drug resistance is essential for survival from advanced hepatoblastoma – a report from the German Cooperative Liver Tumor Study HB-89. J Pediatr Surg 1995;30:845-852.
22. Hata Y, Ishizu H, Ohmori K, et al. Flow cystometric analysis of the nuclear DNA content of hepatoblastoma. Cancer 1991;68:2566-2570.
23. Boechat MJ, Kangarloo H, Ortega J, et al. Primary liver tumors in children: comparison of CT and MR imaging. Radiology 1988;169:727-732.
24. Finn JP, Hall-Craggs MA, Dicks-Mireaux C, et al. Primary malignant liver tumors in children: assessment of resectability with high field MR and comparison with CT. Pediatr Radiology 1990;21:34-38.
25. King SJ, Babyn PS, Greenberg ML, et al. Value of CT in determining resectability of hepatoblastoma before and after chemotherapy. AJR 1993;160:793-798.
26. Vos A. Primary liver tumors in children. Eur J Surg Oncol 1995;21:101-105.
27. Reynolds M, Douglass E, Finegold M, et al. Chemotherapy can convert unresectable hepatoblastoma. J Pediatr Surg 1992;27:1080-1084.
28. Ehrlich P, Greenberg M, Filler R. Improved long-term survival with preoperative chemotherapy for hepatoblastoma. J Pediatr Surg 1997;32:999-1003.
29. Ortega JA, Douglass E, Feussner J, et al. A randomized trial of Cisplatin, Vincristine, 5 Fluorouracil vs Cisplatin, Doxorubicin IV continuous infusion for the treatment of hepatoblastoma: results from the Pediatric Intergroup Hepatoma Study,(CCG8881/POG8945). Proc Am Soc Clin Oncol 1994;13:416.
30. Oue T, Fukuzawa M, Kusafuka T, et al. Trancatheter arterial chemoembolization in the treatment of hepatoblastoma. J Pediatr Surg 1998;33(12):1771-1775.

31. Yoshinari M, Imaizumi M, Hayashi Y, et al. Peripheral blood stem cell transplantation for hepatoblastoma with microscopic residual: a therapeutic approach for incompletely resected tumor. Tohoku J ExpMed 1998;184:247-254.

32. Von Tornout JM, Buckley JD, Quinn JJ. Timing and magnitude of decline in alpha feto protein levels in treated children with unresectable or metastatic hepatoblastoma are predictors of outcome: a report from the Children's Cancer Group. J Clin Oncol 1997;15:1190-1197.

33. Black CT, Luck SR, Musemeche CA, Andrassy RJ. Aggressive excision of pulmonary metastasis is warranted in the management of childhood hepatic tumors. J Pediatr Surg 1991;26:1082-1086.

34. Passmore SJ, Noblett HR, Wisheart JD, Mott MG. Prolonged survival following multiple thoracotomies for metastatic hepatoblastoma. Med Pediatr Oncol 1995;24:58-60.

35. Feussner J, Krailo M, Haas J, et al. Treatment of pulmonary metastases of initial stage I hepatoblastoma in childhood. Report from the Children's Canger Group. Cancer 1993;71:859-863.

36. Koneru B, Flye M, Busuttil R, et al. Liver transplantation for hepatoblastoma: the American experience. Ann Surg 1991;213:118-121.

37. Tagge E, Tagge D, Reyes J, et al. Resection, including transplantation for hepatoblastoma and hepatocellular carcinoma: impact on survival. J Pediatr Surg 1992;27:292-297.

38. Bilik R, Superina R. Transplantation for unresectable liver tumors in children. Transplant Proc 1997;29:2834-2835.

39. Busuttil R, Farmer D. The surgical treatment of primary hepatobiliary malignancy. Liver Transplant Surg 1996;2(5 Supp 1):114-130.

40. Ammann R, Plaschkes J, Leibundgut K. Congenital hepatoblastoma: A distinct entity? Med & Pediatr Oncol 1999; :466-468.

41. Newman KD. Hepatic tumors in children. Semin Pediatr Surg 1997;6:38-41.

42. Douglass E, Ortega J, Feusner J, et al. Hepatocellular carcinoma (HCA) in children and adolescents. Results from the Pediatric Intergroup Study (CCG8881/POG 8945). Proc Am Soc Clin Oncol 1994;13:420 (Abstract 1439).

43. Awan S, Davenport M, Portmann B, Howard ER. Angiosarcoma of the liver in children. J Pediatr Surg 1996;31:1729-1732.

44. Babin-Boilletot A, Flamant F, Terrien-Lacombe MJ, et al. Primitive malignant nonepithelial hepatic tumors in children. Med Pediatr Oncol 1993;21:634-639.

45. Jimenez-Hefferman JA, Lopez-Ferver P, Burgos E, Viguer JM. Pathological case of the month: primary malignant tumor with rhabdoid features. Archiv Ped & Adolesc Med 1998;152(5):509-510.

INDEX